CALLING THE SHOTS

Immunization Finance
Policies and Practices

Committee on Immunization Finance Policies and Practices

Division of Health Care Services and
Division of Health Promotion and Disease Prevention

INSTITUTE OF MEDICINE

NATIONAL ACADEMY PRESS
Washington, D.C.

NATIONAL ACADEMY PRESS • 2101 Constitution Avenue, N.W. • Washington, D.C. 20418

NOTICE: The project that is the subject of this report was approved by the Governing Board of the National Research Council, whose members are drawn from the councils of the National Academy of Sciences, the National Academy of Engineering, and the Institute of Medicine. The members of the committee responsible for the report were chosen for their special competences and with regard for appropriate balance.

Support for this project was provided by the Centers for Disease Control and Prevention (Award No. 200199900023). The views presented are those of the Institute of Medicine's Committee on Immunization Finance Policies and Practices and are not necessarily those of the funding organization.

Library of Congress Cataloging-in-Publication Data

Calling the shots : immunization finance policies and practices / Committee on Immunization Finance Policies and Practices, Division of Health Care Services and Division of Health Promotion and Disease Prevention, Institute of Medicine.
    p. cm.
Includes bibliographical references and index.
ISBN 0-309-07029-5
    1. Immunization—Government policy—United States. 2. Immunization of children—Government policy—United States. 3. Immunization—United States—Finance. 4. Imminization—United States—Planning. 5. Medicine, Preventive—United States. I. Committee on Immunization Finance Policies and Practices (U.S.). II. Institute of Medicine (U.S.). Division of Health Care Services. III. Institute of Medicine (U.S.). Division of Health Promotion and Disease Prevention.

RA638. C35 2000
614.4'7'0973—dc21

00-046277

The full text of this report is available on line at **www.nap.edu.**

Additional information about this report and America's vaccine safety net is available online at **www.nationalacademies.org/includes/shots.htm.**

For more information about the Institute of Medicine, visit the IOM home page at **www.iom.edu.**

Printed in the United States of America

The serpent has been a symbol of long life, healing, and knowledge among almost all cultures and religions since the beginning of recorded history. The serpent adopted as a logotype by the Institute of Medicine is a relief carving from ancient Greece, now held by the Staatliche Museen in Berlin.

"Knowing is not enough; we must apply.
Willing is not enough; we must do."
—Goethe

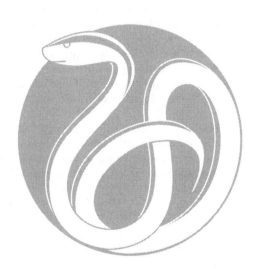

INSTITUTE OF MEDICINE

Shaping the Future for Health

THE NATIONAL ACADEMIES

National Academy of Sciences
National Academy of Engineering
Institute of Medicine
National Research Council

The **National Academy of Sciences** is a private, nonprofit, self-perpetuating society of distinguished scholars engaged in scientific and engineering research, dedicated to the furtherance of science and technology and to their use for the general welfare. Upon the authority of the charter granted to it by the Congress in 1863, the Academy has a mandate that requires it to advise the federal government on scientific and technical matters. Dr. Bruce M. Alberts is president of the National Academy of Sciences.

The **National Academy of Engineering** was established in 1964, under the charter of the National Academy of Sciences, as a parallel organization of outstanding engineers. It is autonomous in its administration and in the selection of its members, sharing with the National Academy of Sciences the responsibility for advising the federal government. The National Academy of Engineering also sponsors engineering programs aimed at meeting national needs, encourages education and research, and recognizes the superior achievements of engineers. Dr. William A. Wulf is president of the National Academy of Engineering.

The **Institute of Medicine** was established in 1970 by the National Academy of Sciences to secure the services of eminent members of appropriate professions in the examination of policy matters pertaining to the health of the public. The Institute acts under the responsibility given to the National Academy of Sciences by its congressional charter to be an adviser to the federal government and, upon its own initiative, to identify issues of medical care, research, and education. Dr. Kenneth I. Shine is president of the Institute of Medicine.

The **National Research Council** was organized by the National Academy of Sciences in 1916 to associate the broad community of science and technology with the Academy's purposes of furthering knowledge and advising the federal government. Functioning in accordance with general policies determined by the Academy, the Council has become the principal operating agency of both the National Academy of Sciences and the National Academy of Engineering in providing services to the government, the public, and the scientific and engineering communities. The Council is administered jointly by both Academies and the Institute of Medicine. Dr. Bruce M. Alberts and Dr. William A. Wulf are chairman and vice chairman, respectively, of the National Research Council.

Project Staff

ROSEMARY CHALK, Study Director
SUZANNE MILLER, Research Assistant
WILHELMINE MILLER, Ph.D., Senior Program Officer
HEATHER SCHOFIELD, Senior Project Assistant

Division Staff

JANET CORRIGAN, Ph.D., Division Director, Health Care Services
ROSE MARIE MARTINEZ, Sc.D., Division Director, Health Promotion
  and Disease Prevention
KATHLEEN STRATTON, Ph.D., Senior Program Officer, Health
  Promotion and Disease Prevention
TRACY McKAY, Senior Program Assistant, Health Care Services

Consultants

SARAH J. CLARK, M.P.H., Department of Pediatrics, University of
  Michigan Medical Center
ANNE E. COWAN, M.P.H., Department of Pediatrics, University of
  Michigan Medical Center
GERRY FAIRBROTHER, Ph.D., Associate Professor of Epidemiology
  and Social Medicine, Montefiore Medical Center, New York City
AMY FINE, M.P.H., Consultant, Washington, DC
ROBIN FLINT, M.P.H., Consultant, Santa Monica, CA
GARY FREED, M.D., M.P.H., Department of Pediatrics, University of
  Michigan Medical Center
ROY HOGAN, M.P.A., Consultant, Austin, TX
KAY JOHNSON, Ed.M., Johnson Group Consultant, Inc., Hinesburg, VT
HANNS KUTTNER, School of Public Policy Studies, University of
  Chicago
EAMON MAGEE, Consultant, Kensington, MD
HEATHER McPHILLIPS, M.D., M.P.H., Department of Pediatrics,
  University of Washington
VICTOR MILLER, M.P.P., Consultant, Washington, DC
GREGORY A. POLAND, M.D., F.A.C.P., Chief, Mayo Vaccine Research
  Group, Mayo Clinic and Foundation, Rochester, MN
BARBARA RICHARDS, M.P.P., Consultant, Washington, DC
KATHY STROUP, Consultant, Riverside, CA

INDEPENDENT REPORT REVIEWERS

This report has been reviewed by individuals chosen for their diverse perspectives and technical expertise, in accordance with procedures approved by the National Research Council's Report Review Committee. The purpose of this independent review is to provide candid and critical comments that will assist the authors and the Institute of Medicine in making the published report as sound as possible and to ensure that the report meets institutional standards for objectivity, evidence, and responsiveness to the study charge. The content of the review comments and draft manuscript remain confidential to protect the integrity of the deliberative process. We wish to thank the following individuals for their participation in the review of this report:

The individuals listed above have provided many constructive comments and suggestions, but responsibility for the final content of this report rests solely with the authoring committee and the Institute of Medicine.

Preface

The U.S. immunization system is a national treasure that is too often taken for granted. Through an intricate maze of public- and private-sector activity, vaccines are delivered to thousands of children, adolescents, and adults each day. The process by which each of us achieves up-to-date immunization status for ourselves and our children differs in large part by the circumstances of birth. Geographic and economic differences in these circumstances can contribute to disparities in access to vaccines and lead to reduced levels of immunization coverage within a general population. Such disparities are not as important, for the purpose of immunization coverage, if they occur within populations that largely achieve complete immunization status. If such disparities are concentrated with certain groups, however, outbreaks of infectious disease that have tragic consequences can occur.

Today we are involved in a national experiment with health care reform. The delivery of immunizations for disadvantaged populations, which once occurred primarily through public health clinics, has shifted in large part to the private sector. This shift has occurred swiftly and unevenly over the past decade, stimulated by changes in Medicaid policies and practices, the creation of new governmental programs such as Vaccines for Children (VFC), and the adoption of a new federal–state partnership known as the State Children's Health Insurance Program (SCHIP). These changes have occurred against a backdrop of traditional public health practices that served disadvantaged families for many decades in each state.

The privatization of primary health care services for the nation's disadvantaged children has caused many individuals to question the scope and scale of federal assistance for state immunization programs. Childhood immunization coverage levels are currently high, and outbreaks of vaccine-preventable infectious disease are low. Adult immunization coverage rates are low, and programs designed to improve coverage levels are rare at the federal or state level. Given these conditions, is the federal government spending too much or too little to support immunization programs within each state? What role should state governments play in this area? And how important are the data collection, assessment, and outreach efforts of public health agencies if most immunization services are being delivered in the private sector?

In this context, the U.S. Senate Appropriations Committee and the Centers for Disease Control and Prevention (CDC) asked the Institute of Medicine to examine the roles and responsibilities of the state and federal governments in supporting immunization programs and services. The Committee on Immunization Finance Policies and Practices was formed to conduct this study. The committee was asked to give attention to a specific program administered by CDC, known as Section 317, that makes annual awards to the states to help them purchase vaccines and support infrastructure efforts. The committee was asked to consider the history of this program, as well as its relationship to newer federal health initiatives such as VFC and SCHIP.

In conducting this study, the 15-member committee met five times during the period February 1999 through January 2000. We commissioned a state survey and eight case studies to inform our deliberations, and we hosted a workshop on issues related to pockets of need, held in September 1999 in Washington, D.C.* Several committee members, consultants, and staff participated in site visits conducted during the period September 1999 through January 2000 in four areas: Detroit, Michigan; Houston, Texas; Newark, New Jersey; and Los Angeles and San Diego, California. We received testimony from a distinguished group of federal, state, and local health officials; representatives of state organizations; congressional staff; and researchers engaged in studies of the national immunization system.

The committee benefited from a series of reports and briefings provided by the staff of the National Immunization Program within CDC, which is responsible for administering the Section 317 grants and the VFC program. CDC staff attended many of the committee meetings and par-

---

*Selected materials from the case studies, state survey, and background papers commissioned by the committee will appear in a special supplemental issue of the *American Journal of Preventive Medicine*, Vol. 19, No. 3S, in October 2000.

ticipated in the September workshop. We are grateful to each of these officials for their thoughtful contributions and expertise over the course of the study: Angie Bauer, Kristin Brusuelas, Jose Cordero, Russell Havlak, Glen Koops, Joel Kuritsky, Martin Landry, Edward Maes, Dean Mason, James Mize, William Nichols, Dennis O'Mara, Walter A. Orenstein, Lance Rodewald, Jeanne M. Santoli, Abigail Shefer, Allyson Shoe, and Nicole Smith.

State health officials also contributed perspectives and information in meetings and conversations with committee members, staff, and consultants. We are especially grateful to the immunization project directors, program managers, and other health officials in each of the states who made themselves available for lengthy phone interviews as part of the project's state survey and case studies. We would particularly like to thank the following individuals for their efforts: Christine Grant, New Jersey Department of Health and Human Services; David Johnson, Michigan Department of Community Health; Brad Prescott, Texas Department of Health; Natalie Smith, Immunization Branch, California Department of Health; and Donald Williamson, Alabama Department of Public Health. Several federal officials assisted in arranging meetings with key agency personnel who provided background information relevant to the study, and we are grateful for their assistance: Patricia MacTaggart, Health Care Financing Administration; Doris Barnette and Rita Goodman, Health Resources and Services Administration; and Barbara Hallman, U.S. Department of Agriculture.

Data collection and analysis and the development of the final study report required an extensive staff effort. Study Director Rosemary Chalk organized our discussions and prepared several drafts of the study report to guide our analysis and recommendations. Senior Program Officer Wilhelmine Miller was responsible for overseeing the development of the case studies and preparation of the site visit reports and provided much of the analysis for Chapter 3 of this report. Two senior program assistants provided valuable assistance over the course of the study. Suzanne Miller prepared materials for Chapter 2, coauthored two papers on adult immunization and the role of immunization registries, and contributed to the production of the numerous charts and figures in this report. Heather Schofield ably administered the myriad activities associated with each meeting, briefing book, workshop, and site visit, and also prepared our public access files over the course of the study. Other staff made important contributions during the initial or final stages of data collection: Division Director Janet Corrigan prepared the initial project proposal, Senior Program Officer Jane Durch prepared descriptive materials and an analysis of the carryover problem in the Section 317 grant awards, Research Assistant Stacey Patmore conducted initial bibliographic searches on behalf of the committee, and Senior Program Assistant Tracy McKay completed final edits of the report and assisted with bringing the manuscript into production. We also thank our editors Rona Briere, Kristin Motley, and Mike Edington; Sally Stanfield and Estelle Miller from the National Academy Press; and Stayce Bush from the reprographics unit, whose efforts all made significant contributions to the organization and presentation of the committee's views.

The committee was extremely fortunate in obtaining the services of a talented and dedicated group of consultants who prepared background papers and case studies to guide and inform the committee's deliberations: Gerry Fairbrother, Amy Fine, Robin Flint, Roy Hogan, Kay Johnson, Hanns Kuttner, Eamon Magee, Heather McPhillips, Victor Miller, Greg Poland, Barbara Richards, and Kathy Stroup. Gary Freed, Sarah Clark, and Anne Cowan in the Division of General Pediatrics, University of Michigan, prepared the state survey that provided much of the data supporting our analysis of state immunization policies and practices. Other individuals, including Harris Berman from Tufts Health Plan; Steven Boedigheimer from the Delaware Health and Social Services; Victoria Freeman from the University of North Carolina at Chapel Hill; Alan Hinman from the Task Force for Child Survival and Development; Vince Hutchins from the National Center for Education in Maternal and Child Health; Kala Ladenheim of the National Conference of State Legislatures; Donald Mattison from the March of Dimes; and William Roper from the University of North Carolina offered useful suggestions and perspectives at critical times in the development of the report. We also benefited from the expertise of staff from professional organizations that are concerned with immunization and the vitality of the nation's public health system. These include Karen Hendricks, American Academy of Pediatrics; Craig Carlson, American Association of Health Plans; Catherine Hess, Association of Maternal and Child Health Programs; Claire Hannan, Association of State and Territorial Health Officers; Tom Musco, Health Insurance Association of America; Cynthia Phillips, National Association of City and County Health Officers; and Doug Greenaway, National Association of Women, Infants, and Children (WIC) Directors. Additional materials regarding state roles in public health were provided by Joan Henneberry of the National Governors' Association and Mary Smith from the National Conference of State Legislatures. We thank each of these individuals and organizations for their assistance and advice over the course of this study.

Bernard Guyer, M.D., M.P.H., *Chair*
David R. Smith, M.D., *Vice Chair*
Committee on Immunization Finance
Policies and Practices

Contents

Boxes, Tables, and Figures

BOXES

TABLES

FIGURES

CALLING THE SHOTS

Executive Summary

ABSTRACT Federal, state, and private-sector investments in vaccine purchases and immunization programs are lagging behind emerging opportunities to reduce the risks of vaccine-preventable diseases. Although federal assistance to the states for immunization programs and data collection efforts rapidly expanded in the early part of the 1990s, significant cutbacks have occurred in the last 5 years that have reduced the size of state grant awards by more than 50 percent from their highest point. During this same period, the vaccine delivery system for children and adults has become more complex and fragmented.

A combination of new challenges and reduced resources has led to instability in the public health infrastructure that supports the U.S. immunization system. Many states have reduced the scale of their immunization programs and currently lack adequate strength in areas such as data collection among at-risk populations, strategic planning, program coordination, and assessment of immunization status in communities that are served by multiple health care providers. If unmet immunization needs are not identified and addressed, states will have difficulty in achieving the national goal of 90 percent coverage by the year 2010 for completion of the childhood vaccination series for young children. Furthermore, state and national coverage rates, which reached record levels for vaccines in widespread use (79 percent) in 1998, can be expected to decline, and outbreaks of vaccine-preventable diseases may occur as a result, particularly among persons who are vulnerable to these diseases because of their undervaccination status.

The Institute of Medicine (IOM) Committee on Immunization Finance Policies and Practices has therefore concluded that a renewal and strengthening of the federal and state immunization partnership is necessary. The goal of this renewed partnership is to prevent infectious disease; to monitor, sustain, and improve vaccine coverage rates for child and adult populations within more numerous and increasingly diversified health care settings; and to respond to vaccine safety concerns. To achieve this renewal, states require a consistent strategy, additional funds, and a multiyear finance plan that can help expedite the delivery of new vaccines; strengthen the immunization assessment, assurance, and policy development functions in each state; and adapt childhood immunization programs to serve the needs of new age groups (especially adults with chronic diseases) in different health care environments.

The IOM committee recommends that federal and state governments adopt a national finance strategy that would allocate $1.5 billion in federal and state resources over the first 5 years to strengthen the infrastructure for child and adult immunization—an annual increase of $175 million over current spending levels. These resources would consist of $200 million per year in state infrastructure grants awarded by the Centers for Disease Control and Prevention (CDC) (the Section 317 program) and an additional $100 million per year in increased state contributions. The committee also recommends that Congress replace the current discretionary Section 317 grants with a formula approach for state immunization grant awards to improve the targeting and stability of federal immunization grants. The formula should provide a base level of support to all states, as well as additional amounts related to each state's need, capacity, and performance. The committee further recommends that Congress introduce a state match requirement for the receipt of increased federal funds to help strengthen and stabilize the infrastructure that supports long-term public health assessment, assurance, and policy development efforts.

Along with the development of a strategic investment plan to support immunization infrastructure, the committee recommends that the federal government provide $50 million in additional funds to help states purchase pneumococcal and influenza vaccines for adults under age 65 who are not eligible for other forms of public health insurance and who have chronic illnesses such as heart and lung disease or diabetes. The committee further recommends that states increase their own vaccine purchases by $11 million annually for adults who cannot afford vaccines but are not eligible for federal assistance (the "underinsured"). Finally, the committee recommends that federal and state agencies develop a set of consistent and comparable measures to monitor the immunization status of children and adults enrolled in public and private health plans.

BACKGROUND

During the 1990s, the U.S. federal and state governments built a dynamic and flexible immunization system that has adapted to extensive changes in the science of vaccines, in demographic patterns, and in service-delivery patterns, in places ranging from remote rural counties to densely populated metropolitan areas. This highly decentralized system is shaped by local circumstances, resources, and needs, as well as by national goals and policies. Though complex and cumbersome, the federal–state immunization partnership has demonstrated an extraordinary capacity to ensure the reliable delivery of an increasing number of vaccine antigens for an expanding range of age groups, including newborns, preschool and school-aged children, adolescents, and adults in a growing number of private and public health care settings.

At present, however, the public health infrastructure that supports the national immunization system is fragile and unstable. Three trends contribute to this instability:

- rapid acceleration in the science of vaccine research and production,
- increasing complexity of the health care services environment of the United States (represented by trends such as the emergence of private managed care organizations as the primary health care providers for low-income populations), and
- recent reductions in federal immunization grants to the states (reflecting congressional responses to shifting health care roles and responsibilities within the federal government, the states, and private health care providers), which followed on the heels of dramatic increases in the early 1990s.

This instability can create pressure points and service gaps that contribute to vaccine coverage disparities and may result in outbreaks of infectious disease. The resurgence of measles in 1989–1991 in the United States, which included a series of outbreaks that contributed to 43,000 cases and more than 100 deaths, primarily among children younger than 5 years of age, is a constant reminder that the presence of vaccines alone is not sufficient to protect populations against vaccine-preventable disease. Outbreaks can emerge swiftly and unexpectedly during times of complacency if vaccines are not accessible to those who are most vulnerable to infectious disease. The absence of adequate measurement tools and appropriate community assessment studies can result in reduced vigilance within the health care system if missing data foster mistaken beliefs that national or local immunization rates are up to date.

Although record levels of immunization were achieved across the

United States in the 1990s, certain problems persist within the national immunization system. These problems include the following:

- *The need to sustain and document high levels of immunization coverage for a growing number of vaccines delivered within multiple health care settings.* Each day sees a new birth cohort of 11,000 infants in the United States, all of whom require routine immunizations in their first 2 years of life. An enormous effort is required in both private and public health care settings to sustain the 1998 level of 79 percent coverage of completion of the recommended immunization series for 2-year-olds across the United States. Improving coverage levels to reach the national goal of 90 percent will be increasingly difficult as new vaccines are added to the recommended schedule and as uncertainties about the benefits of vaccines increase in the absence of visible harm from infectious disease.
- *Persistent disparities in childhood levels of immunization coverage.* The immunization system has successfully reduced racial and ethnic disparities in childhood immunization levels, but coverage levels in areas of concentrated poverty remain significantly lower than national and state-wide levels. National surveys reveal a gap of 9 percentage points between children above and below the federal poverty level for the complete series of the most critical childhood vaccines. Significant disparities also persist in coverage rates in many metropolitan areas that have large populations of low-income residents. In some cases, childhood vaccination coverage rates are as much as 19 percent lower for metropolitan residents compared with the remainder of the state.
- *Low coverage rates and racial and ethnic disparities for adult vaccines.* Immunization coverage rates for adults are well below those achieved for childhood immunizations. National immunization levels for influenza vaccines (which are needed annually) have increased to 63 percent (1997) for adults age 65 and older, but levels of pneumococcal vaccination (which is usually a one-time event) among this age group are significantly lower: only 42 percent of noninstitutionalized adults over age 65 had ever received a pneumococcal vaccination by 1997. Coverage rates for high-risk adults who suffer from chronic disease (e.g., heart or lung disease or diabetes) are especially poor (26 percent have received an influenza vaccination, while only 13 percent have received a pneumococcal vaccination). Validated coverage estimates for other adult vaccines (e.g., hepatitis A, hepatitis B, tetanus, and varicella) are severely limited or nonexistent. In addition to low coverage levels, significant racial and ethnic disparities continue to persist in adult immunization levels.
- *Mortality and morbidity from preventable infectious disease.* Between 50,000 and 70,000 adults and about 300 children in the United States die annually from vaccine-preventable diseases or their complications. The

preventable illness and subsequent complications that result from missed vaccines carry a high and avoidable cost for individuals and society as a whole.

• *Serious gaps and inconsistencies in the coordination, support, and documentation of immunization efforts.* Stress-related cracks stemming from the complexity of the nation's immunization system show signs of deepening as shifts occur within public and private health care delivery systems. Recent controversies over the use of federally financed vaccines for children who are enrolled in stand-alone (i.e., non-Medicaid) state-sponsored insurance programs, for example, reflect inconsistencies and ambiguities in service-delivery efforts.

The collective result of the above trends is diminishing the public benefit of vaccines, especially for groups of children and adults who do not have routine access to high-quality primary care.

CHARGE TO THE COMMITTEE

Current analyses of federal and state spending for immunization services and programs reveal the absence of a strategic plan that can guide a federal–state partnership in supporting immunization efforts. The absence of a national consensus about the roles and responsibilities of federal and state agencies in fostering immunization also complicates efforts to extend the benefits of immunization to the relatively small population of high-risk children and the larger pool of adults who remain unprotected.

It is for these reasons that the U.S. Senate Appropriations Committee in 1998 asked the Institute of Medicine (IOM) to conduct a study of the Section 317 program administered by the Centers for Disease Control and Prevention (CDC).[1] The study was designed to identify areas in which research-based evidence can guide federal, state, and local immunization policies and practices. The Congress formulated five key questions as the basis for the IOM study:

1. What was the extent of overall spending by all sources for immunizations in the United States during the 1990s?

2. How were new federal funds spent by the states, and to what extent did states maintain their own levels of effort over the past 5 years?

3. What are current and future funding requirements for immunization activities, and how can those requirements be met through a combination of state funding, federal Section 317 immunization grant funding, and funding available through the State Children's Health Insurance Program (SCHIP)?

4. How should federal grant funds be distributed among the states?

5. How should funds be targeted within states to reach high-risk populations without diminishing levels of coverage among the overall population?

In addition, a sixth question was added by CDC during the negotiation of the study contract:

6. What should be the role and financing level for CDC's current program supporting state efforts to vaccinate adults and achieve the nation's goals for influenza and pneumococcal vaccines?

These questions reflect a need for guidance to clarify roles and help balance federal and state contributions in extending the benefits of immunization to unprotected children and adults.

SIX ROLES OF THE NATIONAL IMMUNIZATION SYSTEM

In examining current immunization policies and practices in the public and private health care sectors, the IOM committee identified six fundamental roles of the national immunization system:

- Assure the purchase of recommended vaccines for the total population of U.S. children and adults, with particular emphasis on the protection of vulnerable groups.
- Assure access to such vaccines within the public sector when private health care services are not adequate to meet local needs.
- Control and prevent infectious disease.
- Conduct populationwide surveillance of immunization coverage levels, including the identification of significant disparities, gaps, and vaccine safety concerns.
- Sustain and improve immunization coverage levels within child and adult populations, especially in vulnerable communities.
- Use primary care and public health resources efficiently in achieving national immunization goals.

The last of these roles provides overarching support for the other five, and was the focus of the committee's charge. Figure ES-1 displays these roles as components of the national immunization partnership.

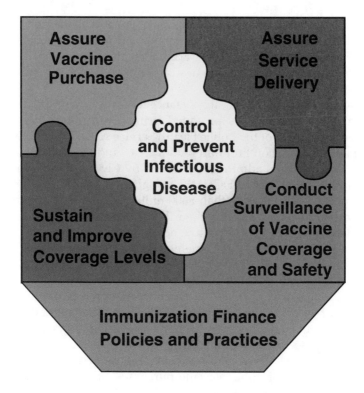

FIGURE ES-1 Six roles of the national immunization system.

A FEDERAL–STATE IMMUNIZATION PARTNERSHIP

Efforts to meet national immunization goals currently involve a set of intricate and separate financial arrangements among federal, state, and local health agencies, as well as collaborative ventures with public and private health care providers. In conducting the study, we gave particular attention to the responsibilities of federal, state, and local health agencies and the burden of effort that is required to support each of the above roles in an integrated manner. State governments are the public health stewards for disadvantaged populations within their borders, and have traditionally been responsible for meeting the health needs of residents who are not served or are underserved by the private health care sector. Each state currently invests in immunization programs through direct or in-kind support, but no state has sufficient resources to support all six of the above immunization roles. Consequently, federal assistance is required to help each state maintain the essential elements of an immunization program, to respond to unexpected circumstances and changing conditions that require enhanced efforts, and to prevent infectious disease transmission across state borders. These arrangements are traditionally divided into two categories: vaccine purchase and infrastructure support.

Vaccine Purchase. Federal assistance for state vaccine purchases and immunization programs is provided primarily through two funding streams: Section 317 of the Public Health Service Act, administered by the National Immunization Program within CDC, and the Vaccines for Children (VFC) program, administered jointly by CDC and the Health Care Financing Administration (HCFA). Through these two efforts, the federal government awarded more than $600 million in vaccine supplies to the states in fiscal year (FY) 1999, primarily for childhood vaccines. In addition, Medicare pays for preventive adult vaccines, which are financed primarily through Medicare payments to physicians. In 1998, HCFA paid Medicare providers $114 million for influenza and pneumococcal immunizations, primarily for adults over age 65.

The vast majority of states depend primarily on federal grants for the purchase of vaccines. Only 10 states rely on state funds for 30 percent or more of the public dollars spent to purchase vaccines. In almost half the states (24), state funds account for less than 10 percent of all publicly purchased vaccines. The remaining states (16) use state funds for between 10 and 30 percent of public vaccine purchases. State-level funds enable the purchase of vaccines for many underinsured children and adults (who are not eligible for federally financed vaccines), especially those who receive vaccines in local public health clinics. Fifteen states have adopted universal purchase policies, whereby they purchase vaccines for all children served by public clinics or participating providers, regardless of their insurance status.

The number of sites administering childhood or adult vaccines purchased with government funds increased dramatically over the past decade—from about 3,000 public health clinics and several hundred Medicaid health care providers in the 1980s to more than 50,000 public and private sites in 1999. The creation of VFC has been extraordinarily successful in encouraging large numbers of private health care professionals to administer vaccines to low-income children as part of their primary health care benefits. But this success in increasing the size and diversity of the vaccine delivery system has complicated the tasks of educating providers, assessing safety, documenting coverage rates, and assuring fairness in providing access to vaccines in public and private settings.

Immunization Infrastructure. Local, state, and federal public health agencies incur significant expense in exercising their responsibilities for monitoring infectious disease outbreaks, vaccine coverage levels, quality of care, and safety concerns. The states differ in the scope and type of public health infrastructure on which they rely to provide both immunization services for disadvantaged individuals and populationwide programs that benefit all citizens within the state.

Some states are better positioned, because of internal administrative arrangements, to use federal funds (e.g., Medicaid, VFC, Section 317 grants, or funds from the newer SCHIP) to support their public health infrastructure. But recent fluctuations in health care programs, reductions in Section 317 grants, and restrictions on the use of federal funds have significantly reduced the ability of many states to develop innovative approaches to program management, data collection, or interactions with private health care providers. Because the Section 317 grants program does not require matching state investments, fiscal incentives for states to share the costs of developing immunization programs that benefit state residents are absent.

The range of per capita contributions among the states is extremely broad: 4 states reported spending more than $10 per capita of their own funds, while the majority of states (31) reported contributions of less than $5 per capita. Only 4 states have direct state funding for a substantial portion (more than 40 percent) of their immunization program infrastructure, and almost half of the states (21) provide no direct state funding for infrastructure needs. When compared with vaccine purchase practices, these estimates indicate a limited commitment within the states to support the public health infrastructure that is required to meet local needs as well as national goals.

Private-Sector Role. The emerging role of the private sector in providing routine medical care for disadvantaged populations requires ongoing attention and oversight to determine whether vulnerable groups are up to date in their immunization coverage. Individual health care providers and health plans have traditionally not been expected to monitor patterns of vaccine coverage or disease within their communities, nor are they currently equipped to assess coverage levels in formats that can facilitate long-term populationwide studies or analysis of local or statewide health patterns.

IMMUNIZATION FINANCE POLICIES AND PRACTICES

Federal funding for state immunization programs underwent a major and rapid rise in response to the 1989–1991 measles epidemic: there was a more than seven-fold increase from $37 million in 1990 to $261 million in 1995. States faced administrative challenges in responding to these initiatives, however, and carried forward large amounts of unspent federal grant monies for several years. As a consequence, federal infrastructure grants declined during 1996–1998. In turn, states had to reduce efforts in such areas as clinic hours and mobile sites; immunization outreach; performance assessment; information and program management; and linkage with community-based programs, such as the Women, Infants, and Children (WIC) clinics. The annual average total of state infrastructure grant awards administered by CDC from 1994 to 1999 was $271 million, compared with an estimated total of $123 million in the year 2000 (see Table ES-1). In the past 5 years (1995–2000), Section 317 infrastructure grants to the states have decreased by more than 50 percent.

The states reported to CDC estimates of state-level annual expenditures for 2000 for vaccine purchase ($109 million) and operations ($231 million). These estimates include support from other federal programs (e.g., Maternal and Child Health grants), state revenues, and private contributions (see Table ES-1).

CONCLUSIONS

Conclusion 1: The repetitive ebb and flow cycles in the distribution of public resources for immunization programs have created instability and uncertainty that impeded project planning at the state and local levels in the late 1990s, and delayed the public benefit of advances in the development of new vaccines for both children and adults. This instability now erodes the continued success of immunization activities.

The instability of funding for state immunization programs discourages the development of strategic responses designed to foster disease prevention, improve immunization coverage levels for specific populations and age groups, reduce coverage disparities between low-income groups and the general population, and ensure vaccine safety.

Conclusion 2: Immunization policy needs to be national in scope. At the same time, the implementation of immunization policy must be flexible enough to respond to special circumstances that occur at the state and local levels.

A comprehensive strategy that clarifies the roles and responsibilities of federal and state agencies as well as private-sector providers and health plans is needed to sustain an important intergovernmental partnership in the midst of change and complexity. Consistent policies and practices at both the state and federal levels are essential to foster productive relationships and reduce overlap among multiple programs and services.

National initiatives that provide immunization coverage for larger numbers of disadvantaged families under private and public health insurance plans require state public health responsibilities to shift from direct service delivery to oversight roles concerned with assessment, assurance, and policy development. Yet certain residual immunization needs will remain that will necessitate reliable access to vaccines within the public health sector. States need flexibility and resources to adapt to these shifts, which occur unevenly across and within state borders.

Conclusion 3: Federal and state governments each have important roles in supporting not only vaccine purchase, but also infrastructure efforts that can achieve and sustain national immunization goals.

The federal government should be the senior finance partner for the national immunization system because of the central importance of vaccines in contributing to the nation's health, and because disease outbreaks in one region can threaten the health of another without respect for political borders. However, the federal role is to supplement and support states, not replace them, in their day-to-day efforts to assure that every child and adult is properly immunized. State legislatures and governments should be expected to sustain an immunization infrastructure that reflects each state's need, capacity, and performance. Because states are the ultimate stewards of public health, they are responsible for delivering services to those whose immunization needs are not met by the private sector. Performance monitoring, including the development of immunization registries, is important to assure that vulnerable groups have access to adequate primary health care and that public resources are used efficiently in meeting residual needs where necessary.

Conclusion 4: Private health care plans and providers have the capacity to do more in implementing immunization surveillance and preventive programs within their health practices, but such efforts require additional assistance, oversight, and incentives. At the same time, comprehensive insurance and high-quality primary care services do not replace the need for public health infrastructure.

The committee believes health plans should not have the option of providing selective coverage for vaccines once they have been recommended for widespread use, as is currently the practice in most states. For example, all health plans (public and private) that offer primary care benefits for children and adults should bear the costs of integrating all vaccines recommended for widespread use into their basic health care package. Federal mandates for insurance coverage may be necessary to

TABLE ES-1 Recommended Finance Levels for the National Immunization System (Section 317, Vaccines for Children [VFC] Program, and state-level contributions) ($ in millions)

Funding Source	Baseline Annual Avg.[a] (FY 1994–1999)	FY 2000 Award[a]	IOM Committee Recommendation		FY 2002 Appropriation
			Rationale for FY 2002 Appropriations		
FEDERAL					
A. Section 317					
1. Vaccine purchase awards	160	162	1. Sustain current spending levels to meet residual needs		160
Expenditures (child)	115	N/A			
Expenditures (adult)	4	N/A	2. Increase federal assistance to the states to purchase adult vaccines to improve coverage rates		50
2. Infrastructure awards	271[b]	123	3. Increase annual award to reflect state capacity as reflected in historical expenditure levels		200
Expenditures	187	111	4. Increase allocation of federal funds to states that have significant immunization needs		
			5. Maintain a "hold harmless" condition for existing state awards		
Total Section 317 Awards	**431**	**285**			**410**
B. VFC (vaccine purchase and operations)	397	548			548[c]
Total Federal Contribution (excluding Medicaid, Medicare)	**828**	**833**			**958**

STATE				
1. Vaccine purchase estimates	N/A	109[d]	6. Sustain and increase state vaccine purchases, especially for adults	120
2. Infrastructure funds and program operations estimates	N/A	231	7. Build support for infrastructure within each state	331
			8. Add state match requirement for new federal funds	
Total State Contribution	**N/A**	**340**		**451**
TOTAL (federal/state combined)	**Unknown**	**1,173**		**1,409**

[a]Source: Centers for Disease Control and Prevention (CDC), National Immunization Program. State-level data based on self-reports by the states submitted to CDC in August 1999, estimating state-level expenditures for the year 2000.

[b]Includes $261 million in Financial Assistance and $10 million in Direct Assistance; also includes carryover funds as well as new awards.

[c]This figure is likely to increase when new recommendations of the Advisory Committee on Immunization Practices are incorporated into the vaccine schedule. For example, the pneumococcal conjugate vaccine was approved in February 2000 for all infants < 2 years of age and for high-risk children < 5 years of age.

[d]State report data include funds from multiple sources, including state revenues and in-kind support, local funds, other federal funds applied to immunization efforts (e.g., Title V, Preventive Health Services Block Grants), and private funds.

reduce serious disparities between public and private health plan benefits. Public health agencies should not be expected to supplement immunization benefits within public or private health insurance plans except under short-term conditions, such as emergency outbreaks or "catch-up" conditions following the licensing of new vaccines.

In addition to vaccine coverage benefits, health plan providers can assess immunization coverage rates among their enrollees in ways that can contribute to accurate community health profiles at the state and local levels. These efforts require independent oversight, however, to assure that all groups are included in such assessments, including those populations that are not currently enrolled in public and private health plans. Public health agencies can provide important measurement and audit services, such as assessment and feedback for private providers, as an investment in the quality of community health.

RECOMMENDATIONS

The financial components of the following six recommendations are summarized in Table ES-1.

Recommendation 1: The annual federal and state budgets for the purchase of childhood vaccines for public health providers appear to be adequate, but additions to the vaccine schedule are likely to increase the burden of effort within each state. Therefore, the committee recommends that CDC be required to notify Congress each year of the estimated cost impact of new vaccines that have been added to the immunization schedule so that these figures can be considered in reviewing the vaccine purchase and infrastructure budgets for the Section 317 program.

The committee believes the annual allocation of federal funds for the purchase of vaccines through the VFC program ($505 million for FY 2000) and the Section 317 state grant program ($162 million per year for FY 2000) is sufficient to meet state requests for child vaccines within the immunization schedule recommended by ACIP as of January 2000.[2] But additions to the ACIP schedule will expand the burden of preventive health care costs to state and federal health agencies as well as private health plans.

Congress should anticipate such cost increases by requiring that CDC notify Congress each year of two trends: (1) the estimated cost impact of new vaccines (including administration fees) that are scheduled for consideration as additions to the recommended immunization schedule, and

(2) the length of time that may be involved from the point at which such vaccines are recommended by the Advisory Committee on Immunization Practices (ACIP) to the establishment of a VFC contract. Federal and state vaccine purchase budgets should then be adjusted as necessary.

Recommendation 2: Additional funds are needed to purchase vaccines for uninsured and underinsured adult populations within the states. The committee recommends that Congress increase the annual Section 317 vaccine budget by $50 million per year to meet residual needs for high-risk adolescents and adults under age 65 who do not qualify for other federal assistance. The committee further recommends that state governments likewise increase their spending for adult vaccines by $11 million per year.

These estimates are based on calculations of the residual vaccine needs for uninsured at-risk populations, including adults who are younger than age 65 and suffer from chronic disease; for hepatitis B coverage among adolescents; for adults who are at risk because of sexual behavior or occupational settings; and for tetanus coverage for unprotected adults. Both federal and state vaccine purchase budgets will require annual adjustments as vaccine costs change or new vaccines or age groups are added to the adult immunization schedule. Therefore, CDC notification of the impact of such changes should be required annually, as indicated in Recommendation 1.

The improvement of adult immunization rates will require more than increased vaccine purchases. A comprehensive and coordinated adult immunization program needs to be initiated within each state, with leadership at the national, state, and local levels, to encourage the participation of private and public health care providers in offering immunizations to adults under the guidelines established in the ACIP schedule.

Recommendation 3: State immunization infrastructure programs require increased financial and administrative support to strengthen immunization capacity and reduce disparities in child and adult coverage rates. The committee recommends that states increase their immunization budgets by adding $100 million over current spending levels, supplemented by an annual federal budget of $200 million to support state infrastructure efforts.

The committee believes state immunization programs could achieve stability and carry out their roles adequately through the adoption of a national finance strategy that involves investing a total of $1.5 billion in federal and state funds in the first 5 years to support infrastructure efforts within the states. The federal budget figure of $200 million per year is derived from three calculations: (1) annual state expenditure levels during the mid-1990s, (2) the level of spending necessary to provide additional resources to states with high levels of need without reducing current award levels for each state (known as a "hold harmless" provision), and (3) additional infrastructure requirements associated with adjusting to anticipated changes and increased complexity in the immunization schedule. The additional state contribution of $100 million per year above current spending levels is necessary to reduce current disparities in state spending practices and to address future infrastructure needs in such areas as records management, development of appropriate performance measures and immunization registries, and outreach and education for adult vaccines.

Federal reporting requirements for immunization grants should be reduced to six key areas that reflect the six fundamental roles of the national immunization system discussed in this report. Grant budgetary cycles should be extended to 2 years to give states greater discretion and flexibility to plan and implement multiyear efforts in each area.

Recommendation 4: Congress should improve the targeting and stability of Section 317 immunization grant awards to the states by replacing the current discretionary grant award mechanism with formula grant legislation.

The formula should reflect a base level as well as factors related to each state's need, capacity, and performance. A state match requirement should be introduced so that federal and state agencies share the total costs of supporting the infrastructure required to operate a national immunization program and respond to the needs of disadvantaged populations.

Recommendation 5: CDC should initiate a dialogue with federal and state health agencies, state legislatures, state governors, and Congress immediately so that legislative and budgetary reforms can be proposed promptly when Section 317 is up for reauthorization in FY 2002.

The construction of a grant formula and the calculation of weights as recommended above is a complex analytical process that requires estimating the appropriate size of the federal base grant; determining the conditions that would facilitate redistribution of federal resources to areas of need but also maintain an adequate level of investment within each state (the hold harmless conditions); developing an appropriate set of proxy measures that reflect need, capacity, and performance in the field of immunization; and choosing the appropriate multiyear finance mechanism for the allocation of federal funds. This work should begin immediately if its results are to be available when needed.

> **Recommendation 6: Federal and state agencies should develop a set of consistent and comparable immunization measures for use in monitoring the status of children and adults enrolled in private and public health plans.**

Assessments of these rates should allow state and federal governments to monitor immunization levels and identify disparities in need, capacity, and performance over time and among regions, including small geographic areas and selected health plans (e.g., Medicaid, SCHIP, and private insurance). A small set of comparable measures that can harmonize the Health Plan Employer Data and Information Set and the National Immunization Survey, for example, will allow federal and state agencies to monitor state need, capacity, and performance without imposing unnecessarily burdensome reporting efforts on the states that would restrict their ability to use federal funds productively in responding to local circumstances. Such measures can also facilitate efforts by state and federal health officials to assess the quality of primary-care health services within private-sector health plans, so that public health agencies can direct appropriate resources to areas in which private-sector plans do not have sufficient capacity to meet health care needs. The use of consistent immunization measures offers benefit not only for immunization efforts, but also for other national programs that require national investments in primary health care.

ENDNOTES

1. Section 317 of the Public Health Service Act authorizes federal grants to the states to assist them in meeting the costs of preventive health services programs for immunization. The program includes grants for vaccine purchase as well as for the development of state infrastructure efforts. This study was requested in U.S. Senate Report 105-300 to accompany S. 2440 (Departments of Labor, Health and Human Services, and Education and Related Agencies Appropriations Bill), which directed CDC to contract with the Institute of Medicine to conduct an evaluation of the recent successes, resource needs, cost structure, and strategies of immunization efforts in the United States.

2. ACIP approval of the pneumococcal conjugate vaccine occurred after the IOM committee formulated its vaccine purchase recommendations and is not reflected in this calculation.

1

Introduction

The future of the national immunization partnership, especially the status of the public health infrastructure for immunization within the states, is the focus of this report of the Institute of Medicine (IOM). We propose a national strategy to guide the federal and state partnership in supporting immunization efforts, improving coordination, and allocating costs between the public and private health care sectors. We also consider how the roles and responsibilities for this partnership should be shared among federal and state agencies.[1]

BACKGROUND

Immunizations that protect children and adults from the dangers of vaccine-preventable diseases are one of the genuine triumphs of basic medical science and the health care delivery system within the United States. Disease morbidity rates declined dramatically for nine vaccine-preventable diseases (smallpox, polio, diphtheria, pertussis, tetanus, measles, mumps, rubella, and *Haemophilus influenzae* type b) during the 20th century (Centers for Disease Control and Prevention [CDC], 1999a). According to current data, smallpox has been eradicated, the number of polio cases has been reduced to 5,500 worldwide, and each of the other seven diseases occurs only sporadically throughout the United States (CDC, 1999a) (see Table 1-1 for disease mortality trends).

Three key strategies have contributed to this success in disease prevention: (1) the discovery and commercial production of vaccines; (2) the

TABLE 1-1 Comparison of 20th-Century Baseline and Current Morbidity, Vaccine-Preventable Diseases

Disease	20th Century	1999 Provisional	Percent Decrease
Smallpox	48,164	0	100.0
Diphtheria	175,885	1	100.0
Measles	503,282	86	100.0
Mumps	152,209	352	99.8
Pertussis	147,271	6,031	95.9
Polio (paralytic)	16,316	0	100.0
Rubella	47,745	238	99.5
Congenital Rubella Syndrome	823	8	99.0
Tetanus	1,314	33	97.5
Haemophilus influenzae Type b and unknown (< 5 years)	20,000	146	99.2

SOURCES: CDC, 1999a; Cochi et al., 1985.

integration of immunization services (including vaccine purchase and delivery) within private and public systems of personal health care services; and (3) the development of a public health infrastructure that can monitor disease patterns and improve immunization coverage rates, especially among vulnerable populations. The combination of these three strategies has resulted in unprecedented high levels of vaccination coverage for a growing number of vaccines for both children and adults within the United States (see Table 1-2). The U.S. immunization system has also demonstrated an ability to achieve high immunization coverage levels among all age groups, across economic and social class lines, and spanning all racial and ethnic populations (CDC, 1998a). To sustain this success is difficult, however, requiring constant vigilance to detect signs of erosion and decline in coverage rates among vulnerable populations.

Costs of Achieving Current Levels of Immunization Coverage

Enormous effort is required within the U.S. health care system to maintain high levels of immunization coverage for a growing number of vaccines and among various age groups. The effort is especially challenging since a new birth cohort of 11,000 infants born each day requires attention within the routine immunization schedule. The first 2 years of life is perhaps the most vulnerable period for transmission of infectious diseases; thus it is crucial that this population be brought up to date as quickly as possible with regard to immunization status. Indeed, immuni-

TABLE 1-2 Vaccination Coverage Levels Among Children Aged 19–35 Months, by Selected Vaccines (1995–1999[a])

Vaccine/Dose	1995 %	(95% CI[b])	1996 %	(95% CI)	1997 %	(95% CI)	1998 %	(95% CI)	1999[c] %	(95% CI)
DTP[d]										
≥ 3 Doses	94.7	(± 0.6)	95.0	(± 0.4)	95.5	(± 0.4)	95.6	(± 0.5)	95.9	(± 0.4)
≥ 4 Doses	78.5	(± 1.0)	81.1	(± 0.7)	81.5	(± 0.7)	83.9	(± 0.8)	84.0	(± 0.8)
Poliovirus										
≥ 3 Doses	87.9	(± 0.8)	91.1	(± 0.5)	90.8	(± 0.5)	90.8	(± 0.7)	90.0	(± 0.6)
Haemophilus influenzae Type b (Hib)										
≥ 3 Doses	91.7	(± 0.6)	91.7	(± 0.5)	92.7	(± 0.5)	93.4	(± 0.6)	93.7	(± 0.5)
Measle-Containing Vaccine (MCV)										
≥ 1 Doses	89.9	(± 0.7)	90.7	(± 0.5)	90.5	(± 0.5)	92.1	(± 0.6)	92.0	(± 0.6)
Hepatitis B										
≥ 3 Doses	68.0	(± 1.0)	81.8	(± 0.7)	83.7	(± 0.6)	87.0	(± 0.7)	87.9	(± 0.7)
Varicella Vaccine										
1 Dose	N/A[e]		16.0	(± 0.7)	25.9	(± 0.7)	43.2	(± 1.0)	52.1	(± 1.0)
Combined Series										
4 DTP/3 Polio/1 MCV[f]	76.2	(± 1.0)	78.4	(± 0.8)	77.9	(± 0.7)	80.6	(± 0.9)	86.2	(± 0.7)
4 DTP/3 Polio/1 MCV/3 Hib[g]	74.2	(± 1.0)	76.5	(± 0.8)	76.2	(± 0.8)	79.2	(± 0.9)	78.8	(± 0.9)

[a]Children were born during February 1992–May 1994 (1995 survey), February 1993–May 1995 (1996 survey), February 1994–May 1996 (1997 survey), and February 1995–May 1997 (1988 survey).

[b]CI = confidence interval.

[c]First two quarters of 1999 and last two quarters of 1998. Data can be found at http://www.cdc.gov/nip/.

[d]Diphtheria and tetanus toxoids and pertussis vaccine/diphtheria and tetanus toxoids.

[e]Not available; data collection for varicella began in July 1996.

[f]Four or more doses of DTP/DT, three or more doses of poliovirus vaccine, one or more doses of MCV.

[g]Four or more doses of DTP/DT, three or more doses of poliovirus vaccine, one or more doses of MCV, and three or more doses of Hib.

SOURCE: Information provided by CDC.

zation coverage assessments commonly focus on 2-year-olds because older children are usually well immunized as a result of child care or school requirements, because most childhood vaccines must be administered within 24 months after birth, and because the immunization status of this population can reveal shifting health care patterns in different geographic areas and health care settings.

The current vaccine schedule (see Figure 1-1 and Table 1-3) recommends that each infant born today receive between 19 and 23 doses of vaccine, most of which should be administered by 18 months of age, to be fully immunized. In 1987, the cost of fully immunizing a child was $116 in the private sector and $34 in the public sector. One decade later, in 1997, the total costs for the vaccines recommended for children had increased to $332 in the private sector and $176 in the public sector (Orenstein et al., 1999).[2] These costs can escalate rapidly. The manufacturer's list price for the new pneumococcal conjugate vaccine (which is effective against meningitis, bacteremia, pneumonia, and otitis media) is $58 per dose, and the Advisory Committee on Immunization Practices (ACIP) has recommended that infants receive 4 doses of the vaccine before age 2 to complete their immunization (Lieu et al., 2000).

Finally, while vaccine purchase costs have increased in both the public and private sectors, it is important to note that the public sector now bears a larger share of the cost of vaccines. The public-sector discount declined from 75 percent of catalog prices in 1987 to 50 percent in 1997 (Orenstein et al., 1999). A smaller number of vaccines recommended for adults differ by age group (see Table 1-3). Annual influenza vaccine is currently recommended for two categories of adults: (1) all persons aged 50 and older, and (2) all persons younger than 50 with certain chronic conditions, such as diabetes, heart disease, and lung disease (CDC, 2000a). One-time pneumococcal vaccines are recommended for adults aged 65 and older and for younger adults with chronic health conditions. ACIP is considering lowering the age range for this vaccine as well, but as of this writing had not made a revised recommendation. ACIP has also made recommendations regarding adult immunization for hepatitis B, hepatitis A, tetanus, diphtheria, measles, mumps, rubella, varicella, polio, and Lyme disease.

National cost data for adult vaccines are generally not available. According to one estimate, the cost for influenza vaccine ranges from $4.16 to $4.87 in the New York City area and for pneumococcal vaccine from $11.54 in upstate New York to $13.02 in Queens (Poland and Miller, 2000).

In addition to the costs of purchasing vaccines, payers must support many other expenses, including the costs of administering the vaccines (which may or may not be billed separately), and record-keeping costs

22

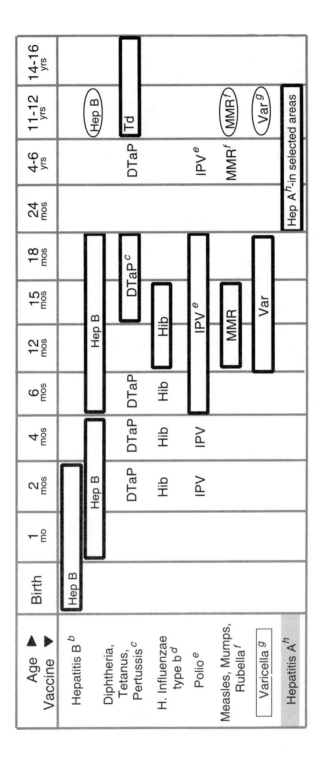

FIGURE 1-1 (Opposite) Recommended childhood immunization schedule—United States, January–December 2000.[a] Vaccines are listed under routinely recommended ages. Bars indicate range of recommended ages for immunization. Any dose not given at the recommended age should be given as a "catch-up" immunization at any subsequent visit when indicated and feasible. Ovals indicate vaccines to be given if previously recommended doses were missed or given earlier than the recommended minimum age. Approved by the Advisory Committee on Immunization Practices (ACIP), the American Academy of Pediatrics (AAP), and the American Academy of Family Physicians (AAFP). *On October 22, 1999, the Advisory Committee on Immunization Practices (ACIP) recommended that Rotashield® (RRV-TV), the only U.S.-licensed rotavirus vaccine, no longer be used in the United States (MMWR, Volume 48, Number 43, Nov. 5, 1999). Parents should be reassured that their children who received rotavirus vaccine before July are not at increased risk for intussusception now.*
[a]This schedule indicates the recommended ages for routine administration of currently licensed childhood vaccines as of 11/1/99. Additional vaccines may be licensed and recommended during the year. Licensed combination vaccines may be used whenever any components of the combination are indicated and its other components are not contraindicated. Providers should consult the manufacturers' package inserts for detailed recommendations.
[b]**Infants born to HBsAg-negative mothers** should receive the 1st dose of hepatitis B (Hep B) vaccine by age 2 months. The 2nd dose should be at least one month after the 1st dose. The 3rd dose should be administered at least 4 months after the 1st dose and at least 2 months after the 2nd dose, but not before 6 months of age for infants.

Infants born to HBsAg-positive mothers should receive hepatitis B vaccine and 0.5 mL hepatitis B immune globulin (HBIG) within 12 hours of birth at separate sites. The 2nd dose is recommended at 1–2 months of age and the 3rd dose at 6 months of age. **Infants born to mothers whose HBsAg status is unknown** should receive hepatitis B vaccine within 12 hours of birth. Maternal blood should be drawn at the time of delivery to determine the mother's HBsAg status; if the HBsAg test is positive, the infant should receive HBIG as soon as possible (no later than 1 week of age). **All children and adolescents (through 18 years of age)** who have not been immunized against hepatitis B may begin the series during any visit. Special efforts should be made to immunize children who were born in or whose parents were born in areas of the world with moderate or high endemicity of hepatitis B virus infection.
[c]The 4th dose of DTaP (diphtheria and tetanus toxoids and acellular pertussis vaccine) may be administered as early as 12 months of age, provided 6 months have elapsed since the 3rd dose and the child is unlikely to return at age 15–18 months. Td (tetanus and diphtheria toxoids) is recommended at 11–12 years of age if at least 5 years have elapsed since the last dose of DTP, DTaP or DT. Subsequent routine Td boosters are recommended every 10 years.
[d]Three *Haemophilus influenzae* type b (Hib) conjugate vaccines are licensed for infant use. If PRP-OMP (PedvaxHIB® or ComVax® [Merck]) is administered at 2 and 4 months of age, a dose at 6 months is not required. Because clinical studies in infants have demonstrated that using some combination products may induce

a lower immune response to the Hib vaccine component, DTaP/Hib combination products should not be used for primary immunization in infants at 2, 4, or 6 months of age, unless FDA-approved for these ages.

*e*To eliminate the risk of vaccine-associated paralytic polio (VAPP), an all-IPV schedule is now recommended for routine childhood polio vaccination in the United States. All children should receive four doses of IPV at 2 months, 4 months, 6–18 months, and 4–6 years. OPV (if available) may be used only for the following special circumstances: 1. Mass vaccination campaigns to control outbreaks of paralytic polio. 2. Unvaccinated children who will be traveling in <4 weeks to areas where polio is endemic or epidemic. 3. Children of parents who do not accept the recommended number of vaccine injections. These children may receive OPV only for the third or fourth dose or both; in this situation, health-care providers should administer OPV only after discussing the risk for VAPP with parents or caregivers. 4. During the transition to an all-IPV schedule, recommendations for the use of remaining OPV supplies in physicians' offices and clinics have been issued by the American Academy of Pediatrics (see *Pediatrics*, December 1999).

*f*The 2nd dose of measles, mumps, and rubella (MMR) vaccine is recommended routinely at 4–6 years of age but may be administered during any visit, provided at least 4 weeks have elapsed since receipt of the 1st dose and that both doses are administered beginning at or after 12 months of age. Those who have not previously received the second dose should complete the schedule by the 11- to 12-year-old visit.

*g*Varicella (Var) vaccine is recommended at any visit on or after the first birthday for susceptible children, i.e., those who lack a reliable history of chickenpox (as judged by a health care provider) and who have not been immunized. Susceptible persons 13 years of age or older should receive 2 doses, given at least 4 weeks apart.

*h*Hepatitis A (Hep A) is shaded to indicate its recommended use in selected states and/or regions; consult your local public health authority. (Also see *MMWR* Oct. 01, 1999/48(RR12); 1–37).

SOURCE: CDC, 2000b.

(sometimes including the cost of registry development and maintenance). Other costs, such as outreach, education, training, data collection, and surveillance of coverage rates and vaccine safety, are incurred by public health agencies (as discussed later in this chapter). The American Academy of Pediatrics has estimated that its members charge approximately $15 per dose for vaccine administration (Fleming, 1995). Vaccine administration fees for adults are significantly lower, and range from $3.95 to $5.38 within the Medicare program, depending on the provider's location (Health Care Financing Administration, 1999a). Such expenses are difficult to monitor, however, because they may or may not be billed separately within well-child visits or other office procedures, depending on

TABLE 1-3 Universally Recommended Vaccinations

Population	Vaccination	Dosage
All young children	Measles, mumps, rubella	2 doses
	Diphtheria-tetanus toxoid and	
	pertussis vaccine	5 doses
	Poliomyelitis	4 doses
	Haemophilus influenzae type b[a]	3–4 doses
	Hepatitis B	3 doses
	Varicella	1 dose
	Hepatitis A (in selected areas)[b]	2 doses
Previously unvaccinated or partially vaccinated adolescents	Hepatitis B[c]	3 doses total
	Varicella	If no previous history of varicella, 1 dose for children aged < 12 years, 2 doses for children aged ≥ 13 years
	Mumps, measles, and rubella	2 doses, total
	Tetanus-diphtheria toxoid	If not vaccinated during previous 5 years, 1 combined booster during ages 11–16 years
All adults	Tetanus-diphtheria	1 dose administered every 10 years
All adults aged ≥ 65[d]	Influenza	1 dose administered annually
	Pneumococcal	1 dose

[a]Only children below age 5 receive *Haemophilus influenzae* type b.
[b]Hepatitis A was added to the schedule after the original table's publication.
[c]An optional two-dose schedule for adolescents aged 11 to 15 was recently approved by the Food and Drug Administration.
[d]The Advisory Committee on Immunization Practices has recommended that all adults aged ≥ 50 receive an influenza vaccination.

SOURCE: Briss et al., 2000.

insurance requirements and local practice guidelines. Some health practices may also charge separate fees for the production and copying of immunization records, fees that are commonly not reimbursed by health plans. Moreover, the shift in many states from fee-for-service to managed care plans (which has occurred swiftly within Medicaid), makes it more difficult to track vaccine administration fees as a separate cost indicator because such fees now are generally included in the capitated payments.

The U.S. federal government currently spends more than $1 billion annually to purchase vaccines for disadvantaged children and adults and to support immunization programs within the 64 grantees, which include the 50 states, 6 municipal regions,[3] and 8 U.S. political jurisdictions (see Table 1-4).[4] These funds are allocated primarily by two federal agencies: CDC, which administers the National Immunization Program, established by Section 317 of the Public Health Service Act (see Appendix A); and the Health Care Financing Administration (HCFA), which administers the Medicaid and Medicare programs and the new State Children's Health Insurance Program (SCHIP) in collaboration with the states. In addition, the Vaccines for Children (VFC) program, created in 1993 through an amendment to the Social Security Act, is financed through HCFA and administered by CDC. CDC supplies VFC vaccines and provides Section 317 vaccines and financial assistance awards to the states annually in response to state requests for assistance and estimates of vaccine need (see Boxes 1-1 and 1-2).

In fiscal year (FY) 1998, the VFC program, which provides federally financed vaccines for four categories of disadvantaged children, spent $437 million in federal funds for vaccines and operational costs; Medicaid program expenditures for immunization in this same year were an additional $127 million, $70 million of which was federal. In addition, CDC provided $418 million in support of vaccine purchase for the states, financial assistance for state immunization programs, and CDC program

TABLE 1-4 Total Federal Immunization Funding, FY 1999 ($ in millions)

Program	Federal	State	Total
Section 317[a]	448	Unknown	448
VFC[b]	467	Not applicable	467
Medicaid	70	57	127
Medicare	115	Not applicable	115
TOTAL	1,100	57	1,157

[a]Total Section 317 federal immunization funding, FY 1999 (actual) as reported in the Department of Health and Human Services FY 2001 Centers for Disease Control and Prevention *Justification of Estimates for Appropriations Committees.*
[b]Total VFC federal immunization funding, FY 1999 (enacted), as reported in the Department of Health and Human Services FY 2001 Centers for Disease Control and Prevention *Justification of Estimates for Appropriations Committees.*

SOURCE: Information provided by CDC.

BOX 1-1
Funding of State Activities Under Section 317 Grant Program

CDC provides annual immunization project grants to 64 separate grantees, including 50 states, the District of Columbia, New York City, Chicago, Houston, San Antonio, Puerto Rico, the Virgin Islands, American Samoa, Guam, the Commonwealth of the Northern Mariana Islands, the Federated States of Micronesia, the Republic of Belau, and the Republic of the Marshall Islands. Immunization grant funds are intended to supplement but not supplant ongoing state and local immunization efforts. Each grantee's funding level is contingent on a number of factors, including historical funding levels, the population size, the size of the state and local public health infrastructure, the size of the grantee's immunization program, the geographical area of the grantee, the proportion of the childhood population served by the public sector, the level of state and local support for the immunization program, the occurrence of vaccine-preventable disease outbreaks, and the grantee's ability to develop programs and expend funds.

Vaccine is available as *Direct Assistance* (in lieu of cash), as requested by the applicant, in the form of a "credit line." Grantees may order childhood or adult vaccines until the credit line is exhausted. CDC also considers requests for CDC personnel (and their travel) and other forms of direct assistance to purchase goods and services through General Services Administration contracts in order to develop and implement immunization registries.

Grant funds in the form of *Financial Assistance* may be used for costs associated with planning, organizing, and conducting immunization programs. Grantees use financial assistance to pay for project personnel, travel, supplies, contracts, other miscellaneous costs, and indirect charges. Grantee personnel carry out programmatic functions such as conducting audits and surveys; investigating vaccine-preventable disease outbreaks; assisting with outbreak control measures; coordinating program efforts with other federal, state, and local governments and private and community-based organizations; and carrying out a variety of professional and community educational efforts.

CDC has always specified that immunization grants are intended to supplement and may not supplant state and local resources. The immunization grants are "discretionary," and no formula exists for the allocation of CDC funding to grantees. Each grantee's funding level is contingent primarily on the grantee's need as expressed in the amount requested annually. Matching funds from the states or territories are not required for the federal grants, and grantees need not allocate any of their own funds to purchase or distribute vaccines or pay for other operational costs. CDC does rely on some grantees to assume a larger share of the responsibility so that a greater proportion of the available funds can be allocated to other grantees.

CDC adjusts the grant awards to meet each grantee's operational needs and unique circumstances in each project area. In general, CDC is unable to provide grantees with as much funding as they request. In the past, the funds have been distributed among geographic regions and earmarked for specific program activities, such as perinatal hepatitis B prevention.

Since 1998, CDC has determined the size of grant awards for each state by applying a uniform percentage reduction to all grantees' operational funding needs.

continued

BOX 1-1 Continued

The requested amounts are adjusted, if necessary, during CDC's review of the applications to exclude budget items outside the scope of the grants and to adjust any amounts considered excessive or unreasonable. The resulting amounts constitute a funding base to which grantee-specific incentive funds are added. In recent years, Senate appropriations language has instructed CDC to distribute $33 million of the grant funds (termed "incentive funding") using a formula that rewards grantees with the highest vaccine coverage rates.

Grantees usually receive funding in two or three installments, although the bulk of operational funds has been awarded in the initial installment since 1996. Vaccine funds continue to be awarded in several large installments.

SOURCE: Information provided by CDC.

BOX 1-2
Section 317 Grant Guidance

Annually, CDC's National Immunization Program (NIP) publishes guidance for immunization grant applications. This guidance describes activities the grantees are required to undertake, as well as those NIP recommends if resources are available. The year 2000 grant application guidance includes 38 required activities and 28 recommended activities. In their applications, grantees describe how they will carry out these activities and provide a detailed budget and budget justification. Grantees are always instructed to request in their applications the amount of funding they will need, at a minimum, to implement the activities required in the guidance regardless of the federal budget situation.

At present funding levels, CDC is not able to provide enough federal funds to support full implementation of all programmatic activities required by the grant guidance (see Box 1-1). Therefore, grantees are allowed the flexibility to pursue activities that are considered most appropriate and effective in their jurisdiction.

Grantees must submit the following reports to CDC:

- Vaccine Adverse Event Reports
- Supplemental Measles/Pertussis/Tetanus/Rubella/Congenital Rubella Syndrome/*Haemophilus influenza* type b Case Reports
- Reports of Discarded Measles Cases (quarterly)
- Program Progress Reports (annually)
- Immunization Registry Status Reports (annually)
- Reports of Perinatally Related Hepatitis B Prevention Data (annually)
- School and Day Care Entry Assessment Surveys (annually/biennially)
- School and Day Care Validation Surveys (report not required)
- VFC Population Estimate Surveys (annually)

SOURCE: Information provided by CDC.

operations in such areas as research and polio eradication. Medicare paid providers almost $115 million in 1998, including $87 million for influenza immunizations, $27 million for pneumococcal immunizations, and $800,000 for hepatitis B immunizations (information provided by HCFA).

In addition to these federal investments, many states and some local governments contribute funds to the support of the national immunization system. The total cost of the state contribution to the purchase of vaccines and the operation of immunization programs, based on estimates provided by state immunization program managers, is estimated at $340 million for FY 2000 (information provided by CDC). This estimate includes funds provided by state and local governments, as well as other federal funds (e.g., Maternal and Child Health Title V grants) that support immunization efforts.

Limitations of Current Efforts

The current levels of public and private investment in immunization efforts have been successful in controlling infectious diseases and improving levels of immunization coverage. But persistent problems remain within the U.S. immunization system:

- *Mortality and morbidity from preventable infectious disease.* Between 50,000 and 70,000 adults die annually in the United States from vaccine-preventable diseases (VPDs) or their complications, compared with approximately 300 U.S. children who die from VPDs each year (National Foundation for Infectious Disease, 1999).
- *Low coverage rates for adult vaccines.* National levels for influenza coverage have increased from 58 percent (1995) to 63 percent (1997) for adults aged 65 and older, but the percentage immunized among adults aged 55 to 64 is still considerably lower, with a median of 38.2 percent nationwide (National Center for Health Statistics [NCHS], 1997). Pneumococcal coverage levels for persons 65 and older are also low—only 42 percent of noninstitutionalized adults aged 65 and over had ever received a pneumococcal vaccination by 1997 (NCHS, 1997). Coverage rates for high-risk adults (under age 65) are especially poor. Recent surveys indicate that 26 percent of this group received an influenza vaccination, while only 13 percent received a pneumococcal vaccination (NCHS, 1997).
- *Persistent disparities in levels of immunization coverage.* Immunization coverage levels within areas of concentrated poverty or among mobile populations are significantly lower than national and statewide levels.[5] National surveys reveal a gap of 9 percentage points between children above and below the federal poverty level for completion of the 4:3:1:3 vaccine series,[6] which includes some of the most critical childhood vaccines

(information provided by CDC). Although improvements have occurred over the past decade, patterns of disparity have persisted between state-level coverage levels and the levels in major metropolitan areas (see Table 1-5). A recent and troubling development is that coverage levels in a few cities (most notably Houston and Chicago) have begun to decline

TABLE 1-5 Estimated Vaccination Coverage of 4:3:1:3[a] Among Children 19–35 Months of Age by Selected Geographic Areas— United States, National Immunization Survey, 1995–1999

Area	1995		1996	
	Geographic Area	Rest of State[c]	Geographic Area	Rest of State[c]
Jefferson County, AL	85 (± 4.9)	74 (± 5.5)	77 (± 4.8)	75 (± 4.8)
Maricopa County, AZ	69 (± 7.2)	71 (± 6.1)	71 (± 5.1)	69 (± 5.8)
Los Angeles, CA	70 (± 7.2)	68 (± 7.3)	79 (± 4.9)	73 (± 4.8)
San Diego County, CA	73 (± 6.4)	—	77 (± 4.4)	—
Santa Clara, CA	74 (± 5.7)	—	79 (± 4.4)	—
District of Columbia	67 (± 6.9)	n/a	78 (± 5.0)	n/a
Dade County, FL	77 (± 6.1)	75 (± 5.9)	76 (± 5.2)	78 (± 4.9)
Duval County, FL	71 (± 6.8)	—	76 (± 5.1)	—
Fulton/DeKalb, GA	79 (± 5.8)	76 (± 5.9)	74 (± 5.5)	82 (± 4.3)
City of Chicago, IL	69 (± 6.8)	83 (± 5.1)	74 (± 5.6)	75 (± 4.8)
Marion County, IN	75 (± 6.0)	74 (± 5.5)	72 (± 5.4)	70 (± 4.7)
Orleans Parish, LA	75 (± 6.1)	76 (± 5.4)	71 (± 5.9)	80 (± 4.5)
City of Boston, MA	87 (± 4.9)	79 (± 4.9)	84 (± 4.2)	86 (± 3.6)
Baltimore City, MD	75 (± 6.9)	79 (± 5.2)	81 (± 4.8)	78 (± 4.7)
Detroit, MI	57 (± 7.6)	69 (± 5.6)	63 (± 6.1)	76 (± 4.5)
Newark, NJ	67 (± 7.3)	73 (± 5.8)	62 (± 6.2)	78 (± 4.8)
NY—5 Counties (NYC)	78 (± 6.5)	76 (± 5.7)	75 (± 5.5)	82 (± 4.5)
Cuyahoga County, OH	71 (± 6.8)	73 (± 5.5)	80 (± 4.7)	77 (± 4.3)
Franklin County, OH	74 (± 5.9)	—	78 (± 5.4)	—
Philadelphia, PA	67 (± 7.4)	77 (± 5.5)	75 (± 5.4)	80 (± 4.3)
Davidson County, TN	73 (± 5.7)	74 (± 5.6)	77 (± 4.7)	80 (± 4.1)
Shelby County, TN	68 (± 6.2)	—	70 (± 5.3)	—
Bexar County, TX	74 (± 6.3)	74 (± 5.4)	74 (± 5.2)	74 (± 5.1)
City of Houston, TX	70 (± 6.7)	—	68 (± 5.9)	—
Dallas County, TX	70 (± 6.1)	—	71 (± 5.8)	—
El Paso County, TX	77 (± 5.1)	—	62 (± 5.6)	—
King County, WA	82 (± 4.7)	75 (± 5.7)	81 (± 4.2)	77 (± 4.6)
Milwaukee, WI	68 (± 6.0)	76 (± 4.8)	70 (± 5.2)	78 (± 4.2)

[a]4:3:1:3 = four or more doses of diphtheria, tetanus, and pertussis vaccine; three or more doses of poliovirus vaccine; one or more doses of a measles-containing vaccine; and three or more doses of *Haemophilus influenzae* type b vaccine.
[b]First two quarters of 1999 and last two quarters of 1998.

(information provided by CDC). The disparities encompass the range of vaccines received by each child or adult; the age of onset and completion of immunization; and the extent of unnecessary, duplicative immunization that occurs because of insufficient documentation. Given these gaps, the National Vaccine Advisory Committee (NVAC) has stated that a com-

1997		1998		1999[b]	
Geographic Area	Rest of State[c]	Geographic Area	Rest of State[c]	Geographic Area	Rest of State[c]
82 (± 4.3)	86 (± 3.7)	85 (± 4.8)	82 (± 5.0)	87 (± 4.1)	75 (± 5.6)
72 (± 4.8)	74 (± 4.8)	77 (± 5.8)	74 (± 6.2)	75 (± 6.0)	77 (± 5.4)
71 (± 5.5)	76 (± 4.6)	76 (± 6.0)	75 (± 5.8)	77 (± 5.7)	75 (± 5.5)
78 (± 4.3)	—	77 (± 5.1)	—	76 (± 5.4)	—
73 (± 4.8)	—	84 (± 4.7)	—	82 (± 5.1)	—
73 (± 5.4)	n/a	71 (± 6.2)	n/a	72 (± 5.9)	n/a
75 (± 5.0)	78 (± 4.5)	75 (± 6.0)	80 (± 5.3)	82 (± 5.1)	81 (± 5.1)
70 (± 5.1)	—	79 (± 6.0)	—	79 (± 5.1)	—
75 (± 4.9)	80 (± 4.3)	71 (± 6.9)	82 (± 4.8)	80 (± 5.9)	81 (± 5.1)
68 (± 5.5)	77 (± 4.8)	64 (± 7.4)	83 (± 5.5)	70 (± 6.1)	84 (± 4.6)
81 (± 4.5)	70 (± 4.4)	78 (± 5.3)	77 (± 5.6)	79 (± 5.2)	72 (± 5.6)
69 (± 6.0)	77 (± 4.6)	79 (± 5.7)	78 (± 5.6)	77 (± 5.7)	76 (± 5.4)
86 (± 3.6)	86 (± 3.4)	89 (± 3.6)	86 (± 4.3)	86 (± 4.5)	89 (± 3.7)
83 (± 4.7)	79 (± 4.2)	81 (± 5.7)	76 (± 5.6)	77 (± 5.9)	78 (± 5.2)
65 (± 5.6)	76 (± 4.2)	70 (± 6.4)	79 (± 5.4)	67 (± 6.3)	75 (± 5.6)
66 (± 6.3)	77 (± 4.5)	64 (± 8.7)	83 (± 6.5)	67 (± 7.3)	85 (± 4.6)
75 (± 5.1)	77 (± 4.7)	81 (± 5.8)	86 (± 4.5)	76 (± 5.9)	84 (± 4.8)
73 (± 5.3)	73 (± 4.6)	75 (± 6.0)	79 (± 5.2)	72 (± 5.5)	74 (± 5.6)
74 (± 5.0)	—	78 (± 6.2)	—	79 (± 5.3)	—
78 (± 5.1)	80 (± 4.3)	80 (± 5.8)	84 (± 4.3)	83 (± 4.7)	85 (+± 4.2)
77 (± 4.6)	80 (± 4.2)	80 (± 5.3)	85 (± 4.6)	77 (± 5.7)	78 (± 5.6)
70 (± 5.3)	—	71 (± 6.5)	—	68 (± 6.0)	—
79 (± 4.8)	76 (± 4.6)	79 (± 5.5)	77 (± 5.5)	74 (± 6.0)	76 (± 5.3)
64 (± 6.1)	—	61 (± 7.5)	—	57 (± 6.9)	—
74 (± 5.4)	—	71 (± 6.7)	—	73 (± 6.5)	—
65 (± 5.3)	—	78 (± 5.0)	—	79 (± 4.9)	—
77 (± 4.6)	79 (± 4.1)	86 (± 4.8)	79 (± 5.0)	82 (± 4.6)	74 (± 5.4)
70 (± 4.9)	81 (± 3.7)	73 (± 6.0)	79 (± 4.9)	75 (± 6.2)	83 (± 4.5)

[c]For states with more than one selected geographical area, "rest of state" data do not include any of the selected areas.

SOURCE: CDC, 2000c.

prehensive, efficient national immunization system is incomplete and remains "a work in progress" (NVAC, 1999a).

• *Serious gaps and inconsistencies in the coordination, support, and documentation of immunization efforts.* As the number and types of vaccines recommended for both adults and children have increased, the systems in place for ensuring their availability, monitoring immunization coverage rates, and improving coverage among vulnerable populations have remained the same. These systems are showing signs of stress in the form of inconsistent measurement, bureaucratic delays, excessive paperwork, and administrative burdens that reduce program efficiencies in private and public health agencies. Efforts to improve coverage rates in areas of social and economic disadvantage are further complicated by two factors: (1) uneven benefits coverage for vaccines within private health plans; and (2) strict eligibility requirements for federally financed vaccines that deny access to similarly situated children on a state-by-state basis (see, for example, HCFA and CDC correspondence regarding the use of VFC vaccines for children enrolled in non-Medicaid SCHIP programs [Richardson and Orenstein, 1999]).

• *Unstable finance patterns.* Budgetary shifts in the support for vaccine purchase and immunization programs have created a climate of uncertainty and instability within the states that discourages the implementation of preventive interventions to improve immunization coverage rates. As a result, states report that they have reduced efforts to link immunization services with other health and social service programs, such as the Women, Infants, and Children (WIC) nutritional supplement program; that they lack sufficient documentation of immunization records; and that they have been hampered in their efforts to audit immunization coverage levels within private provider practices.

The collective result of the above problems is a significant delay in the public benefit of vaccines, especially for groups of children and adults who are not closely connected with high-quality primary care services. Closing the gaps that persist in child and adult immunization levels will require sustained as well as additional efforts within state and federal public health agencies. At the same time, however, these agencies currently confront serious difficulties in achieving stable funding streams, as well as uncertainties about their roles and responsibilities for immunization activities in the United States.

CHARGE TO THE COMMITTEE

Current analyses of immunization investments reveal the absence of a strategic plan that can guide the federal and state partnership in supporting immunization efforts. The lack of such a plan makes it difficult to establish program priorities or estimate the scale of investments necessary to sustain current levels of immunization coverage for children and adults. The absence of a national consensus about the roles and responsibilities of federal and state agencies in fostering immunization also complicates efforts to extend immunization benefits to the relatively small population of high-risk individuals who remain unprotected. Uncertainties about how the costs of such efforts should be allocated across the different levels of government lead to inefficiencies in the use of public resources, including redundant efforts, gaps in services, and unnecessary paperwork.

It is for these reasons that the U.S. Senate Appropriations Committee in 1998 asked IOM to conduct a study of the Section 317 program.[7] The study was designed to identify areas in which research-based evidence can guide federal, state, and local immunization policies and practices. The Congress formulated five key questions as the basis for the IOM study:

1. What was the extent of overall spending by all sources for immunizations in the United States during the 1990s?
2. How were new federal funds spent by the states, and to what extent did states maintain their own levels of effort over the past 5 years?
3. What are current and future funding requirements for immunization activities, and how can those requirements be met through a combination of state funding, federal Section 317 immunization grant funding, and funding available through SCHIP?
4. How should federal grant funds be distributed among the states?
5. How should funds be targeted within states to reach high-risk populations without diminishing levels of coverage among the overall population?

In addition, a sixth question was posed by CDC during the negotiation of the study contract:

6. What should be the role and financing level for CDC's current program supporting state efforts to vaccinate adults and achieve the nation's goals for influenza and pneumococcal vaccines?

These questions reflect a need for guidance regarding the level of national effort necessary to achieve immunization objectives, as well as strategies that can balance federal and state contributions in extending the benefits of immunization to unprotected children and adults.

STUDY CONTEXT: THE NATIONAL
IMMUNIZATION PARTNERSHIP

The U.S. achievement in reducing the burden of infectious disease and increasing immunization coverage rates throughout the states has been accomplished through a series of incremental initiatives over the past 50 years (see Appendix B). An ongoing partnership between the public and private health sectors has emerged that includes extensive collaboration among federal, state, and local health agencies. The result is a dynamic and flexible immunization system that has adapted to evolving science and new vaccines; changing social conditions; and shifting health care finance patterns within all settings, from remote rural counties to metropolitan areas.

In contrast with many other industrialized nations, the United States has a health care system that is highly decentralized and depends primarily on the private sector to deliver services. Each regional health care system is shaped by local circumstances, resources, and needs, as well as by national goals and policies. Though cumbersome, this system has demonstrated an extraordinary capacity to ensure the reliable delivery of an increasing number of vaccine antigens in a growing number of private and public health care settings for an expanding range of age groups, including newborns, preschool and school-aged children, adolescents, and adults.

At present, however, federal and state roles within the national immunization partnership are unstable. Several trends contribute to this instability: rapid acceleration in the science of vaccine research and production, systemic changes in the health care environment of the United States (especially the emergence of managed care organizations), and shifts in thinking within the Congress about the roles and responsibilities of federal and state health agencies in building and supporting public health services. The instability is worrisome because it can create pressure points and blind spots that can swiftly contribute to outbreaks of infectious disease, as was seen in the 1989–1991 measles epidemic in the United States that contributed to 43,000 cases and resulted in more than 100 deaths, particularly among children below age 5 (see Box 1-3) (NVAC, 1991).

The persistence of low immunization coverage rates for routine vaccines (especially measles, rubella, diphtheria, and pertussis) within metropolitan areas is cause for serious concern. Constant vigilance is required to protect the gains that have been made, and to prevent gaps that could result from the addition of new or improved vaccines to the recommended schedules, as well as from changes in health care services for under-immunized populations of adults and children. Unprotected sectors can unexpectedly become sources of infectious disease outbreaks and can

BOX 1-3
The Measles Epidemic, 1989–1991

Measles reached a record low in 1983 (1,497 cases), a 97 percent reduction from the more than 57,000 cases reported in 1977. The Carter Administration's Measles Elimination Program had the goal of eradicating measles in the United States by 1982. However, measles was not eliminated, and this success was not sustained. In 1984 and 1985, outbreaks occurred among older children, including college-age youth who had entered school before the vaccine was in routine use. A new pattern emerged in 1986 when outbreaks occurred among preschool age children and were concentrated in inner city, low-income neighborhoods in 20 U.S. counties.

Sporadic outbreaks of disease became a measles epidemic between 1989 and 1991. During 1989 more than 18,000 cases and 41 deaths were reported, rising to an additional 25,000 cases and at least 60 deaths in 1990 (CDC, 1991). With a reservoir of unimmunized and underimmunized preschool-aged children, the disease spread rapidly through several cities, including Chicago, Houston, and Los Angeles, which accounted for one-third of all cases in 1989. CDC's findings on selected cities (Chicago, Dallas, Los Angeles, Milwaukee, and New York) were used to develop a response to contain the epidemic, as well as new strategies to raise immunization rates. CDC found that half of the children who had had measles were not immunized, even though many of them had seen a health provider. Researchers dubbed these visits "missed opportunities" for immunization, and reducing missed opportunities became a priority. CDC also found that more than one in five of the unvaccinated children who contracted measles were also enrolled in Aid to Families with Dependent Children (AFDC), Medicaid, or the Supplemental Nutrition Program for Women, Infants, and Children (WIC). It became clear that underimmunized children could be identified through other publicly funded programs, and CDC developed demonstration projects to improve immunization levels among WIC clients.

While CDC conducted the laboratory and epidemiological studies of the measles epidemic, the federal response to the epidemic also was shaped by a new force in policy analysis, the National Vaccine Advisory Committee (NVAC). Created by Congress in 1986 as part of the National Vaccine Program, this body was designed to be an independent advisor to the Assistant Secretary for Health. By 1990, an active group of advisors had been appointed by the Bush Administration, and the measles epidemic led them to take unprecedented leadership (*A Shot in the Arm for Vaccine Advocates*, 1990). With the support of CDC and National Vaccine Program Office (NVPO) staff, NVAC prepared a measles white paper, which made key recommendations for responding to the measles epidemic (National Vaccine Advisory Committee, 1991).

Following release of the white paper, a federal Interagency Coordinating Committee was formed to outline an implementation plan involving eleven federal agencies. This committee met on a quarterly basis for 18 months, creating a "Public Health Service Action Plan to Improve Access to Immunization Services." In testimony before the Senate Appropriations Committee in June 1991, Dr. William Roper, Director of CDC, stated that the measles "epidemic still affects predomi-

continued

BOX 1-3 Continued

nantly unvaccinated preschool racial and ethnic minority children in inner cities" (U.S. Senate, 1991). Other witnesses expressed the view that low-income working families living in communities across the country faced financial barriers to immunization.

A year later President Bush announced the Infant Immunization Initiative, targeted at improving the low immunization rates of certain populations, including those under age 2. The model immunization plans were the beginning of a national effort to ensure adequate and timely immunization of infants and young children. This ultimately resulted in the preparation of Immunization Action Plans (Orenstein et al., forthcoming). The Childhood Immunization Initiative, a major effort launched in the early years of the Clinton Administration, subsequently strengthened this effort to include the creation of the Vaccines for Children program and the expansion of the Section 317 program in the early 1990s.

serve as hosts for preventable pathogens such as pertussis. The continued presence of large groups of children and adults that do not have regular access to immunization services also represents an important indicator for those monitoring the performance of the U.S. health care system in meeting the basic health care needs of an increasingly diverse population.

It is ironic that the United States is now in the situation of creating an impressive array of vaccines that can reduce and perhaps eliminate the dreaded diseases that threatened prior generations of Americans, while at the same time relying on a patchwork system for purchasing, distributing, and administering these powerful drugs that undermines the effectiveness of the nation's disease prevention strategy. It is time, therefore, for a strategic vision that can clarify the roles and responsibilities of state and federal agencies in achieving national immunization goals and provide the resources to support this effort.

Role of the Section 317 Program

In the first few decades of the formation of the national immunization partnership, the federal role was limited primarily to the purchase of vaccines that would allow the states to meet the needs of disadvantaged children (see Appendix B for a chronology of the U.S. immunization system). Over time, the federal role gradually expanded to include three key features: (1) financial assistance that allows the states to purchase vaccines collectively under a federal contract at discount prices; (2) infrastructure grants that provide funds for both direct services and other components of the state's immunization program; and (3) federal personnel and technical expertise, especially in such areas as information collection, data analysis, and long-term planning. Section 317, established in 1963, was the first in a series of late 20th-century federal initiatives related to immunizations and primary health care services for disadvantaged families.

Creation of the VFC Program

In 1994, the VFC program was launched as a new entitlement for Medicaid and uninsured children and other groups specified by law. Section 13631 of the Omnibus Budget Reconciliation Act of 1993 created VFC as a means of providing free vaccine to children aged 18 and younger who are uninsured, are eligible for Medicaid, or are Alaska Natives or American Indians. Underinsured children (those whose insurance does not cover childhood vaccinations) are also eligible for VFC vaccines, but may receive them only in federally qualified health centers or rural health clinics (see Chapter 3 for further discussion of the program).

VFC is a vaccine purchase program designed to encourage the provision of immunizations to children within a "medical home" that provides basic primary care services. VFC was created on the premise that the cost of vaccine for parents constituted a major barrier to children's timely immunization, an assumption that was not supported in an evaluation study prepared by the General Accounting Office (GAO) in 1995. GAO concluded that strategies other than VFC may better improve timely vaccination among children, potentially at lower public cost, by reducing missed opportunities for immunization through Medicaid, public health clinics, and other providers with whom underimmunized children already have contact (GAO, 1995a:3). Furthermore, GAO observed that CDC cannot ensure that VFC will reach pockets of need—areas or populations in which immunization rates are low and the risk of disease is consequently high. The legislation creating the VFC program limits VFC expenditures to vaccine purchase and narrowly defined operational costs, such as expenses associated with ordering, inventory maintenance, vaccine distribution, and provider enrollment. VFC lacks any built-in evaluation mechanism that could measure its performance in providing vaccine to at-risk children or attribute changes in age-appropriate immunization rates to the program's operation.

Despite these limitations, VFC has been successful in attracting the participation of public and private health care providers. In 1998, an estimated 44,000 public and private providers were eligible to receive VFC vaccines.

State Children's Health Insurance Program

In 1998, SCHIP was initiated to provide grants to the states to help finance health care services for children in low-income families without health insurance. As discussed in Chapter 3, SCHIP is a block grant program that provides federal resources allowing states to extend services to low-income children who are ineligible for Medicaid but otherwise uninsured (e.g., the "working poor"). States are required to cover all ACIP-recommended vaccines and their administration to children as part of the annual federal SCHIP allotment.

Interaction of Federal Immunization Efforts

The creation and implementation of the VFC and SCHIP programs have raised questions about the mission and role of the Section 317 program. During the first half of the 1990s, the budget for Section 317 state immunization infrastructure grants grew substantially, but funding levels for state infrastructure awards have declined significantly in the past 4 years (see Figures 1-2 and 1-3). Since the federal government now relies heavily on the private sector to administer programs such as VFC and SCHIP to improve the quality of health care for disadvantaged children, the potential for overlap and duplication of effort between these programs and Section 317 awards may exist and requires consideration and oversight. Opportunities may exist to leverage public and private investments and integrate programs to achieve multiple goals or to diminish unnecessary bureaucracy associated with the administration of separate funding streams. At the same time, if different federal programs perform separate but related missions, appropriate measures need to be in place that can be used to assess the performance of individual units in contributing to national goals and objectives.

The separate federal immunization initiatives undertaken over the past several decades have responded to new problems and addressed new dimensions of the immunization system. But certain features have remained consistent over time. One historical review of federal immunization policy identifies the following as critical components of federal immunization policy in the 20th century (Johnson et al., forthcoming):

• From the beginning, immunization financing was explicitly structured to be a federal–state–private-sector partnership.
• Federal policy makers never expected federal funds to be sufficient to cover the full cost of vaccine purchase and delivery for disadvantaged groups.

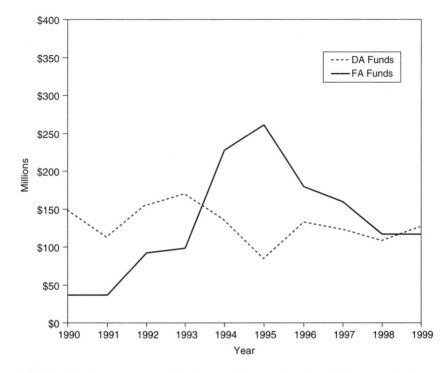

FIGURE 1-2 Amount of new funding awarded as Section 317 Direct Assistance (DA)[a] and Financial Assistance (FA),[b] 1990–1999. [a]DA funds include funds for vaccine purchase and operations. [b]FA funds include funds for state infrastructure programs. SOURCE: Information provided by CDC.

- Federal funds are designed to be used within the states for specific purposes to target specific problems.
- Federal funds are provided to supplement, not supplant, state investments in immunization programs.

Assessment, Assurance, and Policy Development in the National Immunization Strategy

When infectious disease was widespread during the first half of the 20th century, vaccine services generally consisted of community-based, stand-alone, self-contained efforts designed to achieve universal coverage in schools or other community settings within a relatively short period of time. Local health agencies often funded and publicized programs such as "Shots on Sunday" or "Back-to-School Shots." As these programs expanded

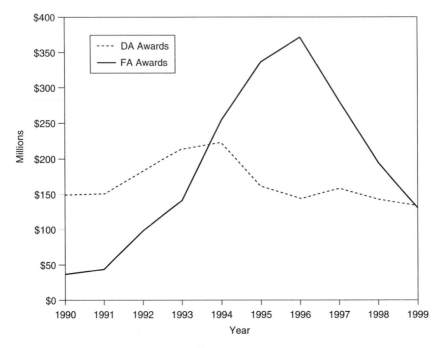

FIGURE 1-3 Amount of total annual awards[a] of Section 317 Funds, Direct Assistance (DA)[b] and Financial Assistance (FA),[c] 1990–1999. [a]Total funds include new funds plus carryover. [b]DA funds include funds for vaccine purchase and operations. [c]FA funds include funds for state infrastructure programs. SOURCE: Information provided by CDC.

to include year-round clinic services, outreach, education, and data collection responsibilities, costs were shared between the states and the federal government. Investments were often financed through emergency appropriation bills or vaccine purchase budgets that drew strong bipartisan support in the interest of controlling outbreaks of infectious disease.

Public health clinics have traditionally provided free vaccines for disadvantaged families and are commonly the first line of defense during outbreaks or epidemics. Special community-based immunization programs such as "Back to School Shots" still continue in many disadvantaged neighborhoods. Today, however, immunizations are routinely acquired within the set of clinical services associated with primary preventive care and well-baby health care. Third-party coverage of immunization services, financed through private and public insurance plans, is more common, resulting in declining use of public health clinics to deliver immunization services. Vaccines purchased with state or federal funds are increasingly delivered through private health care practices, except in states that continue to rely heavily upon public health clinics for primary health care services.

Completion of an immunization series requires multiple interactions with providers over a lengthy period of time, and determining the immunization status of an individual at any particular time can be difficult for both clients and health professionals. More than half of all infants and children aged 0 through 5, for example, are covered by private health insurance, but not all health plans include immunization coverage.[8] In contrast, all Medicaid health plans include comprehensive immunization benefits within the Early and Periodic Screening, Diagnosis and Treatment program (as described in Chapter 3). SCHIP plans must also include immunizations as a basic benefit, comparable to Medicaid standards.

As noted earlier, however, the costs of achieving national immunization goals are not limited to the purchase and administration of vaccines. Other costs are incurred by public health agencies as part of their community-wide immunization programs, both universal and targeted (see Box 1-4). Disease prevention and control efforts, public information campaigns, provider education, reminder and recall systems, and immunization registry programs are all examples of universal programs whose costs are generally borne by the public sector. Immunization budgets are frequently combined with other public health programs at the state and local levels, supporting both core efforts and targeted initiatives. For individuals who do not have insurance or whose insurance does not cover immunization services, for example, targeted community assistance efforts are often required to assess their immunization status, and to connect individual children and adults with recommended immunization services and immunization records. Immunization assessment and referral services have also been added to Head Start centers, welfare assistance programs, and WIC clinics that provide nutritional supplement programs. Such efforts are commonly distributed across a broad spectrum of public and private agencies and are part of mission efforts within such fields as primary care, maternal and child health services, migrant health, and public health. As a result, their costs are generally not measured in estimating the expenses associated with immunization. Later in this report we examine whether the basic components of these costs can be identified, along with how they are allocated across different levels of government.

In summary, the role of the public health sector in immunization has shifted in the 1990s from a service-delivery function to one that is more directly involved with assessment, assurance, and policy development. This shift is consistent with trends in other public health programs, as described in earlier IOM reports (IOM, 1988, 1997). Yet federal immuniza-

BOX 1-4
Immunization Infrastructure: The Michigan Example

Michigan received $6.4 million for "infrastructure" in 1999, about $20 per child under age 3. These funds support efforts associated with direct service delivery, infectious disease prevention, surveillance and assessment, efforts to improve coverage rates, and programs to strengthen system performance. Additional federal support pays for the state health department's immunization program staff. That staff includes two public health advisers (employees of CDC)—one on the Michigan state central staff and one assigned to the city of Detroit.

More than half the infrastructure grant funds support service delivery. The state allocates funds to 43 local health departments based on the number of young children who live in the area. Local health departments are free to pursue the strategy they choose to ensure timely immunization. The most common use of the funds is to pay staff to administer vaccines.

The infrastructure grant supports a central immunization program staff and two four-person field staffs—one that works with local health departments and another that works with the VFC providers who work in the private sector. Both field staffs work with providers on the logistics of obtaining vaccines and proper vaccine storage and handling. The field staff working with local health departments assists when outbreaks occur. It also reviews assessments of coverage levels among children immunized by local health departments. This group is responsible as well for working with schools to ensure compliance with school entry immunization requirements. The field staff that deals with other VFC providers tries to retain and recruit new providers.

The core of the central staff comprises the program manager, a series of individuals with specialized functions, and support staff. A surveillance coordinator focuses on epidemiology and surveillance through activities such as visiting localities experiencing outbreaks and gathering reports of vaccine-preventable diseases. An outreach and education manager and staff work broadly through a newsletter with a circulation of 8,000 and annual immunization workshops conducted around the state that attract 800 people a year. This group targets efforts to improve service delivery, such as a peer-to-peer physician education network and distribution of an immunization provider toolkit.

The assessment coordinator oversees two contracts designed to provide immunization assessments—one for clinics and physician offices in the Detroit area and the other in 22 community and migrant health centers. This individual also conducts assessments outside Detroit. Assessments use the CDC-developed Assessment, Feedback, Incentives, and eXchange of information (AFIX) methodology. This activity has produced an average of 10 percent higher coverage levels at the time of the second follow-up assessment. The state staff also includes an immunization registry coordinator, although the costs of operating the registry are paid with state funds. One person focuses on reducing perinatal hepatitis B transmission, following up on possible cases of transmission by mothers to their newborn children.

Federal funding for infrastructure supports other outreach efforts as well. These include contracts to answer calls to a toll free number for immunization information, and to conduct outreach to day care providers in an urban area with a history of outbreaks in day care centers.

tion policy is still concentrated primarily on service-delivery roles; VFC, for example, is narrowly restricted to vaccine provision and some small amount of operational costs. The VFC program does not have the flexibility to supply resources to the states that could be used to support oversight of public- and private-sector performance in meeting the immunization needs of vulnerable groups. Section 317 appears to be the only federal program, at present, that provides opportunities and resources to support the states in developing performance measures that can help in managing the immunization system itself and responding to shortcomings within the private sector, rather than simply providing vaccines to individuals who request them or conducting short-term outreach programs.

SIX ROLES OF THE NATIONAL IMMUNIZATION SYSTEM

To address the questions under its charge, the IOM committee constructed a new analytic framework to represent the fundamental roles of the national immunization system. At present, this system is often described in terms of the federal and state agencies that administer immunization services and programs (see, e.g., Figure 1-4) or the components of the state programs that are administered with Section 317 funds (termed "core functions" by CDC) (see Figure 1-5). The committee found that these representations inadequately illustrate the dynamics of the national immunization system because they do not address the interactions among public and private roles and responsibilities. Most important, the presence or absence of private health care services (including insurance coverage and benefits that encompass immunization services for children, adolescents, and adults at reasonable cost) influences the burden of effort required within the public sector to assure access to vaccines recommended for widespread use. Changes in the recommended vaccine schedule, as well as shifts in the quality of and access to primary care services for disadvantaged groups in any community, necessitate responses by the public sector to "gear up" or "gear down," often in the face of static or declining resources.[9]

In examining current policies and practices in the public and private health care sectors, the committee identified six fundamental roles of the national immunization system:

- Assure the purchase of recommended vaccines for the total population of U.S. children and adults, with a particular emphasis on the protection of vulnerable groups.
- Assure access to such vaccines within the public sector when private health care services are not adequate to meet local needs.
- Control and prevent infectious disease.
- Conduct populationwide surveillance of immunization coverage

44

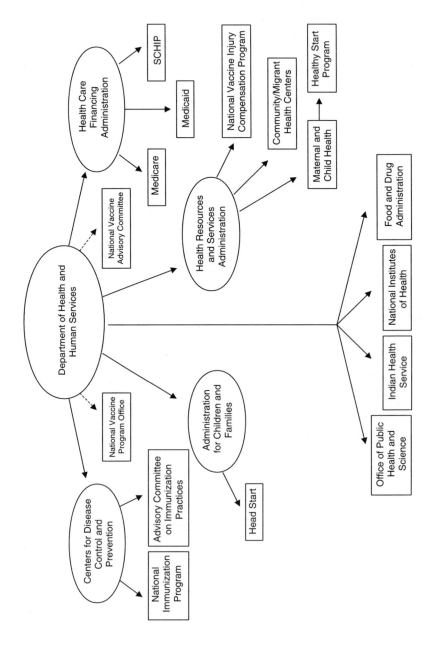

FIGURE 1-4 Federal agencies that support immunization services and programs.

Public Health Function	Essential Services	Immunization Core Functions	Immunization Program Components
Assessment	Evaluate effectiveness, accessibility, and quality of personal and population-based health services.	Assessment	• General assessment • Public clinic AFIX[a] • Private-sector AFIX • Registry • Perinatal hepatitis B prevention
	• Monitor health status to identify community health problems.	Surveillance	• Surveillance of vaccine-preventable disease adverse events • Perinatal hepatitis B prevention
Policy Development	• Develop policies/plans that support individual and community health efforts.	Management	• Program management • Partnerships
	• Enforce laws/regulations that protect health.		
	• Research new insights and innovative solutions to health problems.	Research	• Program management
Assurance	• Diagnose and investigate health problems in the community.	Outbreak control	• Control of infectious disease
	• Ensure the availability of a competent public health and personal health care workforce.	Assuring service delivery	• Service delivery • Perinatal hepatitis B prevention • WIC[b] linkage • Outreach • AFIX • Registry • VFC[c]
	• Inform, educate, and empower people about health issues.	Public information/ education	• Public education • Outreach
	• Mobilize community partnerships to identify and solve health problems.		
	• Link people to needed personal health services, and ensure the provision of health care when it is not otherwise available.	Provider training	• Professional information/education • Public clinic AFIX • Private-sector AFIX • Perinatal hepatitis B prevention
		Vaccine supply	• Vaccine management • VFC

FIGURE 1-5 Immunization core functions. [a]Assessment, Feedback, Incentives, and eXchange of information. [b]Special Supplemental Nutrition Program for Women, Infants, and Children. [c]Vaccines for Children. SOURCE: Information provided by CDC.

levels, including the identification of significant disparities, gaps, and vaccine safety concerns.

• Sustain and improve immunization coverage levels within child and adult populations, especially in vulnerable communities.

• Use primary care and public health resources efficiently in achieving national immunization goals.

The last of these roles provides overarching support for the other five, and was the focus of the committee's charge. In conducting the study, we gave particular attention to the responsibilities of federal and state health agencies and the burden of effort required to support each of the above roles in an integrated manner. Figure 1-6 displays these roles as components of the national immunization partnership.

We recognize that the U.S. immunization infrastructure involves a broader set of activities than can be incorporated within the six roles described above. For example, the separate cycles of research, development, licensing, and production of vaccines and the selection of vaccines

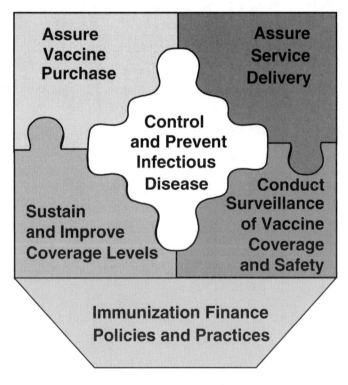

FIGURE 1-6 Six roles of the national immunization system.

for the recommended schedule of child and adult immunizations are important parts of the national immunization partnership; however, such efforts are not addressed in this report.[10] Efforts to monitor vaccine safety and provide adequate compensation for adverse events related to vaccine use through special government trust funds represent an additional area of concern that lies beyond the framework for this study, although public concerns about the safety of vaccines have major implications regarding the level of resources necessary to sustain high immunization coverage rates.[11]

The six roles of the national immunization system are complex for three reasons. First, each encompasses an array of specific programs and functions (see Figure 1-7). Programs to improve immunization coverage rates, for example, include interventions to reduce vaccine costs, expand access to immunization services, address missed opportunities, improve documentation of immunization status, increase community demand for vaccinations, and establish requirements and incentives for providers. Likewise, the surveillance of immunization coverage rates may include a variety of tools and methods, including the National Immunization Survey, national surveillance studies, pocket-of-need assessment studies, regional and state immunization registries, and local-area surveillance studies that focus on specific populations.[12]

Second, the six roles of the national immunization system are not rigid or fixed, and certain other factors add to their complexity. Although they share common features, they are also elastic and decentralized, expressed in different ways over time within the broad array of public health efforts throughout the United States. A successful national immunization system requires that each role be present within each state, but their form, scope, and intensity will vary. For example, certain populations are easier to track than others, and the extent of monitoring efforts required will be proportional to the level of heterogeneity within the population and the complexity of the health service plans that serve their immunization needs. Likewise, the public costs of immunizing the first 10 percent of a large population, who often have private insurance and are motivated to request immunizations from their health care providers, are significantly lower than the costs of immunizing the final 10 percent, who rely fully on public assistance to cover their health care costs and vaccine purchases. The final 10 percent includes significantly larger numbers of individuals who are not routinely connected to health care service centers, who experience consistent disruptions in changes in residence and in health care coverage (and whose health records are consequently scattered across multiple sources), and who are socially isolated or distrustful of services that do not demonstrate a tangible or immediate health benefit. Targeted community assistance efforts are required to connect

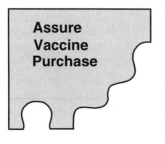

- ACIP recommendations
- Private and public insurance coverage (Medicaid and Medicare)
- Federal contracts for selected vaccines
- VFC coverage
- State coverage under SCHIP
- State supplemental purchases

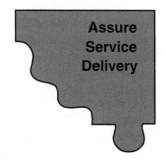

- Private insurance benefits
- Public insurance benefits (Medicaid, Medicare, and SCHIP)
- VFC administration in private sector
- Public health clinics
- Maternal and Child Health/WIC/community health clinics

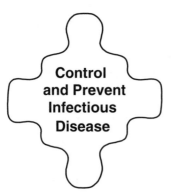

- National Notifiable Disease Surveillance System
- Public health laboratories
- State epidemiology centers
- Emergency vaccination programs
- Educational programs

FIGURE 1-7 Six roles of the national immunization system, broken down by role (continues on next page).

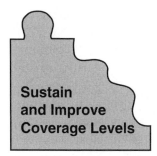

- Reducing cost barriers
- Expanding access to immunization services
- Addressing missed opportunities
- Improving awareness and documentation of immunization status

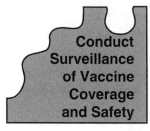

- National Immunization Survey
- Retrospective school entry surveys
- Special area/population surveys
- CASA surveys
- Managed care/HEDIS surveys
- Registries
- Vaccine Adverse Event Reporting System

Immunization Finance Policies and Practices

- Private-sector roles and responsibilities
- Public-sector roles and responsibilities
- Use of outcome measures/performance standards
- Linkages among health plans and immunization programs
- Strategic investments in infrastructure
- Funding levels

these groups with immunization services and to sustain that connection over time. Financing that effort is expensive, and pay-offs may be small in terms of absolute numbers of individuals who are brought up to date in immunization coverage. Yet even small improvements in immunization coverage in high-risk areas have broad positive impacts within the general community, since they reduce the risk of outbreaks (and the costs of hospitalization or injury that may result), improve general health status, and demonstrate improvements in the quality of health care services within a selected region.

Third, the level of resources required for each state to perform each role effectively is not well understood, since immunization coverage rates are influenced by a broad mix of factors that include national health trends, local demographics and social conditions, and public and private health finance patterns. For example, some states (e.g., Alabama) rely heavily on public health clinics to immunize more than 80 percent of their disadvantaged populations. Such states may spend large amounts on vaccine purchase and direct services and invest little effort in assessing rates of immunization coverage among private providers because vulnerable groups are served directly by the public health system. In contrast, states (e.g., New Jersey) that rely primarily on private managed care plans to supply vaccines to Medicaid clients or other at-risk groups may spend less on direct services, but need to create incentives, regulations, or performance measures that establish accountability within the private health sector for achieving high levels of immunization coverage.

The complexity of the national immunization system should not discourage efforts to address the finance policies and practices that can ensure high levels of performance and direct resources to areas of need. Achieving consistency of effort in both service delivery and assessment of performance and coverage patterns is especially important, because history has demonstrated that when levels of protection begin to decline, disease outbreak occurs, and remedial action becomes necessary (NVAC, 1991). As noted earlier, unprotected sectors can unexpectedly become sources of infectious disease outbreaks and can serve as hosts to preventable pathogens such as pertussis. These lapses in public health preparedness have tremendous negative impacts involving loss of life, preventable morbidity, and financial cost. A strong and vigilant infrastructure is necessary to sustain coverage rates in the face of the changes in science, social conditions, and health care systems discussed above.

STUDY APPROACH

To respond to the six questions listed above, IOM formed the Committee on Immunization Finance Policies and Practices in December 1998.

The committee was tasked to conduct an 18-month study that involved both extensive data collection and careful deliberations about the nature, scope, impact, and cost of the national immunization partnership for both children and adults. The committee met five times to consider relevant research data and expert testimony (see Appendix C for a list of sources that contributed to the committee's deliberations). The committee heard testimony from congressional staff; officials of federal, state, and local health agencies; and organizations representing public and private health care professionals.

In May 1999, the committee released an interim report that addressed two key concerns posed by CDC: (1) the experience with carryover (unobligated funds) in the administration of the Section 317 program, and (2) the impact of SCHIP on the need for federal Section 317 funds for both infrastructure initiatives and vaccine purchase (IOM, 1999a).

Recognizing that local circumstances and economic and social factors strongly influence the levels of need and the quality and scope of immunization services within the states, the committee organized two major fact-finding efforts to illustrate and compare the ways in which states allocate resources for health care services and infrastructure. These efforts included (1) a national survey of 50 states and the District of Columbia conducted by a research team at the University of Michigan,[13] and (2) a set of eight case studies (Alabama, Maine, Michigan, New Jersey, North Carolina, Texas, Washington State, and a two-county comparison of San Diego and Los Angeles counties in California), prepared by a team of project consultants.[14] Four site visits were organized to supplement the national survey and case study materials.[15] State-level data were also drawn from background materials and data analyses provided by CDC's National Immunization Program, including proposals submitted by case study states for Section 317 funds in FY 1992, 1995, 1999, and 2000.[16] In addition, the committee sponsored a workshop on pockets-of-need issues, held in September 1999.

Committee members and staff met frequently with state health officials over the course of the study[17] and received materials pertaining to state and private immunization efforts from the American Academy of Pediatrics, the American Association of Health Plans, the Association of Maternal and Child Health Programs, the Association of State and Territorial Health Officers, the Health Insurance Association of America, the National Association of City and County Health Officers, and the National Association of WIC Directors. Additional materials regarding state roles in public health were provided by the National Governors' Association and the National Conference of State Legislatures. Information on public- and private-sector investments in immunization services was also obtained through literature searches.

ORGANIZATION OF THE REPORT

Five chapters follow this introduction. Chapter 2 explains how today's U.S. immunization system differs from that of 1990 and earlier decades, and identifies emerging challenges and scientific opportunities in the decades ahead that have finance implications for the national immunization system. Chapters 3, 4, and 5 address the six roles of the national immunization system: vaccine purchase and service delivery (Chapter 3); infectious disease prevention and control, surveillance of vaccine coverage and safety, and efforts to improve and sustain coverage rates (Chapter 4); and immunization finance policies and practices (Chapter 5). Throughout Chapters 2 through 5, the committee's findings are in italics. In Chapter 6, the committee uses these findings to respond to the six questions posed under our charge and to formulate a final set of conclusions and recommendations.

ENDNOTES

1. Local health agencies play important public health roles, but they are usually not involved in financing vaccine purchase or immunization infrastructure efforts. The analyses in this study also do not include current or former U.S. territories (American Samoa, Guam, Republic of the Marshall Islands, Federated States of Micronesia, the North Mariana Islands, Republic of Belau, Puerto Rico, and the Virgin Islands), even though they are grantees within the National Immunization Program. The analyses are confined to state-level efforts because the committee's charge focused explicitly on state budgetary roles.

2. Costs are not adjusted for inflation.

3. The six municipalities are Chicago, Illinois; New York City, New York; Philadelphia, Pennsylvania; Houston and San Antonio, Texas; and the District of Columbia.

4. These jurisdictions are American Samoa, Guam, the Marshall Islands, Micronesia, the North Mariana Islands, Belau, Puerto Rico, and the Virgin Islands.

5. The term *mobile populations* refers to a variety of groups that have no fixed residence or frequently change residences within a limited period of time. They include immigrants (both legal and illegal), migrant workers, and the homeless.

6. The 4:3:1:3 series includes four doses of DTaP; three doses of polio; one dose of measles, mumps, and rubella (MMR); and three doses of *Haemophilus influenzae* type b (Hib). The coverage status of 2-year-olds is measured between 18 and 35 months of age.

7. The IOM study was requested in U.S. Senate Report 105-300 to accompany S. 2440 (Departments of Labor, Health and Human Services, and Education and Related Agencies Appropriations Bill), which directed CDC to contract with IOM to conduct an evaluation of the recent successes, resource needs, cost structure, and strategies for immunization efforts in the United States.

8. NVAC (1999a:364), citing research from the Employee Benefit Research Institute (Fronstin, 1996), observes that 54 percent of infants and 62 percent of children aged 1 through 5 are covered by private health insurance.

9. See the ACIP recommendation for pneumococcal vaccine (CDC, 2000d).

10. Other IOM committees have addressed some of these issues. See, for example, *Vaccines for the 21st Century* (IOM, 1999b).

11. Vaccine safety issues have been addressed by several IOM reports, including *Research Strategies for Assessing Adverse Events Associated with Vaccines: A Workshop Summary* (IOM, 1994a), *Adverse Events Associated with Childhood Vaccines: Evidence Bearing on Causality* (IOM, 1993), and *Adverse Effects of Pertussis and Rubella Vaccines* (IOM, 1991).

12. In addition, vaccine safety reporting systems (e.g., the Vaccine Adverse Events Reporting System), add another dimension to the role of surveillance.

13. The survey was conducted by a team that included Gary Freed, MD, MPH, principal investigator; Sarah Clark, MPH; and Anne Cowan, MPH, all in the Division of General Pediatrics at the University of Michigan. See Appendix D for a brief overview.

14. See Appendix E for a detailed description of the case study selection and preparation methods.

15. Site visits were conducted within four of the case study states: Detroit, Michigan; Newark, New Jersey; Houston, Texas; and Los Angeles and San Diego, California.

16. As noted, one case study involved a two-county comparison in California. County-level data were included in California's statewide grant proposal.

17. These meetings included a CDC meeting with national partners in March 1999 (Atlanta), a CDC meeting with state immunization directors in April 1999 (Atlanta), and the National Immunization Conference in June 1999 (Dallas). In addition, the following state and local health officers presented testimony at meetings of the IOM committee: David Johnson, Deputy Director and Chief Medical Executive, Michigan Department of Community Health, Lansing; Donald Williamson, State Health Officer, Alabama Department of Public Health, Montgomery; Christine Grant, Acting Commissioner, New Jersey Department of Health and Social Services, Trenton; Steven Friedman, Assistant Commissioner, New York City Health Department; Eleni Sfakianaki, Medical Executive Director, Dade County Health Department, Miami, Florida; Akiko Kimura, Medical Director, Immunization Program, Los Angeles, California; Babatunde A. Jinadu, Kern County Health Department, Bakersfield, California; Edd Rhoades, Chief, Maternal and Child Health Service, Oklahoma State Department of Health, Oklahoma City; and Natalie Smith, Chief, Immunization Branch, California State Health Department, Berkeley.

2

Change and Complexity in the National Immunization System

s noted in Chapter 1, significant changes have occurred within the national immunization system in the past decade, including continual changes in the immunization schedule, the nature of infectious disease, and the basic demographics of the U.S. population. Immunization was once associated with emergency public health programs designed to stop the spread of infectious disease through mass campaigns conducted within a fairly short time period. Today, the process of immunization involves a series of inoculations spread out over an individual's lifetime. This transformation has expanded the roles and responsibilities of public health agencies beyond direct service delivery to encompass records management and performance monitoring. Transformations have also occurred in the organization of U.S. health care that have redefined the responsibilities of the public and private health care sectors. These changes have added new layers of complexity to the national immunization system that must be examined with regard to their impact on coverage rates and service-delivery patterns.

Despite the stresses imposed on the system by these changes, important successes have been achieved, such as reductions in the incidence of vaccine-preventable diseases (VPD) and national increases in immunization coverage levels. Nevertheless, as discussed in Chapter 1, significant problems remain, including disparities in coverage levels for children, low adult coverage rates and ethnic disparities in adult immunization rates, and concerns about the quality of measurement tools and programmatic efforts. This chapter first describes the markers of change and complexity that affect the national immunization system, and then reviews examples of success and problem areas.

KEY CHANGES

Key areas of change affecting the national immunization effort include (1) the immunization schedule, (2) the nature of infectious disease, and (3) population demographics.

Immunization Schedule

Ever since the American Academy of Pediatrics (AAP) offered the first immunization guidelines in the 1930s, scientific developments have led to regular changes in the recommended immunization schedule. The rate of change has increased dramatically in the last decade and is likely to continue accelerating in the next 20 years (see Figure 2-1). Between 1938 and 1985, five vaccines (three childhood and two adult) comprising nine different antigens were available. In the next 15 years, the number of recommended vaccines more than doubled.

To complete the current harmonized childhood immunization schedule,[1] children must receive 15 to 19 doses of vaccine before 18 months of age and a total of 19 to 22 doses to be fully immunized by the age of 6 (see Figure 1-1 and Table 1-3 in Chapter 1). During some office or clinic visits, the administration of 3 or 4 separate injections is indicated. Adolescents are to receive a tetanus shot between ages 11 and 15, as well as measles, mumps, and rubella (MMR), varicella, and hepatitis B vaccinations if these were not administered at a younger age.

Immunization recommendations for adults have recently changed. The Advisory Committee on Immunization Practices (ACIP) currently recommends that all adults over age 50 receive an annual influenza vaccine (CDC, 2000a). One-time pneumococcal immunizations are recommended for all adults age 65 and over (although ACIP is considering a proposal to lower this recommendation to age 50). Both influenza and pneumococcal immunizations are recommended for anyone below age 65 with certain high-risk conditions, such as heart and lung disease, diabetes, and a compromised immune system. In certain situations, depending on age and health status, adults are also advised to receive hepatitis A, hepatitis B, tetanus, diphtheria, measles, mumps, rubella, and varicella vaccinations (see Table 1-3). Meningococcal vaccine is now recommended for college students, especially those living in dormitories.

Repeated changes to the immunization schedule in the last 5 years foreshadow the exponential changes anticipated in the future. These recent changes include the following:

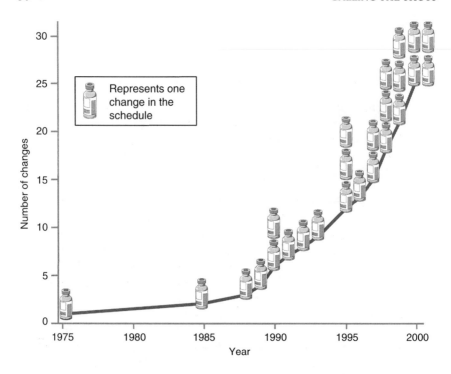

FIGURE 2-1 Changes in the childhood vaccination schedule, 1975–2000. SOURCE: Information provided by CDC.

- Varicella vaccine was licensed in March 1995 and recommended for limited use the same year (CDC, 1995).
- Hepatitis A vaccine gained recommended status in 1996 (CDC, 1996).
- ACIP added rotavirus vaccine to the childhood schedule in August 1998 and then removed it in July 1999 because of indications of increased risk of bowel obstruction during the first few weeks after its administration (CDC, 1999b).
- DTaP, with an acellular form of pertussis, has replaced DTP as the recommended vaccine against diptheria, tetanus, and pertussis (CDC, 2000b).
- In 1999, inactivated poliovirus vaccine (IPV) was recommended for the first two doses of poliovirus vaccine instead of oral poliovirus vaccine (OPV) (CDC, 1999c). As of January 2000, IPV was recommended for all four doses (CDC, 2000b).

In addition to novel vaccines, new age groups for which vaccines are recommended have been identified. A new pediatric pneumococcal conjugate vaccine received approval for children under age 2 and high-risk children under age 5 in February 2000 (CDC, 2000d). In 1996, ACIP, AAP, the American Academy of Family Physicians, and the American Medical Association (AMA) jointly recommended immunizing all adolescents aged 11 to 12 with hepatitis B (CDC, 1998b). As mentioned above, ACIP lowered the recommended age for adult influenza vaccination from 65 to 50 years (CDC, 2000a). Many of the vaccines now in the research pipeline will be targeted at adults, and new initiatives will be required to adapt the vaccine delivery system to serve new age groups.

In the next 20 years, the number of vaccines available could triple relative to those recommended today, almost a ninefold increase since the 1950s (when only polio, diphtheria, tetanus, and pertussis vaccines were recommended) (IOM, 1999b) (see Table 2-1). While all of the vaccines that become available may not be recommended for universal use, the schedule's complexity is certain to increase, although the creation of combination vaccines may minimize the required number of vaccine administrations and office visits.[2] Moreover, in addition to the creation of new vaccine types, new forms of administration are being tested, such as the use of live, attenuated influenza virus administered by intranasal spray (Nichol et al., 1999; Poland and Couch, 1999).

With the introduction of new vaccines and changes to the immunization schedule, the cost of vaccination has fluctuated, generally increasing. A majority of new vaccines are considerably more expensive than those used previously. The catalog price for DTP increased from $11.22 in 1987 to $17 for DTaP in 1997, primarily as a result of inflation (Orenstein et al., 1999). In contrast, varicella vaccine has a per-dose catalog price of $45.56, and adolescent hepatitis B costs $20 to $24 per dose (information provided by CDC). The pediatric pneumococcal conjugate vaccine, which will prevent pneumonia, meningitis, and a limited number (about 8 percent) of ear infections, is expected to be relatively expensive, costing about $232 for a four-dose series (Lieu et al., 2000; Stolberg, 2000). In 1987, the combined catalog price for all childhood vaccines was $116; by 1997, the total price had increased to $332–$370 (Orenstein et al., 1999).

Nature of Infectious Disease

The national immunization system is also affected by the changing nature of infectious disease. Pathogens, like human populations, undergo genetic evolution. Such evolution has allowed some viruses to jump from species to species. For example, many scientists believe that smallpox made a trans-species jump into humans between 3,000 and 12,000 years

TABLE 2-1 Vaccines in Widespread Use, 1985–2020

1985	2000	2020[a]
Adult influenza	Adult influenza	Adult influenza[c]
Adult pneumococcal polysaccharide	Adult pneumococcal polysaccharide	Adult pneumococcal polysaccharide
Diphtheria, pertussis, tetanus, and components	Diphtheria, tetanus, acellular pertussis, and components [b]	DTaP[c]
Measles, mumps, and rubella	MMR[b]	Measles, mumps, rubella, and varicella[c]
Oral poliovirus	Inactivated poliovirus[b]	Eradication of polio expected
	H. influenzae type b[b]	Hib[c]
	Hepatitis A[b]	Hepatitis A[c]
	Hepatitis B[b]	Hepatitis B[c]
	Varicella[b]	Varicella with MMR
	Pediatric conjugate of pneumococcal polysaccharide	Pediatric conjugate of pneumococcal polysaccharide[c]
	Borrelia burgdorferi	Borrelia burgdorferi
	Meningococcal polysaccharide A,C,Y,W-135	Conjugated meningococcal polysaccharide A,B,C,Y,W-135[c]
		Adult tetanus, diphtheria, acellular pertussis, and components[c]
		Chlamydia
		Coccidioides immites
		Cytomegalovirus
		Enterotoxigenic E.coli
		Epstein-Barr
		Helicobacter pylori[c]
		Hepatitis C[c]
		Herpes simplex
		Histoplasma capsulatum
		Human papillomavirus[c]
		Child influenza[c]
		Insulin-dependent diabetes mellitus (therapeutic)
		Melanoma (therapeutic)
		Multiple sclerosis (therapeutic)
		Mycobacterium tuberculosis
		Neisseria gonorrhea
		Neisseria meningitidis B
		Parainfluenza[c]
		Respiratory syncytial virus[c]
		Rheumatoid arthritis (therapeutic)
		Rotavirus[c]
		Shigella
		Streptococcus, Group A[c]
		Streptococcus, Group B

[a]Priority candidate vaccines, drawn from IOM, 1999b.
[b]Vaccines covered by Vaccines for Children (VFC) as of February 2000.
[c]Vaccines likely to be recommended for universal use (including VFC coverage for childhood vaccines).

ago in one of the Mesopotamian river valleys (Preston, 1999). In addition, population migrations and new areas of human habitat during the past century have led to the emergence and reemergence of pathogens unaffected by current medical treatments (IOM, 1992). The phenomenon of antibiotic resistance is alarming because antibiotic-resistant pathogens are cumulative and accelerating (IOM, 1998a; Feikin et al., 2000). The loss of treatment alternatives makes the prevention of communicable disease through immunization ever more critical.

In addition to pathogen evolution, increased global travel has changed disease patterns throughout the world. In 1998, more than 53 million individuals flew on U.S. carriers to domestic and international locations. Travelers, businesspeople, immigrants, and migrants make national and state boundaries ineffectual barriers to disease in the United States. The IOM report *Emerging Infections: Microbial Threats to Health in the United States* summarizes the threat posed by the increased global movements of people:

> As the human immunodeficiency virus (HIV) disease pandemic surely should have taught us, in the context of infectious disease, there is no-where in the world from which we are remote and no one from whom we are disconnected. Consequently, some infectious diseases that now affect people in other parts of the world represent potential threats to the United States because of global interdependence, modern transpor-tation, trade, and changing social and cultural patterns (IOM, 1992:v).

The September 1999 outbreak of a West Nile-like virus in New York serves as a reminder of how easily disease can spread across the global community. This was the first time the West Nile-like virus, contracted from mosquitoes that have bitten infected birds, had ever been reported in the Western Hemisphere (CDC, 1999d).

Population Demographics

The worldwide movement of people, especially through immigration and migration, continually changes U.S. population demographics, affect-ing susceptibility to infectious diseases and placing increased demands on the national immunization effort. For example, immigrants accounted for 35 percent (7,930) of total U.S. tuberculosis cases in 1995 (IOM, 1998b). One of every five children under age 18 in the United States (14 million) is an immigrant or has immigrant parents (IOM, 1998b). Since foreign birth has been identified as a barrier to immunization, immigrant children and adults are likely to fall further behind in vaccination coverage unless special efforts are made to integrate them into the U.S. health care system (Findley et al., 1999).

Immunizing the U.S. migrant population presents special challenges as well. Approximately 750,000 migrants live in the United States (Mountain, 1999). Since many migrants cross state borders, they are literally a moving target for health financing, service delivery, and state-based surveillance systems. In addition, a considerable number of migrants may be undocumented persons, creating ethical and political dilemmas regarding the financing of their immunizations (Mountain, 1999).

In addition to immigration and migration, the aging of the U.S. population merits consideration in the development of strategies for immunization policy and practice. As larger numbers of individuals enjoy increased life spans, the importance of vaccines such as influenza and pneumococcal will increase.

The Challenge of Change

The above changes in vaccine development, the nature of disease, and population demographics create challenges for the U.S. immunization system. First, delays and gaps in the uptake of new vaccines occur. For example, the negotiation of a federal contract price with manufacturers of varicella vaccine required 1 year, causing significant delays in the availability of publicly purchased varicella vaccine following its appearance on the market (N. Smith, CDC, personal communication, February 10, 2000). Even with this major financial barrier removed, the national pediatric coverage rate for varicella was only 43.2 percent in 1998 (CDC, 1998a). Second, the addition of new vaccines to the schedule has broadened discrepancies among state standards and coverage practices. State immunization requirements for school children vary considerably (see Appendix G). In addition, some states mandate insurance coverage of pediatric immunizations, but the policies affected and specific vaccines covered differ greatly (Freed et al., 1999). Third, a more complex immunization schedule has made it more difficult to confirm the immunization status of special groups. Identifying pockets of need has become problematic because records are scattered among public and private providers even as the number of vaccines that require surveillance has increased. Finally, the dramatic, almost exponential increase in vaccines on the horizon creates concerns about adverse reactions. As the general public becomes less familiar with the nature and threat of infectious disease, reports of adverse events associated with the use of vaccines are likely to acquire greater significance.

Finding 2-1. The rate of change in the immunization schedule, the nature of infectious disease, and population demographics increased dramatically in the 1990s and is likely to accelerate in the future. At the same time, determining the immunization status of individuals and groups has become more difficult, especially among vulnerable populations. The complexity of the immunization schedule is likely to contribute to more missed opportunities that could decrease coverage levels and reduce the benefits of vaccines.

INCREASING COMPLEXITY

In addition to the challenges resulting from scientific advances and changes in the environment, the national immunization effort must adapt to the increasing complexity of the financing, service delivery, and public health information systems. Many vulnerable populations now receive vaccines from private health care providers, as the well-insured have long done. Yet the public sector still has primary responsibility for financing vaccine purchases and surveillance efforts for at-risk groups. A patchwork of public and private programs and funding streams that is inadequately described and poorly understood has complicated the national effort to supply, deliver, and monitor immunizations.

Vaccine Supply

The public sector currently relies on a combination of Vaccines for Children (VFC), Section 317, and state funds to purchase childhood vaccines. These programs for vaccine purchase are described in Chapter 3. VFC now provides vaccine for approximately 35 percent of the national birth cohort (National Vaccine Advisory Committee [NVAC], 1999a). In 1998, VFC purchased approximately 37 million doses of vaccine, while Section 317 funds were used to purchase about 13 million doses (information provided by CDC). States also use their own funds to buy vaccine. The states purchased a total of approximately 7 million doses through federal purchase contracts in 1998, and purchased an undetermined number of additional doses directly. Altogether, public-sector funds were used to purchase more than 57 million doses of childhood vaccine in 1998. More than half of all vaccine doses purchased in the United States in 1998 (52.4 percent) were publicly purchased through federal contracts (information provided by CDC).

Vaccine Delivery

Although the public sector purchases the majority of vaccine doses, it is not the primary source of vaccine delivery. Historically, virtually all immunizations received by public program beneficiaries were administered in the public sector. With the inception of VFC in 1994 and the rapid growth of managed care enrollment in Medicaid over the past decade, a majority of immunizations are currently administered in the private sector.

In 1998, according to the National Immunization Survey (NIS), 54.6 percent of U.S. children received immunizations from private providers, 16.9 percent from public providers, 7.9 percent from mixed providers (public and private), and 20.5 percent from other providers[3] (CDC, 1999e). In 1998, an estimated 55 percent of all U.S. children were enrolled in employer-sponsored health plans that covered pediatric immunizations (KPMG Peat Marwick, 1998; Bureau of the Census, 1999). Information on the provision of adult immunization benefits by private plans is lacking.

The rise of managed care has caused public health services, such as immunizations, to be increasingly privatized and funded through capitated arrangements, which makes it difficult to document immunization services. For example, the number of Americans that receive health care services from health maintenance organizations (HMOs) increased from 6 million in 1976 to 67.5 million in 1996 (NVAC, 1999a). The proportion of Medicaid beneficiaries enrolled in a managed care arrangement increased from less than 15 percent in 1993 to 54 percent in 1998 (Health Care Financing Administration [HCFA], 1999b). In addition, 2 million low-income children previously ineligible for Medicaid have been enrolled in the State Children's Health Insurance Program (SCHIP) over the past 2 years, and the majority of these children receive their vaccines from private providers (HCFA, 2000a). Consequently, children who were likely to be immunized in the public sector 10 years ago may no longer be eligible for its services.

Over the past decade, both general and immunization-specific pediatric best practices have included immunizations within the child's medical home (AAP, 1992). Administration of immunizations in a timely manner by the child's primary care practitioner is viewed as a quality measure in its own right and as an indicator of access to a broader array of preventive and routine primary care services. There will always be conditions and population groups that require some kind of special effort, such as children attending school for the first time, adolescents who need immunizations recently added to the schedule (e.g., hepatitis B), or migrant children served by mobile clinics. However, the preferred immunization setting is the child's regular source of primary care.

Yet the enrollment of Medicaid and SCHIP beneficiaries in private managed care organizations has led to uncertainties and tensions regarding the appropriate site for delivering publicly financed vaccines. Some clients still rely on public clinics for immunizations, either because the public clinic is more convenient (in terms of hours of service or geographic location) or because of the relatively low cost of vaccines thus acquired. Similarly, some private health care providers find it convenient and less costly to refer their clients to public health clinics for immunizations, even though federal officials have sought to discourage this type of referral practice through advisory notices and consultations (Richardson, 1999; Richardson and Orenstein, 1999). Public health departments are facing decreased revenues from third-party payers, such as Medicaid, for immunizations because of the rapid growth in capitated arrangements. Consequently, public health officials in some areas now negotiate payment plans for immunizations with HMOs or actively discourage private provider referrals through the use of screening questions. The result is a series of mixed signals and increased paperwork for clients and public providers that can result in missed opportunities for immunization within populations with startlingly low coverage levels.

VFC has also contributed to the vaccine delivery system's shift toward the private sector. A total of 43,000 health care provider sites have enrolled in VFC, and the majority of these (approximately 70 percent, or 30,000) are private provider sites (NVAC, 1999a). By providing free vaccine to primary care physicians, VFC attempts to keep children in their medical homes (their regular source of primary care) and decreases private provider referral of patients to public clinics for immunizations (NVAC, 1999a).

Surveillance

The complexity of vaccine supply and immunization delivery arrangements creates a dilemma for surveillance efforts. Private health plans have assumed responsibility for providing personal health services to public program beneficiaries, but are not readily held accountable for ensuring that all of their enrolled clients are kept up to date in their immunization status. Public agencies continue to deliver vaccines to disadvantaged adults and children, and also retain the responsibility for assessing records and auditing data for public program beneficiaries in both private and public health care settings. Yet the enrollment growth among Medicaid beneficiaries in capitated plans that do not bill for individual services has reduced public agencies' ability to monitor service delivery for vulnerable populations. Record scattering and patient movement both on and off Medicaid and between health plans (known as "cycling") have also made immunization records management more difficult. A clearer definition of responsibility for ensuring immunization services and conducting surveillance efforts is needed between the private and public sectors, as well as among public health agencies such as Medicaid, Medicare, and state immunization programs.

Roles and Responsibilities

The multiple public programs and agencies involved with vaccine purchase and administration reflect the dispersion of responsibilities within the national immunization system. This situation raises important questions about the respective leadership roles of federal and state agencies, as well as the appropriate distribution of effort between the private and public health care sectors. For example:

• ACIP recommends vaccines for the U.S. population. ACIP's pediatric recommendations are binding for VFC, Medicaid, and SCHIP. Most commonly, it is only after ACIP has recommended a new vaccine that CDC begins to negotiate a federal contract under which VFC and Section 317 can purchase the vaccine. Even before such contracts are in effect, however, Medicaid programs are required to reimburse providers for the newly recommended vaccine as a shared federal–state cost.

• One strategy states have adopted to encourage private provider participation in VFC and Medicaid has been to increase Medicaid vaccine administration fees after VFC has made vaccines available to private providers at no cost. However, the impact of this strategy has been diminished by the growth of Medicaid managed care plan enrollments because these plans generally do not pay providers separately for vaccine administration.

• Immunization records are maintained by multiple private and public parties. No single record-keeping system exists that can track clients across health care settings. For clients who use multiple providers, records are scattered, making monitoring of coverage levels as well as individual documentation difficult.

• The array of public and private agencies involved with immunization in some manner is extensive. The public organizations include state and local public health agencies, insurance regulators, school systems, ACIP, state Medicaid agencies, HCFA (which administers Medicaid and Medicare), CDC, and Women, Infants, and Children (WIC) programs. Private agencies include individual providers, managed care organizations, health plans, and insurers. Each of these organizations has some responsibility for the immunization process, but no single entity has a universal role that allows it to establish data standards, criteria for record keeping, or performance guidelines, or to make cost allocation decisions. The result is a multifaceted enterprise that encourages diverse arrangements; tolerates discrepancies in policies and practices; and frustrates the analysis of trends and patterns, especially for vulnerable populations that depend on both public and private settings.

The scale and impact of changes in the immunization schedule, the nature of disease, and the health care delivery system have distinct implications for the efforts of various levels of government to monitor and respond to trends and shifts in immunization coverage. The states, largely through local governmental authorities, have the primary responsibility for ensuring public health and the delivery of health care services for their citizens. Infectious disease control and prevention, however, requires a nationwide effort and if only for this reason constitutes a national interest. In addition, many states require extra assistance to meet the needs of their populations, either because those needs are extraordinary or because state resources are especially limited. Finally, it is essential to acknowledge the legitimacy of state and local variations in the organization and financing of immunization services, as these services must be responsive to local needs, populations, and professional and fiscal resources. National immunization policy is better focused on goals, outcomes, and identification of successful interventions that increase immunization coverage than on "how to" prescriptions.

The changing realities of health care organization, financing, and politics have resulted in a concomitant shift in public health policy and strategy. To meet its protective responsibilities, the public health sector must work with a rapidly changing health care system, first to understand its approach, and then to apply a variety of government tools to fulfill public health objectives. These tools include (1) a regulatory environment that protects the public from dangerous or ineffective vaccines, (2) a new level of surveillance information that not only captures the peaks of epidemics but also identifies individuals who require immunization services, and (3) a quality assurance role that applies health services research and technical assistance in ensuring immunization coverage.

State and local public health agencies are taking on health system management roles and developing tools that can help them work with and through managed care to improve practices, reduce missed opportunities, and ensure timely immunization coverage. At the same time, however, public health agencies at all levels of government must remain prepared to combat disease epidemics and provide vaccines when necessary to underserved groups.

Finding 2-2. The magnitude and complexity of the modern immunization system have significant implications in terms of both cost and records management. Protecting the public's health requires attention to multiple components of a complex system composed of numerous public and private agencies. Institutional relationships within this system are loose and disjointed, resulting in ambiguous roles and responsi-

bilities that require coordination and integration through investments in infrastructure.

Finding 2-3. The increasing complexity of the immunization schedule necessitates intensive surveillance and records management for young children, especially for vulnerable populations who may not have a regular source of health care and are therefore at greatest risk of low immunization coverage. This complexity is likely to increase during periods of reform and realignment within the health care delivery system; thus, greater oversight and monitoring are required to ensure that disparities in immunization coverage rates do not grow.

SUCCESSES AND PERSISTENT PROBLEMS

Despite the increasing change and complexity affecting the national immunization effort, the incidence of VPDs has decreased, and important objectives for national coverage were partially met in the 1990s. Yet as noted earlier, persistent problems, such as disparities in childhood coverage levels, low adult immunization rates, ethnic disparities in adult immunization rates, and concerns about the quality of surveillance tools, continue to plague the system.

Successes

The successes of the national immunization effort are most evident in the dramatic decrease in VPD incidence in the 1990s (CDC, 1999a). Only one case of diphtheria was reported in both 1998 and 1999 (CDC, 1999f; information provided by CDC). Polio has been eradicated in the Western Hemisphere, and global polio eradication is expected in this decade (information provided by CDC).

Certain childhood and adult coverage goals have been achieved as well. By 1996, more than 90 percent of American children aged 19 to 35 months had received the first and most critical doses in the primary series for DTP, *Haemophilus influenzae* type b (Hib), polio, and measles vaccines (NVAC, 1999a). The complete immunization of 79.2 percent of 2-year-old children for the 4:3:1:3 series (four or more doses of DTP, three or more doses of poliovirus, one or more dose of any measles-containing vaccine, and three or more doses of Hib) in 1998 is another major accomplishment, made possible by a remarkable federal–state partnership effort (CDC, 1998a), although approximately 1 million 2-year-olds still need one or more vaccine doses to be fully immunized (NVAC, 1999a). Strides have also been made in adult immunizations. In 1997, the national influenza immunization rate for adults aged 65 and older was 63 percent, up from 58 percent in 1995 (National Center for Health Statistics, 1997).

Disparities in Childhood Coverage Levels

Despite increased national coverage levels for children and substantial reductions in disparities among racial and ethnic groups, disparities still exist among and within states, as well as within major metropolitan areas. Between 1970 and 1985, surveys of immunization coverage of preschool-age children revealed racial and ethnic disparities in coverage levels that ranged as high as 26 percentage points (CDC, 1997). The most current available NIS data (July 1998–June 1999) show disparities of 7 to 8.6 percentage points between the immunization coverage levels for non-Hispanic white children and Hispanic and non-Hispanic black children for the 4:3:1:3 series, and lesser disparities for individual vaccine coverage rates among these groups (CDC, 2000e). Much of the difference in coverage levels among racial and ethnic groups is attributable to differences in poverty rates among these groups. Again for the latest annual period, the NIS documented a disparity of 9 percentage points between children living below and those at or above the poverty level for the 4:3:1:3 immunization series (CDC, 2000f). Concentrated poverty, along with the somewhat lower immunization levels for minority children, contributes to the lower coverage levels found in large metropolitan areas.

In 1999, state coverage levels for the 4:3:1:3 series ranged from 71 percent in Arkansas to 89 percent in Vermont, Rhode Island, and Massachusetts (see Figure 2-2). Also in 1999, the coverage levels for the same series were 57 percent in the City of Houston and 73 percent in Dallas County, compared with 76 percent for the rest of Texas. Newark's coverage level was 67 percent, 18 points lower than the rate for the rest of New Jersey. Chicago's rate was 70 percent in 1999, compared with 84 percent for the rest of Illinois (CDC, 2000c) (see Table 1-5 in Chapter 1).

Serious disparities in coverage levels also exist within certain large metropolitan areas. Several studies have demonstrated that the NIS, which collects state and county data, is often not sensitive to small area variations, which reveal significant underimmunization among the most disadvantaged populations. For example:

- In Marion County, Indiana (Indianapolis), a special survey of poor children found their coverage rate to be 53 percent as compared with an NIS estimate of 78 percent for the county as a whole (Bates and Wolinsky, 1998).
- A special survey of children in East Los Angeles found coverage to be 49 percent as compared with NIS data showing a coverage rate of 71 percent for the Los Angeles region (Shaheen et al., 2000).

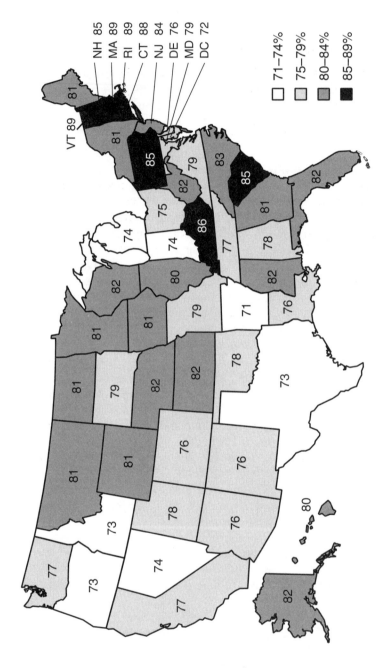

FIGURE 2-2 Immunization coverage levels with the 4:3:1:3[a] series, by state (national coverage = 79%).
[a]4 DTP, 3 polio, 1 MMR, and 3 Hib. SOURCE: Information provided by CDC.

• A Chicago study found coverage rates of 36 percent for African American children in general and 29 percent for African American children in public housing, as compared with the NIS estimate of 59 percent coverage for children countywide (Kenyon et al., 1998).

Low Adult Immunization Coverage Rates

Although the objective that 60 percent of elderly Americans receive an influenza immunization has been met, problems in adult coverage rates persist, especially for chronically ill working-age adults who are at high risk for complications from influenza and pneumococcal disease. Many have argued that a 60 percent influenza coverage rate is too low, and the national goal has been raised to 90 percent for 2010 (Department of Health and Human Services, 2000). Pneumococcal immunization levels for the elderly are particularly low. Nationally, only 42 percent of non-institutionalized adults over age 65 had ever received a pneumococcal vaccination by 1997 (National Center for Health Statistics, 1997). Just 17 states had achieved pneumococcal immunization rates of 50 percent or greater among elderly persons by 1997 (information provided by CDC). In addition, noninstitutionalized high-risk adults aged 18 to 64 have extremely low immunization rates. Data from the 1997 National Health Interview Survey show that only 26 percent of this group had received an influenza vaccination, and just 13 percent had received a pneumococcal vaccination (National Center for Health Statistics, 1997). Data on national coverage rates for adult immunizations other than influenza and pneumococcal are severely limited.

Disparities in Adult Coverage Levels

While the generally low adult immunization coverage levels are disconcerting, disparities in the immunization rates among ethnic populations represent an even more serious situation. In 1997, 66 percent of white adults aged 65 and over received an influenza vaccination, compared with 45 percent of black and 53 percent of Hispanic adults in the same age group (National Center for Health Statistics, 1997). The trend is similar for pneumococcal immunizations. As of 1997, 46 percent of elderly whites had received a one-time pneumococcal vaccination, but only 22 percent of elderly blacks and 23 percent of elderly Hispanics. These disparities result in communities at heightened risk for outbreaks of influenza and pneumococcal disease, in addition to other VPDs. Among persons aged 65 and over, influenza and pneumococcal disease were the fifth leading cause of death for African Americans and Hispanics as well as non-Hispanic whites. Reductions in these deaths are hindered by relatively low vaccine utilization. Because of the association of appropriate health care with an individual's economic status, race, and gender, access to immunization coverage proves difficult for many racial and ethnic minorities. For example, although rubella has been virtually eliminated within the U.S.-born population, rubella outbreaks have occurred sporadically among Hispanic populations in the last 5 years as a result of immigration from countries where rubella vaccine is not part of the childhood immunization schedule (information provided by CDC).

> *Finding 2-4. Important strides have been made in decreasing the incidence of vaccine-preventable diseases and increasing the immunization coverage levels for children and adults. However, sustained efforts are needed to address the troublesome disparities that remain in childhood and adult coverage levels.*

ENDNOTES

1. The harmonized schedule is determined jointly by the American Academy of Pediatrics (AAP), the Advisory Committee on Immunization Practices (ACIP), and the American Academy of Family Physicians (AAFP).

2. For example, researchers are experimenting with a measles, mumps, rubella, varicella (MMRV) vaccine that will include four distinct antigens in one injection (S. Katz, Duke University, personal communication, 1999).

3. "Other" includes community health centers, the military, hospital-based clinics, and those who describe themselves as "other."

3

Financing Vaccine Purchase and Delivery

This chapter examines the roles of public and private programs in financing immunization services and purchasing vaccines, which reflect both the strengths and limitations of the nation's health care financing system. As is true with personal health care generally, immunization coverage policies have changed substantially over the past half-century. Immunizations today represent a significant part of the cost of routine health care for infants and young children. The cost of an immunization reflects both the cost of the vaccine and the cost of administering it (the health professional's time, supplies, and overhead).[1] When an individual needs multiple vaccines over a relatively brief period of time (e.g., a child who has fallen behind in the routine childhood immunization schedule and for whom a "catch-up" schedule is warranted), the cost at the point of service can be considerable.

Immunizations are both a basic public health intervention and a personal health service, benefiting society as well as the protected individual. In contrast with many personal health care interventions, the benefit of immunizations to nearly all individuals is undisputed, and their cost-effectiveness is both documented and widely recognized (Sisk et al., 1997; Cochi et al., 1985; White et al., 1985; Huse et al., 1994; Midani et al., 1995). An additional and relatively unique aspect of immunization services is that, unlike many types of health care, their provision is the subject of widely accepted, evidence-based practice guidelines for both children and adults, promulgated and updated by CDC's Advisory Committee on Immunization Practices (ACIP) (see Figure 1-1 and Table 1-3 in Chapter 1).

71

Despite these national consensus recommendations, however, substantial variations in coverage and payment policies among public and private insurers remain, a consequence of the nation's multipayer approach to health care.

When there were few recommended vaccines, immunizations were financed as a public health service and were typically delivered by public health agency personnel. Most Americans over the age of 40, for example, can probably recall receiving polio vaccine from a public health nurse, typically at school. As the number and cost of immunizations increased, and as insurance expanded to cover primary and preventive services as well as traditional insurable events, the very concept of immunizations also evolved. Immunizations became less of a public health intervention and became increasingly integrated into comprehensive primary health care.

The sheer magnitude of the modern immunization effort has implications for both health care cost and quality, as well as the protection of the public's health. Vaccine purchase and service delivery are essential features of the national immunization enterprise, and immunizations are optimally provided within the context of an ongoing primary care relationship. General health care financing provided through employment-based and other private insurance, Medicaid, the State Children's Health Insurance Program (SCHIP), and Medicare aids in integrating immunizations into routine health care. Yet while these private and public health insurance programs account for the majority of immunizations provided nationally, they do not offer the U.S. population seamless and universal coverage. The federal Section 317 categorical grant program and state vaccine purchase and delivery programs address residual needs created by gaps and uncertainties in these health financing plans (see Box 3-1).

Over the past 50 years, public and private insurance initiatives at both the federal and state levels have expanded insurance coverage for immunizations among both publicly and privately insured children. In 15 states, pediatric immunization coverage has been achieved through the establishment of universal, public vaccine purchase programs that distribute vaccines directly to pediatric health care providers. The Vaccines for Children (VFC) program, enacted by Congress in 1993, created a similar direct purchase and delivery system for certain children on a nationwide basis.

Despite the fact that vaccine-preventable diseases can be spread by and affect individuals of all ages, finance policy with regard to adult immunization is significantly more limited and uneven. Both public and private insurers are less likely to cover recommended immunizations for adults, and adults are not included in universal state vaccine purchase and distribution systems.

BOX 3-1
Examples of Residual Needs That Require
State Vaccine Purchase

The following are examples of the types of children and adults who require assistance for vaccines purchased with both Section 317 and state-level funds:

- Families that are eligible for either Medicaid or SCHIP but are not enrolled in these programs. This group includes families that are unaware of their eligibility or are reluctant to apply for public benefits, as well as families that frequently change residences and recent immigrants who are unfamiliar with or have not yet completed the enrollment process.
- Children enrolled in Medicaid or SCHIP plans whose provider does not participate in the VFC program or otherwise fails to offer reduced-cost immunizations.
- Families with insurance that does not cover vaccines (the "underinsured"). Such families may also have income that disqualifies them for Medicaid or SCHIP but is not sufficient to cover out-of-pocket fees for vaccine services on a routine basis.
- Families with private insurance that lack access to vaccines because of cultural barriers, or difficulties in scheduling appointments or establishing routine medical care.
- Children who are enrolled with a private provider through a freestanding SCHIP plan—one that is not an extension of the state's Medicaid program. Such children do not qualify for VFC since they are considered "insured"; legislation has been proposed to reverse this policy, and clarification on this issue is needed by HCFA.
- School-aged children who have not received vaccines required for school entry and who need swift access to immunization services.
- Families that require ACIP-recommended vaccines not available within the VFC or SCHIP vaccine schedule (such as rabies and meningococcal, and tetanus for persons 7 years of age and older).
- Adolescents and young adults who lack insurance for immunizations and do not meet their state's age requirements for Medicaid or SCHIP or are not qualified for VFC because they are older than 18.
- Adults who lack insurance for immunizations and who do not yet qualify for Medicare coverage, particularly adults with chronic disease (such as diabetes or chronic heart disease) who may be especially vulnerable to infectious disease.

As with many aspects of American health care financing, it is virtually impossible to determine with any precision the extent to which insured persons are covered for immunizations. The nation's multipayer insurance system lacks any single cross-payer database that would provide information on the extent of coverage for particular items or services. Although several national probability studies are designed to measure insurance coverage and utilization of health services, none contains sufficiently detailed information to determine immunization coverage by type of insurance.[2] Even within classes of public and private insurance (e.g., Medicaid, SCHIP, employer-sponsored plans), insurance coverage levels cannot be documented with accuracy, since plan sponsors (individual state Medicaid agencies or sponsoring employers) typically have significant discretion in formulating coverage and payment policies. Despite the limitations of available data, however, certain trends and patterns of coverage can be identified. The first three sections of this chapter examine immunization coverage and payment policies under private health insurance; Medicaid, SCHIP, and VFC; and Medicare. The fourth section reviews vaccine purchase grants under Section 317, while the fifth examines state vaccine purchase policies. The final section addresses current issues in vaccine purchase policy.

PRIVATE INSURANCE COVERAGE OF IMMUNIZATION

In 1998, 227 million Americans had some form of public or private health insurance. Yet more than 44 million people, one-fourth of them children, were uninsured (see Table 3-1). As Table 3-1 shows, about three-fourths of those with private health insurance obtain that insurance through employer-sponsored health plans.

By 1999, 28 states had enacted laws requiring insurers to cover childhood immunization services to at least some degree (Freed et al., 1999). As with any type of state insurance regulation, coverage standards vary considerably from state to state. For example, a state law might:

• Regulate the scope of coverage, requiring that insurers cover immunizations in accordance with ACIP standards or refer to the standards endorsed by a professional society, such as the American Academy of Pediatrics.
• Prohibit deductibles or coinsurance, resulting in what is called "first-dollar" coverage for immunizations.
• Fashion less specific standards, simply requiring that insurers cover "appropriate" pediatric vaccines, with decisions regarding which vaccines to include or the nature of any cost sharing left to the discretion of the insurer.

TABLE 3-1 U.S. Population Health Insurance Coverage, 1998

Population Group	Number (in thousands)	Percentage
All persons	271,743	
Not covered	44,281	16.3
Total covered	227,462	83.7
Private	190,861	70.2
Employer-based	168,576	62.0
Government	66,087	24.3
Medicare	35,887	13.2
Medicaid	27,854	10.3
Military	8,747	3.2
All children (under 18 years of age)	72,022	
Not covered	11,073	15.4
Total covered	60,949	89.6[a]
Private	48,627	67.5
Employer-based	45,593	63.3
Government	16,400	22.8
Medicare	325	0.5
Medicaid	14,274	19.8
Military	2,240	3.1
Poor children (under 18 years of age)[b]	13,467	
Not covered	3,392	25.2
Total covered	10,075	74.8
Private	3,059	22.7
Employer-based	2,586	19.2
Government	7,955	59.1
Medicare	135	1.0
Medicaid	7,784	57.8
Military	223	1.7

[a]Some individuals have multiple sources of coverage (e.g., Medicare and private insurance, or Medicaid and Medicare). Thus the percentages add to more than 100.
[b]Children in families with incomes of less than 100 percent of the federal poverty line.

SOURCE: Bureau of the Census, 1999.

Employers that self-insure are generally exempt from state insurance regulation under the federal Employee Retirement Income Security Act (ERISA).[3] Approximately 50 million privately insured individuals are covered by self-insured plans, and this limits the reach of state insurance laws or regulations governing the coverage of pediatric vaccines (Copeland and Pierron, 1998; Polzer, 2000).

Other federal legislation, however, prohibits employers (regardless of whether they purchase insurance or self-insure) from reducing "coverage of pediatric vaccines (as defined under [the Medicaid program]) below the coverage . . . provided as of May 1, 1993."[4] Thus, employers that provided any vaccine coverage as of that date must continue to provide such coverage. This "maintenance-of-effort" provision was aimed at preventing employer-sponsored plans from reducing coverage following enactment of the VFC program. While the statute does not require a particular level of coverage and does not specify standards regarding deductibles and cost sharing, it establishes some federal standards with respect to childhood immunizations.[5]

There are few data available on insurance practices with respect to immunizations. One national survey of employer-sponsored health coverage reports that coverage of childhood immunizations is common, but it does not provide detailed information about the nature of the coverage, e.g., whether it meets the ACIP standard or whether deductibles and copayments apply (KPMG Peat Marwick, 1998) (see Table 3-2). The results of this survey support an estimate that 92 percent of all children covered by employer-sponsored plans, or 42 million children, have some coverage for immunizations.[6]

Researchers at The George Washington University collected data on the immunization coverage policies of five health care companies (four national and one regional) that suggest significant variation by type of plan, as well as by vaccine (S. Rosenbaum, The George Washington University, personal communication, February 8, 2000). Consistent with the KPMG study, the respondents indicated that coverage varies by type of product. All five companies reported that they generally would cover

TABLE 3-2 Coverage of Pediatric Immunizations by Health Benefit Plans Offered by Employers[a]

Type of Insurance Product	Percentage of Covered Workers with Each Type of Product[b]	Percentage of Employees with Dependent Coverage for Pediatric Immunization Services[c]
Health Maintenance Organizations	28	99
Point-of-Service Plans	25	98
Fee-for-Service Plans	9	79
Preferred Provider Organization Plans	38	86

[a]Insurance coverage does not mean that children actually get vaccinated.
[b]SOURCE: Health Research and Educational Trust, 1999.
[c]SOURCE: KPMG Peat Marwick, 1998.

diphtheria-tetanus-pertussis (DTP); *Haemophilus influenza* type b (Hib) conjugate; hepatitis B; measles, mumps, and rubella (MMR); oral poliovirus (OPV); and varicella. However, coverage was more variable for other pediatric vaccines.[7] Respondents did not indicate whether their coverage was consistent with ACIP standards, nor did they report their cost-sharing policies.

The five companies reported more limited coverage of immunizations for adults. Three reported typical coverage of rubella vaccine for persons aged 25–65, two reported coverage of varicella for working-age adults, and three reported coverage of tetanus and diphtheria toxoids. Three companies reported covering influenza and pneumoccocal vaccines for enrollees over age 65, but not for younger adults.

Capitated managed care plans may realize savings from immunizing elderly and at-risk younger adults for influenza and pneumococcal disease, and are more likely than traditional indemnity insurance plans to cover and actively promote these immunizations. However, no systematic surveys of the extent of such coverage have been conducted.

Finding 3-1. While most private health plans provide some form of immunization coverage, this coverage varies by type of plan, as well as by vaccine. Enrollment in a private plan does not guarantee that immunizations will be provided as a plan benefit.

MEDICAID, VACCINES FOR CHILDREN, AND STATE CHILDREN'S HEALTH INSURANCE PROGRAM

Medicaid and Early and Periodic Screening, Diagnosis, and Treatment Program

Medicaid, the nation's largest public insurance program for low-income and medically indigent persons, covered an estimated 31 million people in 1998, more than half of whom were children (Health Care Financing Administration, 2000c, 2000d). An additional estimated 4.7 million children aged 18 or younger who lacked health insurance and were eligible for Medicaid were not enrolled in it (Selden et al., 1998).

In 1967, 2 years after its inception, Medicaid was expanded to include comprehensive primary health care for children under age 21 through the Early and Periodic Screening, Diagnosis, and Treatment Program (EPSDT).[8] Since then, Medicaid has been a significant source of funding (federal and state) for immunizations, and since 1979, immunizations have been a mandatory service for eligible children. Amendments to the Medicaid law in 1989 specifically codified immunizations as a mandatory component of the Medicaid program for individuals under age 21 and

specified coverage in accordance with ACIP standards. [9] Federal Medicaid policy prohibits the imposition of cost sharing for enrollees under age
18; the extent to which states impose cost sharing for immunizations in
the case of persons aged 18–21 remains uncertain. States have the option
of covering all routine and risk-related ACIP-recommended immunizations for Medicaid-enrolled adults (both elderly and nonelderly), but the
extent of state coverage for adult immunizations is not known.

Prior to VFC, Medicaid paid for both vaccines and administration
fees. Estimates of Medicaid program expenditures for immunization services were $364 million in fiscal year (FY) 1994, the last year before imple-
mentation of VFC; $200 million of this total was federal costs, and the
remainder was state Medicaid matching costs (information provided by
CDC). In FY 1998, when VFC spending for vaccines and operational costs
was $437 million, Medicaid program expenditures—largely for adminis-
tration fees, but including some vaccines not covered by VFC—were
$127 million, $70 million of which was federal (see Table 3-3) (information provided by CDC).

Vaccines for Children Program

In 1993 Medicaid was further amended to include the VFC program,
which is 100 percent federally financed.[10] The program creates a federal
entitlement to immunization services for children aged 18 and under who
are (1) Medicaid-eligible, (2) uninsured, (3) underinsured and receiving
immunizations through a federally qualified health center (FQHC) or
rural health clinic, or (4) Native American or Alaska Native.[11] Figure 3-1
displays the share of VFC spending represented by each eligibility group.
Notably, the legislation establishing the VFC program explicitly prohibits
spending on program administration except for narrowly defined operational costs associated with ordering, inventory maintenance, distribution of vaccines, and provider enrollment and coordination.[12]

The VFC program requires the Secretary of Health and Human Services to negotiate vaccine purchase agreements with manufacturers. VFC
vaccines are available only when administered by "program-registered"
providers.[13] In 1998, an estimated 44,000 public and private providers
were eligible to receive VFC vaccines (information provided by CDC).
The VFC legislation requires "maintenance-of-effort" by states, similar to
the maintenance-of-effort provision for employer-sponsored health plans
included in ERISA. The law provides that, as a condition of receipt of
vaccine under VFC, states must agree to maintain their insurance laws
governing immunization coverage at 1993 levels.[14]

The VFC program does not change the states' basic obligation to cover
all ACIP vaccines for Medicaid children. Significant delays can occur,

however, between the adoption of a new vaccine by ACIP and the completion of federal contract negotiations between CDC and the vaccine manufacturer. For example, an 11-month delay occurred between the time that varicella vaccine was recommended by ACIP (June 1995) and the effective date of VFC coverage (May 1996) (N. Smith, CDC, personal communication, February 10, 2000). In the absence of a VFC contract, state Medicaid agencies must directly cover all ACIP-recommended vaccines as a basic EPSDT service, paying commercial price for the vaccine and sharing the cost of the purchase at the usual Medicaid matching rate. Furthermore, since VFC covers children aged 18 and younger, states remain responsible for the immunization of adolescents aged 18–21 who are enrolled in Medicaid. In sum, the VFC program has reduced, but not eliminated, states' financial obligations with respect to coverage of immunizations for Medicaid-enrolled children.

State Children's Health Insurance Program

SCHIP, enacted in 1997, provides states with "child health assistance" to extend services to "targeted low-income" children who are ineligible for Medicaid but otherwise uninsured.[15] Unlike Medicaid (including the VFC program), which creates a federal entitlement to coverage and is financed on an open-ended basis, SCHIP is a block grant program subject to aggregate federal payment limits.[16] The federal SCHIP allotment formula is more generous than the Medicaid federal financing scheme: the SCHIP state matching requirement is 70 percent of the state's Medicaid matching rate.

States have the discretion to use their annual SCHIP allotments to expand Medicaid; create separate, freestanding children's insurance programs; or design a combination of the two. As of January 2000, 33 states had used their SCHIP allotments in whole or in part to establish freestanding programs (see Table 3-4).

To the extent that states use their SCHIP allotments to expand Medicaid, all Medicaid coverage requirements apply. As with other Medicaid-covered children, those whose enrollment is purchased with federal SCHIP funds are entitled to the full EPSDT benefits, including vaccines purchased through the VFC program.

In the case of freestanding SCHIP programs, immunizations are a mandatory service, and coverage is set according to ACIP standards.[17] However, SCHIP children enrolled in freestanding programs are not entitled to receive vaccines through the VFC program. States are required to cover vaccines and their administration for children in freestanding SCHIP programs as part of their annual federal SCHIP allotment. States may, however, purchase these vaccines through the federal VFC contract

TABLE 3-3 Medicaid and Vaccines for Children (VFC) Program,
FY 1994–1999 (millions of dollars)

Program	FY 1994[a] Enacted[b]	FY 1994 Actual[c]	FY 1995 Enacted	FY 1995 Actual	FY 1996 Enacted	FY 1996 Actual
VFC Program						
Vaccine purchase	20.9	20.9	412.0	213.8	349.3	254.9
Operations	3.8	3.8	45.3	29.8	24.7	24.7
Total	24.7	24.7	457.3	243.6	374.0	279.6
Medicaid		200.0	140.0	140.0	60.0	60.0
TOTAL		224.7	597.3	383.6	434.0	339.6

[a]In FY 1994, $80 million was awarded for phase 1 operations and vaccine purchase.
[b]The enacted level is the amount requested in the president's budget.
[c]Actual expenditures.

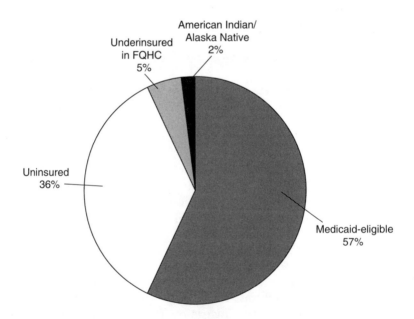

FIGURE 3-1 Children receiving VFC vaccines by eligibility category, calendar year 2000 (estimated). SOURCE: Information provided by CDC.

FY 1997 Enacted	FY 1997 Actual	FY 1998 Enacted	FY 1998 Actual	FY 1999 Enacted	FY 1999 Actual	FY 2000 Estimate
498.6	351.0	408.5	388.6	526.9	434.9	504.2[d]
25.4	24.7	28.6	29.6	39.4	32.6	40.9[d]
524.0	375.7	437.1	418.2	566.3	467.5	545.1
65.0	65.0	70.0	70.0	75.0[d]	75.0[d]	80.0[d]
589.0	440.7	507.1	488.2	641.3	542.5	625.0

[d]Projection.

SOURCE: Information provided by CDC.

(Richardson and Orenstein, 1999). Thus states with freestanding SCHIP programs maintain some level of financial exposure for the cost of immunization services.

Figure 3-2 shows the combined potential reach of Medicaid, the VFC program, and SCHIP. Assuming full coverage of all eligible children, Medicaid and SCHIP would reach about one-third of all American children aged 18 and under.[18] The addition of VFC entitlement for non-Medicaid children increases by another 6 million the number of children

TABLE 3-4 State Children's Health Insurance Programs, 2000[a]

Type of Program	Number of States
Medicaid Expansion Only	18 plus District of Columbia (16 operational for full year)
Separate SCHIP	15 (7 operational for full year)
Combination Program	18 (Medicaid expansion portion operational for full year in 16 states; separate programs operational in 9 states)

[a]Of the 33 states with some form of separate SCHIP, 23 offer 12 months of continuous eligibility in their separate programs; 15 states provide 12-month continuous coverage to children enrolled in Medicaid.

SOURCE: Health Care Financing Administration, 2000b.

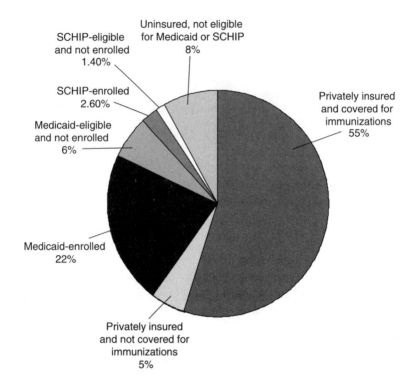

76 million children under age 19, 1998

FIGURE 3-2 U.S. children's insurance coverage for immunizations. SOURCES: Medical Expenditure Panel Survey estimates of those Medicaid-eligible and enrolled, and SCHIP-eligible (Agency for Healthcare Research and Quality, 1996); SCHIP enrollment (Health Care Financing Administration, 1999b); U.S. Bureau of the Census 1998 population estimates; private insurance coverage for immunizations (KPMG Peat Marwick, 1998).

entitled to vaccine coverage as a matter of federal law.[19] Thus as of 1999, federal policies allowed for the potential coverage of roughly 30 million children for immunization services.

SCHIP enrollment had reached a total of almost 2 million children by September 30, 1999, double the number covered in the first full year of the program, calendar year 1998 (Health Care Financing Administration [HCFA], 1999b). States have streamlined applications for SCHIP and increased outreach efforts. An additional 600,000 to 1.1 million children are eligible for SCHIP but not covered, according to projections based on the

Medical Expenditure Panel Survey (Selden et al., 1999). In some states, Medicaid enrollment has increased as a result of SCHIP outreach efforts (HCFA, 1999a). Finally, 23 states offer 12-month continuous eligibility in their separate SCHIP programs, as do 15 states for Medicaid (HCFA, 1999a). This longer minimum eligibility period should improve the continuity of primary care, including immunizations, received by enrolled children. Table 3-5 summarizes federal coverage policies for children under Medicaid, VFC, and SCHIP.

Enrollment in Medicaid in particular remains below the potential reach of the program, however, with 22 percent of all eligible children (4.7 million out of 21.2 million) not enrolled (Selden et al., 1998). This underenrollment appears to be the result of many factors, ranging from a lack of awareness of programs on the part of families to systemic barriers that make enrollment difficult (Ellwood, 1999).

Managed Care and Medicaid, VFC, and SCHIP

In 1998, all but four states mandated enrollment in managed care by some or all Medicaid beneficiaries as a condition of coverage for at least a portion of Medicaid benefits (information provided by HCFA). As of 1998, 16.6 million Medicaid enrollees (54 percent of the total), were enrolled in some form of managed care arrangement, a more than three-fold increase in Medicaid managed care enrollment since just 1993 (information provided by HCFA).

Freestanding SCHIP programs often involve managed care arrangements, with providers or provider groups, such as independent practice associations, being "at risk" for the services used by their enrollees. Because children enrolled in freestanding SCHIP programs are "insured" and therefore not eligible for VFC vaccines, the capitation rates paid to SCHIP plans ostensibly cover both the cost of purchasing required vaccines and the cost of administering them, unless the state makes other arrangements (see Box 3-2). In California, a state with a combination SCHIP program, some providers argue that the capitation rates in the freestanding SCHIP plans are set too low to compensate them for vaccine purchases, and some capitated providers have referred patients to public health clinics to receive free vaccinations (Fairbrother et al., forthcoming).

States that require beneficiaries to enroll in a managed care plan may require these plans to provide additional benefits and services not normally offered to Medicaid beneficiaries receiving care in the fee-for-service system.[20] Thus even if immunizations were not otherwise covered for adults, a state Medicaid agency could specify such coverage in its managed care service agreements.

Very limited information is available on the extent of adult immuni-

TABLE 3-5 Federal Immunization Coverage Policies for Children Under Medicaid, Vaccines for Children (VFC), and State Children's Health Insurance Programs (SCHIP)

Program	Eligibility[a]	Federal Financing
Medicaid	Children up to age 6: 133% FPL[b]	50–78%
	Children aged 6–18: 100% FPL (through age 21 in the EPSDT[c] program)	
	State option to cover additional children up to state-defined eligibility levels	
VFC	Children aged 0-18 who are:	
	Medicaid-eligible	100%
	Uninsured	100%
	Native American / Alaska Native	100%
	Underinsured	Only if vaccinated at FQHCs[d]
SCHIP (Medicaid)	State sets level using Medicaid coverage flexibility	Enhanced FFP[e] (65–85%)
SCHIP (freestanding)	Children with incomes above Medicaid but < 50% over Medicaid eligibility levels who are uninsured and ineligible for Medicaid	Enhanced FFP (65–85%)

[a]The Advisory Committee on Immunization Practices establishes general vaccine schedule recommendations and then prepares a separate resolution for coverage through the VFC Program. CDC publishes the recommendations and negotiates a vaccine contract(s). Funds are awarded to the states, and the vaccine is purchased and supplied by the states to health care providers.
[b]Federal poverty level.
[c]Early and Periodic Screening, Diagnosis, and Treatment Program.
[d]Federally qualified health center.
[e]Federal financial participation.

SOURCE: Health Care Financing Administration, 2000c.

zation coverage under Medicaid managed care. A study of contracts between state Medicaid agencies and managed care organizations furnishing comprehensive services revealed that 19 standard contracts in effect as of January 1998 specified coverage of immunizations for adults (Rosenbaum et al., 1998). All contracts specified coverage of childhood immunizations, although the nature of the specifications ranged from

> **BOX 3-2**
> **New Jersey: Carving the Vaccine**
> **Administration Fee Out of Capitation Rates**
>
> New Jersey has designed "NJ KidCare," its mixed-model SCHIP, to be as seamless as possible, from both the providers' and the patients' point of view, across its Medicaid expansion program and three additional freestanding plans. Immunization payment policy is the same for all children in either Medicaid or NJ KidCare. Children in Medicaid receive vaccines from VFC. The state uses a portion of its state SCHIP contribution to purchase vaccines at the CDC contract price for distribution to all physicians in the three freestanding SCHIP plans. Thus physicians receive vaccines up front for all children in state-sponsored insurance programs.
>
> Physicians in New Jersey participate in Medicaid/SCHIP largely through the six managed care organizations (MCOs) with which the state contracts. Instead of allowing these MCOs to capitate primary care providers for the provision of immunizations to their pediatric patients, New Jersey has negotiated with them to "pass through" the state's vaccine administration fee of $11.50, which the state built into the MCOs' actuarially-based capitation payments. To receive this fee, providers must send the MCO a notice of the immunization, essentially a bill for rendering the service. Not only does the payment encourage providers to immunize, but it also improves the reporting and documentation of immunizations delivered for the MCOs, which can build their HEDIS reports from these notices.

language that paralleled federal requirements (e.g., coverage at the ACIP level) to broader specifications.

Finding 3-2. Medicaid, VFC, and SCHIP are important components of the national immunization effort, with the potential to finance immunizations for more than one-third of the nation's children. Yet eligibility for any of these programs does not guarantee enrollment, and enrollment does not guarantee the receipt of up-to-date immunizations. Medicaid eligibility is determined monthly in most states, and discontinuities in coverage interfere with timely immunization. SCHIP has expanded access to primary health care, including immunizations, for a growing number of uninsured children. However, the administrative requirements of this program have added new complexities to vaccine purchase and delivery that require additional oversight, monitoring, and compliance activities on the part of state public health agencies. Because of the scale of the VFC program and the narrow statutory definition of administrative costs for that program, states must draw upon Section 317 grants and state revenues to implement the VFC effort fully in public and private health care settings.

MEDICARE

Medicare is a completely federal social insurance program that entitles eligible persons to coverage for a defined set of benefits, including certain immunizations.[21] All Medicare-eligible individuals enrolled in Part B of the program, whether entitled to coverage on the basis of age, disability, or coverage for end-stage renal disease (ESRD), are entitled to immunizations for influenza and pneumococcal disease, as well as for hepatitis B if determined to be at risk for that disease. Since the original 1965 Medicare statute excluded coverage of all preventive services, other vaccines or inoculations are excluded as "preventive immunizations" unless directly related to the treatment of an injury or direct exposure to diseases or conditions.[22] Pneumococcal and influenza immunizations are covered by Medicare without deductible and coinsurance.

In 1998, 32.3 million persons aged 65 and older were covered by Medicare Part B. An additional 5 million persons under age 65 were covered as disabled or ESRD beneficiaries. Originally designed in 1965 as a health insurance program to cover the expenses of acute and rehabilitative medical care, Medicare explicitly excluded coverage of preventive services until Congress authorized the coverage of pneumococcal vaccine in 1981. In 1984, hepatitis B vaccine was covered for ESRD patients, and it is now covered for any beneficiaries who are at risk of the disease. Annual influenza immunizations were added to Medicare benefits in 1993, following a 4-year demonstration program. In 1994, the first full year in which both influenza and pneumococcal vaccines were covered, Medicare spent an estimated $100 million on the vaccines and their administration (General Accounting Office, 1995b). In 1998, Medicare paid providers $87 million for influenza immunizations, $27 million for pneumococcal immunizations, and $800,000 for hepatitis B immunizations (information provided by HCFA).

Medicare began paying providers a separate fee for vaccine administration as a uniform national policy in 1993. Prior to that time, payment for immunizations was inconsistent among Medicare administrative areas, and sometimes only the cost of the vaccine was reimbursed. As for other physician service payments, Medicare's vaccine administration payment rates vary geographically.[23] For the year 2000, vaccine administration fees range from a low of $3.95 in Mississippi to a high of $5.38 in New York City, with a national average of $4.39 (information provided by HCFA).

Some have argued that Medicare administration fees are too low to compensate physicians adequately for the costs of storing and administering vaccines, and that these low fees contribute to low immunization coverage rates among beneficiaries (Poland and Miller, 2000). However, other factors contribute to low influenza and pneumococcal coverage rates for the elderly, including provider practices and knowledge, and patients' beliefs about and understanding of the relative risks and benefits of immunization for these diseases. Coverage of persons aged 65 and older for influenza vaccine climbed steadily during the past decade, from 42 percent in 1991 to 63 percent in 1997 (see Table 3-6). The cumulative (ever vaccinated) coverage levels for pneumococcal vaccine for the elderly between 1991 and 1997 doubled from 21 to 42 percent (see Table 3-6). Yet racial and ethnic disparities in immunization rates for the elderly have persisted. In 1997, the influenza immunization rate for elderly blacks was just two-thirds that for whites (45 as compared with 66 percent), and the pneumococcal immunization rate for both blacks and Hispanics was half that for whites (22–23 percent as compared with 46 percent). For non-institutionalized high-risk adults aged 18–64 (often those with chronic illness such as heart and lung disease or diabetes), coverage rates in 1997 for influenza vaccine were 47 percent for those with Medicare (disabled or ESRD beneficiaries), 29 percent for those with private insurance, and 14 percent for those without insurance. Pneumococcal vaccine coverage rates for high-risk adults aged 18–64 were 28 percent for those with Medicare, 12 percent for those with private insurance, and 10 percent for those without insurance (see Table 3-6).

The number of adults aged 18–65 who are at high risk of complications from influenza and pneumococcal disease, for whom immunization is strongly recommended, is roughly 26 million (11 percent of those aged 18–44 and 24 percent of those aged 45–64 have chronic conditions that put them at risk) (Singleton et al., forthcoming). Of these, about one-fifth, or 5 million high-risk nonelderly adults, lack health insurance, and thus have no coverage for these immunizations. As noted earlier, there is very little information on the extent to which private health plans cover adult immunizations. Although the extent of the high-risk population facing financial barriers to receiving immunizations cannot be estimated precisely, the number is likely to be substantially greater than the 5 million who are completely uninsured (see Box 3-3).

As with Medicaid managed care, Medicare beneficiaries enrolled in Medicare+Choice plans may qualify for additional benefits, including all routine or recommended immunizations. As of February 2000, 6.8 million Medicare beneficiaries were enrolled in prepaid managed care plans— almost five times as many as were enrolled in 1991 (information provided by HCFA).[24] With increasing numbers of Medicare beneficiaries enrolled in managed care, the program costs for immunizations cannot be determined separately, nor can immunization coverage levels be estimated from billing records, as such records are not available for prepaid plan enrollees. Adult influenza coverage levels are currently a Health Plan Employer Data and Information Set (HEDIS)-reported measure, however, and pneumococcal coverage levels may be added in the near future (Poland

TABLE 3-6 Influenza and Pneumococcal Immunization Rates (percent coverage)

Population Group	1991		1993		1995		1997	
	Influenza	Pneumococcal	Influenza	Pneumococcal	Influenza	Pneumococcal	Influenza	Pneumococcal
Adults ≥ 65 years old	42	21	52	28	58	34	63	42
White					61	36	66	46
Black	27	14	33	14	40	22	45	22
Hispanic	34	12	47	13	50	23	53	23
Noninstitutionalized High-Risk Adults								
Aged 18–64							26	13
White							27	13
Black							22	13
Hispanic							19	9
Private health insurance							29	12
Medicare							47	28
Medicaid							26	16
Medicare and Medicaid							45	25
No health insurance							14	10

SOURCE: National Center for Health Statistics, 1997.

BOX 3-3
Calculating the Size of the Adult Population That Relies on State-Purchased Vaccines

No national survey data are available on which to base estimates of the number of privately insured adults between the ages of 18 and 65 who have coverage for immunizations. Consequently, the following estimate of the demand for pneumococcal and influenza vaccines from public health departments is based only on estimates of the uninsured working-age adult population, and does not reflect any low-income underinsured adults, who also may depend on public clinics for free immunizations.

ACIP recommends immunization against pneumococcal disease and influenza for adults under age 65 with heart disease, chronic respiratory system conditions, and diabetes, and influenza vaccine for all those age 50 and older. An estimated 11 percent of the population aged 18 through 49 have these conditions, as do an estimated 24 percent of the population aged 50 through 64 (Singleton et al., forthcoming). Applying these risk rates to 26.6 million uninsured adults aged 18 through 49 and 6.2 million uninsured adults aged 50 through 64, respectively, yields a total of 4.4 million at-risk working age adults without health insurance. Adding in all other uninsured persons (those without these chronic conditions) between ages 50 and 65 would double the demand for annual influenza immunizations to 9 million uninsured persons.

The public purchase price of influenza vaccine is $2.15 per dose. The annual cost of purchasing vaccines for the groups for which immunization is recommended by ACIP who are uninsured and aged 18 through 64 is thus $19 million. The public purchase price for pneumococcal vaccine is $5.50. The one-time cost of immunizing the 4.4 million at-risk uninsured adults is thus about $24.2 million.

---

and Miller, 2000). Health plans' internal tracking and reporting systems for immunizations become more important for population surveillance as less information can be gleaned from third-party billing records.

Finding 3-3. The Medicare program has become the single most important source of financing and service delivery for adult immunization efforts over the past decade, and coverage rates for influenza and pneumococcal vaccines have shown significant increases during this period. Yet these coverage levels remain far below recommended levels, especially for racial and ethnic minorities.

SECTION 317 VACCINE PURCHASE GRANTS

Prior to the implementation of VFC in 1994, Section 317 was the major source of support for public vaccine purchase. Historically, the program's emphasis has been on pediatric immunization, but use of Section 317 funds for adolescents and adults has been permitted since 1994. Section 317 currently supports 64 state, territorial, and municipal health agency immunization programs. These funds enable grantees to purchase vaccines and ensure that other basic functions of an immunization program are carried out.

The Section 317 program supports national-level and centrally operated CDC programs, as well as state grants. Under the category of program operations, CDC develops national goals, plans and assesses strategies for reaching these goals, negotiates consolidated vaccine purchase contracts, provides surveillance of vaccine-preventable diseases and technical assistance to state and local health agencies, and conducts vaccine safety activities. CDC also engages in international eradication efforts targeting polio, measles, and other vaccine-preventable diseases, which account for a growing share of Section 317 funding.

Section 317's discretionary grants to states take two forms: (1) Direct Assistance (DA), which amounts to a line of credit with CDC for the purchase of vaccines as needed, salaries of federal public health personnel who work within state agencies, and support for immunization registries, and (2) Financial Assistance (FA), which the states may use for programmatic activities such as outreach, disease surveillance and outbreak control, professional and public education, and immunization assessment. Legislative history clearly reflects that the 317 program was intended to supplement state and local immunization efforts; grantees are specifically prohibited from using federal grant funds to replace existing state spending on immunization programs.

The level of funding for the Section 317 program is set through annual federal appropriations, and both the total appropriation and the distribution of awards among the states and local grantees are discretionary. The total appropriation is determined by Congress and the individual grant amounts by CDC. Unlike two other major state grant programs that focus on child health—the Maternal and Child Health Services Block Grant and SCHIP—Section 317 awards involve no federal formula and require no financial matching of federal grants with state funds.

Historically, CDC's annual budget request for the Section 317 program has tracked the level of funds appropriated in the previous year. Although it is not an explicit program standard, by the early 1990s CDC had articulated Section 317's programmatic responsibility as the financing of vaccines for roughly half of all children served in the public sector (Kelley et al., 1993). Those children dependent on the public sector for immunizations were estimated to comprise 25 to 30 percent of the national birth cohort, just slightly less than the fraction estimated for the initial polio vaccine program in the 1950s. States and localities were expected to finance immunizations for the remaining half of the children dependent on public-sector services, roughly 12 to 15 percent of their annual birth cohort.

The programmatic objectives of the National Immunization Program administered by CDC are described as follows:

> A goal of the Immunization Grant Program has always been to help ensure that the Nation's citizens have access to and receive all appropriate, routinely recommended vaccines. Throughout the existence of the Program, vaccines for use in the public sector have been purchased with a combination of Federal, State and local funds . . . . overall, the 317 program purchased 50–60 percent of vaccines used in the public sector [prior to VFC]. However, CDC never intentionally established a "goal" of purchasing 50–60 percent of the public sector need. This proportion was arrived at through a combination of circumstances, including what States were able to contribute, which vaccines the 317 funds were buying (usually the higher-priced and newer products), and available appropriations (information provided by CDC).

In the early years of the program, Section 317 grants for vaccine purchase (DA) and program administration (FA) were roughly equivalent. Over time, however, as vaccine costs rose and the schedule of recommended vaccines increased, vaccine purchase accounted for a higher proportion of total funds received (Kelley et al., 1993). This balance within the Section 317 program shifted once again after the VFC program became operational in October 1994 and relieved many of the demands on states' 317 DA grants for pediatric vaccines (see Figures 1-3, 3-3, 3-4, and Appendix F).

Since 1994, at the direction of the Senate Appropriations Committee, CDC has reserved $33 million in FA funds each year for incentive awards to grantees with the highest immunization coverage rates, as measured by the National Immunization Survey (NIS) for 2-year-olds who are up to date with the 4:3:1 immunization series (four DTP, three polio, and one measles). Variable bonuses are available on a per child basis, according to the grantee's completion rate. As the FA grants have declined over the past 5 years, these incentive funds have become an increasingly larger proportion of overall infrastructure funding, representing 28 percent of new FA funds awarded in 1998.

Finding 3-4. The Section 317 vaccine purchase program allows states to purchase vaccines for administration to disadvantaged populations in a timely manner and to avoid missed opportunities when no other coverage is available to support immunization services. Section 317 infrastructure grants also provide funds for service delivery in the public health sector, and afford state immunization programs swift access to

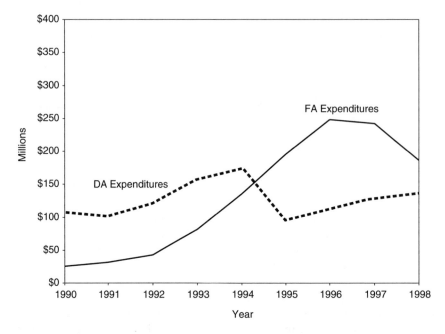

FIGURE 3-3 Section 317 Direct Assistance and Financial Assistance expenditures by grantees, 1990–1998. SOURCE: Information provided by CDC.

newly licensed vaccines at reduced cost. As of January 2000, VFC had become the primary source of funding for public vaccine purchase. However, states continue to use Section 317 funds to address residual needs as part of their safety net role. The dynamics of how states identify and respond to these needs, using federal or state funds, are not well characterized in the research literature.

STATE VACCINE PURCHASE

When immunizations were limited in number and furnished as a nominal-cost public health benefit, the issue of immunization financing was not significant. As the scope of required immunizations has grown and costs have increased, however, serious tensions have emerged that warrant greater scrutiny. Prior to VFC, private health plans and families paid for most of the immunizations provided in private health care settings, although some private providers immunized children covered by Medicaid. Families that were uninsured or underinsured generally received their immunizations in public health clinics, financed by state revenues and Section 317 funds.

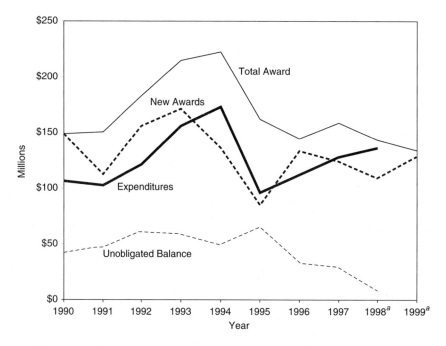

FIGURE 3-4 Total Section 317 Direct Assistance awards, expenditures, and balances, 1990–1999. [a]Estimated. SOURCE: Information provided by CDC.

Today, the purchase of childhood vaccines is a major component of all state immunization programs. The relative contribution of VFC, Section 317, and state revenues to public vaccine purchase depends on the level of each state's needs, as well as the particular constellation of immunization financing policies and service-delivery mechanisms (see Box 3-4). States are highly variable in the extent to which they use state revenues for vaccine purchase. Estimating the state-funded share of publicly purchased vaccines in each state from records of expenditures for all vaccines purchased under federal discounted price contracts yields the following results:

- 24 states plus the District of Columbia provide less than 10 percent of publicly purchased vaccines in their jurisdiction,
- 16 states contribute between 10 and 30 percent of publicly purchased vaccines, and
- 10 states contribute 30 percent or more of all publicly purchased vaccines.

BOX 3-4
Calculating the Size of the Child Population That
Relies on State-Purchased Vaccines

Almost 600,000 children (15 percent) among the annual birth cohort of 3.88 million children in the United States lack health insurance, and an additional 1.2 million (31 percent) are enrolled in Medicaid plans.[1] The committee estimates that the majority within this combined national population of 1.8 million infants (80 percent, or 1.44 million) are served by public and private health care providers that rely on VFC vaccines or SCHIP funds to serve their patients. This calculation leaves a residual need for the population of at-risk children (20 percent of 1.8 million, or 360,000 infants) who for some reason are not identified as VFC-eligible, or who otherwise depend on vaccines provided by local health clinics that are commonly purchased with Section 317 or state funds.[2]

An additional group of children (the "underinsured") are enrolled in private health plans that lack coverage for vaccines. An estimated 8 percent of families with private health insurance do not have coverage for childhood immunizations (KPMG Peat Marwick, 1998). Their providers often refer them to local health clinics if they cannot cover vaccine costs out-of-pocket, but these children are not eligible for VFC, unless seen in federally qualified health centers, because they are insured. This population is estimated to represent between 4 and 5 percent of the annual birth cohort, or 170,000 infants.

The combination of 360,000 children who are eligible for but do not have access to the VFC/SCHIP programs and the 170,000 children who have private insurance but lack vaccine coverage totals 530,000 children (about 14 percent of the annual U.S. birth cohort) who rely on Section 317 or state-purchased vaccines for their immunization needs. This is one component of the safety net population commonly served by public health clinics. Other components include recent immigrants who have not yet met residency requirements that qualify them for Medicaid or SCHIP assistance, and adults aged 18 to 65 who do not have access to vaccines (see Box 3-3).

Immunization costs for children in the first 2 years of life are estimated at $400 (including $175 for vaccine purchase at federal contract rates [and not including pneumococcal conjugate], plus $225 in vaccine administration fees [$15 times 15 antigens]). Multiplying this $400 total immunization cost times the estimated 530,000 residual needs population derived above generates a total annual requirement of $212 million for early childhood vaccines alone.

Special note: An additional population that may be served by public health clinics deserves consideration in this discussion. In many communities, children who are enrolled in a Medicaid or SCHIP managed care plan request immunizations from their local public health clinics either because they have difficulty scheduling appointments with their own providers, because their providers are not participating in the VFC program, because they are responding to certain local outreach initiatives, or because of other special circumstances. However, the managed care plans in most states are priced to include the cost of purchasing and administering vaccines within the early childhood schedule. Several states and communities have successfully negotiated contracts that allow their public health clinics to bill

continued

BOX 3-4 Continued

the client's plan for immunization services provided in the clinical setting. This integration of public health and health financing is important because it reduces missed opportunities for immunization and allows the cost of immunizations to be charged to those who are responsible for the care of public program beneficiaries.

---

[1]This estimate of Medicaid enrollment for children from birth to age 2 is the midpoint between the proportion of children under age 6 (24 percent) who are covered by Medicaid (U.S. Bureau of the Census, 1999) and the proportion of newborns (38 percent) who are covered by Medicaid (Annie E. Casey Foundation, 1999).

[2]This estimate varies by community. In Detroit, for example, health providers indicated that perhaps 50 percent of the children seen in public health clinics were eligible for Medicaid or SCHIP assistance. However, these children did not have access to primary care services because Medicaid managed care contracting in their area was oversubscribed and underfinanced.

Nationally, state vaccine purchases account for 12 percent of all expenditures under the federal contract; VFC accounts for 65 percent, and Section 317 for 22 percent (information provided by CDC).

Since the inception of VFC, state approaches to vaccine purchase and immunization delivery have fit one of three models: VFC only, enhanced VFC, or universal purchase (see Table 3-7).

VFC Only

The VFC program provides federally purchased vaccine for all eligible children (Medicaid enrollees aged 18 and younger, uninsured children, Native American children) at participating public and private sites. Underinsured children may receive VFC vaccine at federally qualified health centers (FQHCs) and rural clinics only. In 19 states, all children, including those not eligible for VFC, may receive state-supplied vaccines at public clinics. Section 317 and state revenues pay for the vaccines administered in public settings to children who do not qualify for VFC (information provided by CDC).

TABLE 3-7 Vaccine Supply Policy, January 2000

VFC Only[a]	Enhanced VFC[b]	Universal Purchase[c]
Alabama	Arizona	Alaska
Arkansas	District of Columbia	Connecticut
California	Florida	Idaho
Colorado	Georgia	Maine
Delaware	Hawaii	Massachusetts
Indiana	Illinois	Nevada
Iowa	Maryland	New Hampshire
Kansas	Michigan	New Mexico
Kentucky	Minnesota	North Carolina
Louisiana	Mississippi	North Dakota
Missouri	Montana	Rhode Island
New Jersey[d]	Nebraska	South Dakota
Ohio	New York	Vermont
Oregon	Oklahoma	Washington
Pennsylvania	South Carolina	Wyoming
Tennessee	Texas	
Virginia	Utah	
West Virginia		
Wisconsin		
Total 19	17	15

[a]These states provide publicly purchased vaccine to private health care providers only for Vaccines for Children eligibles.
[b]These states provide publicly purchased vaccine to all health care providers for both the Vaccines for Children and underinsured populations. "Underinsured" is defined as those who have health insurance that does not include immunizations as a covered benefit.
[c]A universal purchase state offers all vaccines recommended by the Advisory Committee on Immunization Practices to all health care providers to serve all patients, including those who are fully insured.
[d]The Vaccines for Children program was implemented in the private sector on January 1, 1999.

SOURCE: CDC, 1998c.

Enhanced VFC

States with enhanced VFC programs are like those described above, but in addition, state-supplied vaccines are made available to participating private providers for administration to underinsured children, comparable to the VFC policy for underinsured children served in FQHCs. In this case, Section 317 funds vaccines for non-VFC-eligible children served in public settings, and state revenues fund vaccines for underinsured children seen in the private sector. Sixteen states and the District of Columbia have enhanced VFC programs (information provided by CDC).

Universal Purchase

Universal purchase states supply vaccine for all children in the state, regardless of whether administration takes place in public clinics or participating private provider sites. VFC thus becomes one source of funding within a vaccine purchasing system for which all children are eligible, regardless of their insurance status. The 15 states with universal purchase programs, all of which were in existence prior to VFC, commit the highest level of state resources to vaccine purchase and to immunization programs overall (information provided by CDC), although not all universal purchase states buy all recommended vaccines.

ISSUES IN VACCINE PURCHASE

Generally, the introduction of VFC resulted in savings to states, as funding for the purchase of vaccines for most Medicaid-enrolled children could be shifted from the state to the federal level. The extent of those savings depended on several variables, include the following:

- the extent of Medicaid enrollment,
- the prices Medicaid paid for vaccines prior to VFC, and
- whether states required Medicaid providers to enroll in VFC or discontinued reimbursing providers for privately purchased vaccine.

The way states used these Medicaid savings was highly variable. In response to the 1999 IOM state survey, 25 states said that Medicaid payment levels for vaccine administration or other pediatric care had increased, but only 4 states identified those increases as being related to savings from VFC (in one state, for example, the vaccine administration fee increased because the state Medicaid agency misinterpreted HCFA's maximum allowable reimbursement as the minimum). Three states said these savings were used in other ways, such as increasing support for local health departments or purchasing vaccine for groups not covered by VFC. In most states, however, VFC-related savings did not accrue directly to the immunization program.

With Section 317 funds becoming increasingly limited, some states have restricted the availability of vaccine in public clinics. For example, for non-VFC-eligible children, a vaccine may not be available or may be restricted to certain age groups. In some states, public clinics are now required to check insurance status and refer children back to their private provider if they are not VFC- or 317-eligible. Though many states still adhere to the policy that free vaccines are available in the public sector to all children, practices in several urban areas suggest that some states have qualified their distribution of free vaccines by placing greater emphasis on eligibility criteria. States that have tightened their screening and referral procedures have encountered some resistance from local health departments.

The intent of VFC was to eliminate a two-tiered system of care, in which poor children were precluded by cost from receiving immunizations in their medical homes. Yet a growing rift between VCF-eligible and -ineligible children has developed in many states. Recent additions to the primary immunization schedule—varicella, hepatitis A, the now rescinded rotavirus, and the new pneumococcal conjugate vaccine for infants—are relatively expensive vaccines. The recommended switch from OPV to inactivated polio vaccine also carries increased costs. Many states have faced difficult decisions regarding vaccine purchase for non-VFC children:

> Issuance of new or expanded ACIP recommendations is one of our biggest problems. Every time a vaccine is added as an entitlement on VFC, we have to make sure that we don't end up with different classes of children with different levels of protection; that means trying to come up with funding for that new vaccine for non-VFC children. The new recommendation doesn't necessarily come along with extra 317 funds, and it doesn't come with infrastructure funds that are needed to deliver the new vaccine and keep the records. It's a constant juggling act to fund vaccines (Freed et al., 1999).

The problem is most pronounced for universal purchase states:

> When the ACIP makes a recommendation for a new vaccine and they include it in the VFC program, then they are in effect pushing and controlling state budgets for universal purchase states. They do not take into consideration some very specific situations that exist for states. If our state was to lose universal status, it would have a very negative impact. We don't have a lot of managed care, and most fee-for-service insurance does not cover immunizations. In many ways, we're stuck between a rock and a hard place: even though universal status is costing more, it would be a real detriment to lose it. . . .

> We have local health departments that are reluctant to provide the vaccine to VFC kids if they can't do it for everybody. Our philosophy has been to push for the VFC kids to get vaccinated, because very often they are at higher risk for disease complications. We tell local health departments that they are able to vaccinate half the kids and they should do it. That doesn't necessarily translate into universal acceptance of this policy at the local level (Freed et al., 1999).

The significant cost of immunizations may create point-of-service barriers to immunizations among both uninsured and underinsured children and adults. In the case of uninsured children and a small number of underinsured children, federal policy provides a guarantee of coverage under the VFC program for ACIP-recommended immunizations, once a federal vaccine purchase contract has been completed. In addition, as noted earlier, 15 states have established universal purchase programs that provide access to free vaccine regardless of insurance coverage; however, these programs are limited to children.

> *Finding 3-5. Complex eligibility criteria and coverage conditions for the multiple federal and state programs supporting vaccine purchase and delivery have left gaps and omissions in the financial coverage of immunizations for children and adults. States respond to these residual needs by continuing to provide free vaccines in public health clinics, financed by a combination of Section 317 funds and state revenues.*

> *Finding 3-6. The broad mission and general standards of service associated with the Section 317 program result in some overlap with more tightly constructed federal programs (such as VFC and SCHIP), but the amount of overlap is not large, and it should be seen as complementary rather than duplicative. The overlap allows the states to bridge coverage gaps, respond to timely needs, and advance the national goal of preventing disease through immunization.*

SUMMING UP

VFC and SCHIP provide federal support for the purchase of vaccines for increasing numbers of disadvantaged children. However, residual needs remain, causing states to continue to rely on Section 317 vaccine purchase grants to serve at-risk children and adults who are ineligible for other federally supported vaccines. The scope of these residual needs varies among the states, depending on Medicaid eligibility and private health plan participation in meeting the health needs of low-income families.

The following specific factors contribute to the scale of residual needs within each state:

- The eligibility requirements for VFC are more restrictive than those for Section 317 funds. Underinsured families that cannot afford to pay for vaccines or the administration fees charged by private practitioners may be ineligible for VFC but still seek vaccines from a local public health clinic.
- Families enrolled in Medicaid or SCHIP may encounter delays in service or other access barriers in seeking care from private providers and thus return to public clinics for timely immunizations. The latter encoun-

ters are especially important to meet school entry requirements for young children and to address the health needs of recent immigrants.

• The appearance of new vaccines offering valuable and long-awaited protection from additional infectious diseases has caused states to draw on Section 317 funds during transitional periods. This situation occurred, for example, during the 11-month period after ACIP recommended the varicella vaccine and before a federal purchase contract was negotiated.

States vary in the way they respond to their residual needs. A few states rely solely on federal support, since all of the vaccines provided through their public health clinics are financed by Section 317. Others have used state revenues to purchase additional vaccines to meet their residual needs. States have broad discretion in determining whether to use state or federal funds to purchase vaccines, hire staff, or support contractual efforts. Some states use internal funds for personnel and thus rely more heavily on federal vaccine purchases; others draw on federal employees where possible to staff their immunization programs, and reserve their own funds for vaccine purchases and other programmatic needs.

State investments in immunization services appear to have increased during the 1990s, but these increases have not been at the same dramatic levels seen with the creation of VFC or the early growth in Section 317 budgets. States were more likely to extend their efforts through their investments in expanded Medicaid coverage, both by increasing vaccine administration fees and by broadening the base of clients served by Medicaid plans. Evidence is not available to indicate how the states invested in other types of immunization programs during this period.

ENDNOTES

1. Despite their cost-effectiveness, immunizations may be relatively costly at the point of service. Immunization costs vary greatly by vaccine. They reflect the cost of development and manufacturing, the competitive situation (i.e., if there are multiple suppliers of a vaccine, its price tends to be lower), the length of time a vaccine has been on the market, and the federal excise taxes that are levied on vaccines under the Childhood Vaccine Injury Act. The vaccine administration fee includes the actual injection, assessment of any possible risks or counterindications, disclosure of information to parents and individuals to ensure that immunizations are provided only following informed consent, and compliance with record-keeping and reporting requirements under state and federal law.

2. Two of these studies, the Current Population Survey March Supplement, conducted annually by the Census Bureau, and the Medical Expenditure Panel Survey (MEPS), conducted in 1996 by the Agency for Health Care Policy and Research (now the Agency for Healthcare Research and Quality), are the basis for estimates of general insurance coverage used in this report.

3. ERISA (29 U.S.C. §1000 et seq.) was enacted to regulate employer-sponsored pensions. The law contains a so-called "preemption" provision that exempts employer plans from most state laws. State laws that "regulate insurance" are saved; thus, employers that purchase insurance remain subject to state law under the holding in *Metropolitan Life*. ERISA also specifies, however, that employee benefit plans may not be considered insurance (29 U.S.C. §1144). In trying to make sense of this provision, the Supreme Court drew a distinction between employers that buy insurance and those that self-insure under their own ERISA plans. These self-insured plans are immune from the provisions of state law.

4. These were ERISA amendments enacted as part of the same legislation that created the VFC program in 1993 (29 U.S.C. §1169 (d)).

5. The original House VFC proposal would have covered all children uninsured for immunizations (that is, it would have reached underinsured children as well). The final legislation omitted all but a small percentage of underinsured children. The ERISA maintenance-of-effort provision was part of the House bill and was determined to be necessary to protect insured children from employer rollbacks in coverage in the face of the new program. Despite the fact that coverage of underinsured children was dropped in conference, the ERISA amendments survived.

6. This estimate is based on the the KPMG survey's estimate of the proportion of employees with each type of plan coverage (conventional, health maintenance organization [HMO], preferred provider organization [PPO], point of service [POS]), multiplied by the likelihood that each of those types of plans covers childhood immunizations, as shown in Table 3-2. Information from the 1998 Current Population Survey (Table 3-1) provides an estimate of the total number of children with employer-based coverage.

7. Three of five reported coverage of poliovirus vaccine, inactivated (IPV); two of five reported coverage of rubella; four of five reported coverage of tetanus; one of five reported coverage of influenza; one of five reported coverage of pneumococcal vaccine; and two of five reported coverage of diphtheria, tetanus, and acellular pertussis (DTaP).

8. The initial EPSDT statute did not specify particular services.

9. Public Law 101-239, §6403(a), adding §1905(r) to the Social Security Act. Section 1905(r), 42 U.S.C. §1396d(r), sets forth all mandatory EPSDT services, including immunizations.

10. Public Law 103-66, §13621(b), adding §1928 of the Social Security Act, 42 U.S.C. §1396s. The VFC program was originally proposed as the initial phase of the Clinton Administration's national health care reform proposal; this is reflected in another provision of the law, which would terminate the VFC program at the point at which federal law provides for immunization services for all children as part of a "broad-based reform of the national health care system" (§1928(g) of the Social Security Act; 42 U.S.C. §1396s(g)).

11. §1928(h) of the Social Security Act; 42 U.S.C. §1396s(h). Children aged 19 to 21 are thus entitled to vaccines as part of the EPSDT program, but their vaccines are not covered through the VFC program. States remain responsible for immunization services for this age cohort, with federal contributions available at normal federal medical assistance percentage rates.

12. This provision is found at §1903(i)(14) of the Social Security Act; 42 U. S. C. §1396(b).

13. §1928(b)(3) of the Social Security Act; 42 U.S.C. §1396s(b)(3).

14. §1928(f) of the Social Security Act; 42 U.S.C. §1396s(f).

15. These are children under age 18 whose family income exceeds the Medicaid income level for children but does not exceed 50 percentage points above the Medicaid eligibility level (§2110(b)(1)(A) of the Social Security Act; 42 U.S.C. §1397jj(b)(1)(A)).

16. §2104 of the Social Security Act; 42 U.S.C. §1397dd.

17. §2103(c)(1)(D) of the Social Security Act; 42 U.S.C. §1397cc(c)(1)(D). Federal SCHIP guidelines require all SCHIP programs to cover immunizations in accordance with ACIP

requirements (letter from Sally Richardson to State Medicaid Directors dated May 11, 1998, <http://www.hcfa.gov>). SCHIP-enrolled children in freestanding programs are considered insured and thus are ineligible for VFC vaccines.

18. Based on MEPS estimates of eligible but not enrolled children for Medicaid and SCHIP (Selden et al., 1999).

19. Based on 1998 Current Population Survey estimates of the number of persons under 18 who are uninsured (11 million) and MEPS estimates of those eligible for Medicaid and SCHIP but not enrolled (Selden et al., 1998; Selden et al., 1999).

20. States that administer mandatory managed care programs under either §§1115 or 1915(b) of the Social Security Act can offer additional benefits to managed care enrollees.

21. Medicare outpatient benefits, including immunizations, are provided under Part B of the program. Medicare Part A covers hospital and nursing home care.

22. For example, anti-rabies treatment, tetanus antitoxin or booster vaccine, botulin antitoxin, antivenin sera, or immune globulin.

23. There is a single national Medicare relative value scale (RVS) code, or payment weight, for vaccine administration. Like other physician services included in the RVS-based Part B payment system, the actual payment amount for vaccine administration varies according to a Geographic Practice Cost Index that distinguishes 360 localities nationally according to their relative medical practice input prices. These fees are also updated annually for general inflation.

24. See also www.hcfa.gov/stats/mmcc0200.txt.

4

Building, Monitoring, and Sustaining Immunization Capacity

The government role in public health provides the necessary context for private-sector activity. Government is responsible for striving to achieve a balance between the two great concerns embodied in the American public philosophy: individual liberty and free enterprise on the one hand, and just and equitable action for the good of the community on the other (IOM, 1988:46).

This context continues to shape the infrastructure of the public health system. More than a decade ago, the IOM (1988:40) defined the mission of public health as "the fulfillment of society's interest in assuring the conditions in which people can be healthy." This mission has been undertaken by private organizations and individuals as well as by public agencies. However, the government has the singular role of ensuring that the public health mission is sufficiently addressed and that its crucial features are implemented. To this end, the governmental public health system encompasses three key functions: *assurance, assessment,* and *policy development.* As discussed in Chapter 1, the framework for the present study represents these functions somewhat differently, identifying six specific roles of the national immunization system (see Figure 1-6):

- vaccine purchase,
- service delivery,
- infectious disease prevention and control,
- surveillance of vaccine coverage and safety,

103

- efforts to improve and sustain high vaccine coverage levels, and
- immunization finance policies and practices.

This chapter examines in turn the scope and evidentiary base of three of these roles: infectious disease prevention and control, surveillance of vaccine coverage and safety, and efforts to improve and sustain high vaccine coverage levels. The final role—immunization finance policies and practices—is reviewed in Chapter 5. The three roles discussed in this chapter complement the vaccine purchase and delivery arrangements discussed in Chapter 3, and are commonly regarded as infrastructure efforts.

Infrastructure is defined as "an underlying base or foundation" and refers to "the basic facilities, equipment, and installations needed for the functioning of a system" (*Webster's Dictionary*, 1996:569). In the context of this study, infrastructure encompasses the formal set of arrangements that guide the immunization system in the United States. Although we focus principally on the public infrastructure for immunization services at the federal and state levels, we recognize that these efforts interact with local health agencies, private health care providers, and private insurers in a complex manner. Most important, the presence or absence of private health care services, including insurance coverage and standard benefits that provide immunization services for children, adolescents, and adults at reasonable cost, influences the infrastructure burden that is located within the public health sector. The scope and quality of the assessment, educational, and technical assistance efforts required within the public sector to ensure access to recommended vaccines and monitor the performance of health care providers thus depends on the extent to which the private sector can be relied upon to serve the needs of vulnerable populations.

The importance of infrastructure is not always apparent. It is often difficult to grasp, for example, why high levels of immunization coverage cannot be achieved simply by the purchase and delivery of vaccines. But sustaining high levels of immunization coverage for an increasing number of vaccines for the 11,000 children born each day, as well as a growing immigrant population, requires various forms of data collection, identification and analysis of high-risk and underserved populations, and technical assistance to health care providers. Certain roles and responsibilities within the public health sector acquire greater or lesser importance as health conditions shift and private providers acquire new responsibilities for immunization services. As immunization services are integrated into routine primary care, for example, the need for precise measurement and appropriate accountability standards grows, while actual caseloads decline within the public sector. Targeting outreach and reminder services to those most in need requires reliable benchmark, baseline, and performance monitoring data so public resources can be used wisely and efficiently.

INFECTIOUS DISEASE PREVENTION AND CONTROL

When disease incidence and burdens are high, the immunization infrastructure is often concerned with launching prominent national campaigns designed to attack infectious disease and deliver vaccines through special stand-alone and short-term programs. During active stages of disease transmission, infectious disease control includes three key components: (1) campaigns to change behavior to reduce the risk of disease transmission, (2) contact tracing, and (3) mass immunization of high-risk populations in outbreak areas.

In periods when disease burdens are low (as they are today), the use of sentinels that monitor the health of the general population acquires greater importance (IOM, 2000). These sentinels are essential to the prevention of disease outbreaks and transmission because they reveal long-term trends and provide early warnings of new patterns of disease reports. The persistent presence of infectious disease in reservoirs scattered around the world requires constant vigilance within each U.S. community until disease eradication is complete (IOM, 1992).

Although the threat of morbidity and mortality associated with vaccine-preventable diseases has decreased significantly, overall mortality from infectious diseases continues to rise as a result of the appearance of new infectious agents and the reemergence of diseases previously considered to be under control (Department of Health and Human Services [DHHS], 1998). As a group, infectious diseases were the third leading cause of death in the United States in 1992; overall mortality from infectious diseases rose 58 percent in the United States between 1980 and 1992. Although much of this increase reflects the growing burden of HIV-associated disease, the removal of HIV-associated diagnoses still leaves a 22 percent increase in mortality from infectious diseases (DHHS, 1998).

Responsibilities for prevention and control of disease outbreaks are shared among all levels of government. Local jurisdictions have on-site responsibility for dealing with outbreaks of disease in schools and the community. Each state has its own health codes and its own on-site epidemiologist, but federal expertise is often requested during outbreaks and as part of disease monitoring and reporting arrangements. Indeed, several states with unique infectious disease circumstances have disease reporting requirements that exceed those of CDC. When disease outbreaks occur, the three levels of government usually cooperate in their control efforts. States can request technical assistance from CDC to address both acute and chronic disease patterns. CDC also monitors nationwide and international trends that have national implications.

In some cases, outbreaks can be sudden, with deadly effects (see Box 4-1). A single case of meningococcal meningitis, for example, can prompt emergency drills to identify the scores of people with whom the victim came in contact before falling ill so that each can be given immediate antibiotic therapy (Altman, 1999). To counter this threat, the Advisory Committee on Immunization Practices (ACIP) has urged the 520,000 college freshmen who live in dormitories to consider receiving the meningococcal vaccine, even though the vaccine is not expected to prevent more than a few dozen actual cases.

Disease prevention and control efforts are different from the treatment of disease itself. The latter generally falls within the domain of personal medical services and is covered by insurance; personal payments; managed care organizations; and public funding programs such as Medicaid, Medicare, and the State Children's Health Insurance Program (SCHIP). Disease prevention and control, on the other hand, is an intrinsic role of public health agencies, which look beyond individual health to address the risk to whole populations. The major means of evaluating the impact of most vaccine-preventable disease programs is reports of the occurrence of these diseases (Orenstein and Bernier, 1990; Wharton

---

BOX 4-1
Alaskan Measles Outbreak in 1998

In late 1998 an outbreak of 33 confirmed measles cases (ages ranging from 2 to 28 years) occurred in Anchorage, Alaska, including 17 cases among a highly vaccinated high school population (CDC, 1999g). Analysis of the outbreak revealed that Alaskan schools did not require students entering kindergarten or first grade to have two doses of MMR until September 1996. Consequently, in the high school setting of 2,186 students, about half (1,057 students, or 49 percent) had received one dose of MMR, and the remaining half (1,112 students, or 51 percent) had received two or more doses (only 1 of the students had not received at least one dose of MMR before the outbreak). The Alaskan Department of Health and Social Services issued an emergency order requiring all Anchorage schoolchildren to have two doses of MMR by early January 1999. By mid-November 1998, 98.6 percent of the almost 50,000 Anchorage students were able to produce such documentation. Although no endemic measles virus is currently circulating in the United States (the outbreak was traced to importation by a 4-year-old child visiting from Japan), health officials have observed that outbreaks may continue to occur when imported cases are introduced into settings such as schools with incomplete second-dose MMR coverage.

and Strebel, 1994). Disease control and surveillance involves not only responding to such reports, but also maintaining vigilance to ensure that appropriate sentinels are in place within an increasingly fragmented health care delivery system.

The primary mechanism for monitoring disease reports is the National Notifiable Disease Surveillance System (NNDSS), maintained by CDC. The list of reportable diseases is determined and revised collaboratively between the Council of State and Territorial Epidemiologists and CDC. Currently, 52 infectious diseases are designated as notifiable (information provided by CDC). CDC operates several additional surveillance systems as well, including a national registry for congenital rubella syndrome and surveillance systems for paralytic polio and diphtheria (Orenstein et al., 1999). CDC also sponsors efforts to collect data beyond the NNDSS for measles, pertussis, tetanus, *Haemophilus influenzae* type b, and hepatitis B, and relies on laboratory-based surveillance systems to monitor and confirm reports of bacterial meningitis (including *Haemophilus influenzae* type b and pneumococcal disease). Additional influenza surveillance is performed using a laboratory-based system, as well as death certificate data (Orenstein et al., 1999). Traditionally, influenza surveillance involved monitoring the population through the voluntary reporting of communicable diseases by practicing physicians, with no expectation of complete reporting.

Monitoring of disease reports continues to be one of the primary functions of public health across the nation. Although such efforts can be expensive, they represent an important preventive function that can result in significant health benefits and cost savings for both individuals and communities. For example, a typical case of Lyme disease (which can be prevented by vaccine) diagnosed in the early stages incurs about $174 in direct medical treatment costs. However, delayed diagnosis and treatment can result in complications that cost from $2,228 to $6,724 per patient in direct medical costs in the first year alone (DHHS, 1998). The cost of screening patients who report symptoms is an additional expense borne by those who do not experience the disease itself.

Investigations of disease reports often require independent laboratory confirmation to meet clinical case definitions, as well as epidemiological analysis to trace disease origins, pathways, and high-risk settings. Such investigations commonly involve close and swift data collection and exchange among local, state, and federal employees, who often collaborate to educate and alert the professional science and health communities about important disease patterns.

Public health laboratories have an intrinsic role in these investigations. These laboratories support surveillance activities, conduct outbreak inquiries, and monitor for new or emerging infectious diseases. Public health laboratories provide a mechanism for developing new methods to combat disease. Studies conducted in the nation's public health laboratories made possible identification of the organisms that cause diphtheria, cholera, tuberculosis, leprosy, and typhoid fever, which in turn enabled the development of vaccines and other treatments used to prevent and control these diseases.

Today, public health laboratories are faced with numerous challenges resulting from changes within both the public and private sectors that have made it increasingly difficult for the laboratories to fulfill their missions. In the private sector, managed care and independent laboratories are on the rise, hospital laboratories are consolidating, and both clinical and information technologies are changing rapidly. In the public sector, the public health safety net is being redefined, there is increasing reliance on managed care to address public health needs, and state budgets have become further constrained. The strategies used to achieve the goals of public health laboratories need to be altered to reflect these contextual changes. Presently, there is much variation among the states in the way the core activities of public health laboratories are carried out, and there is no unified, common theme among laboratory strategic plans. Centralized leadership will be necessary to help meet these challenges. Increased federal guidance could be particularly useful in assessing the regionalization of some laboratory services, in supporting information infrastructure development, and in facilitating cooperation between public and private concerns.

Finding 4-1. Disease sentinels and surveillance data must be reliable since infectious agents can spread rapidly in a global community. Federal officials collaborate with state and local agencies to monitor routine disease patterns and provide technical assistance during periods of outbreak, during emergency conditions when local systems are overwhelmed, or during the implementation of new surveillance systems. Efforts to collect infectious disease data require stability, consistency, and federal and state collaboration to enhance the monitoring of long-term trends and the analysis of data from different regions of the country.

SURVEILLANCE OF VACCINE COVERAGE AND SAFETY

For the first half of the 20th century, the prevention and control of vaccine-preventable disease were the frontier of the public health infrastructure. Until the 1950s, public health authorities did not monitor levels of vaccine coverage within the general population because few vaccines were available, and because relatively low levels of vaccine coverage were thought to be sufficient to control disease transmission within the general population—a concept known as "herd immunity." Even the national polio campaigns of the late 1950s achieved fairly low levels of vaccine coverage (in the range of 50–60 percent for the general population).

The measles outbreak of 1989–1991 exposed many incorrect assumptions behind the belief that low levels of coverage were sufficient to control the transmission of infectious disease. The changing demographics of society, the mixing of young children in day care settings, new patterns of health care delivery, high rates of uninsured children, and the shrinking size and morale of health departments all fostered circumstances in which disease transmission occurred within major metropolitan areas even though disease reports were low, and state health officials believed statewide immunization coverage was at acceptable levels (see Chapter 2). The measles epidemic demonstrated that new approaches were necessary to protect vulnerable populations from disease—approaches that depended more heavily on surveying the populations at greatest risk to determine their immunization coverage levels and to identify points of vulnerability that might emerge from a variety of causes, including shifts in population trends, disruptions in health care services, and new behaviors among providers or clients.

In the 1990s, small-area immunization coverage studies or assessments of coverage levels within specific populations (including low-income workers with private insurance, Medicaid families served by managed care organizations, and migrant farmworkers) acquired greater importance for the following reasons:

• Small-area coverage studies reflect the quality and impact on immunization levels of national and state health finance programs, especially for programs such as Vaccines for Children (VFC), Medicaid, and SCHIP.
• Small-area studies can demonstrate the effectiveness or limitations of other types of interventions, including outreach, education, reminder–recall, and community partnerships.
• Despite the high rates of national coverage for preschool and school-aged children, selected regions of the United States characterized by extreme disadvantage have consistently reported low levels of coverage for routine immunizations (see Table 1-5 in Chapter 1). Studies of specific population groups can identify systemic features that need to be addressed within local, state, or national health care systems to promote quality health care, prevent the occurrence of disease, and improve immunization coverage rates.
• High statewide coverage levels are generally sufficient to provide protection against infectious disease outbreaks, provided underimmunized individuals are dispersed among the general population. However, the

concentration of underimmunized individuals within specific regions increases the potential for the transmission of disease.

• Children who receive care from more than one health provider may receive too many immunizations. One CDC study reports that 14 percent of young children (aged 19–35 months) were immunized beyond need for the vaccine to prevent polio (Feikema et al., 2000). Children seen only in public health departments were significantly less likely to be extra-immunized. Additional analysis, however, suggests that rates of extra-immunization may be overestimated as a result of documentation errors in medical records (Davis, 2000).

Virtually any and all of the data collection tools discussed below for determining immunization coverage at the national, state, and local levels can be employed or adapted to examine special populations or geographic pockets of need. In addition to these direct measures of immunization coverage, geographic pockets of need can be identified by surrogate measures, including demographic and socioeconomic variables such as average income level, percent of the population receiving Medicaid, and maternal education, all of which are associated with underimmunization (Santoli et al., forthcoming). Surrogate measures have the advantage of being readily available and inexpensive; although they do not provide direct information about immunization coverage, they can be used to identify neighborhoods at high risk for underimmunization.

Measurement of Immunization Coverage

Information about immunization coverage comes from five major sources: the National Immunization Survey (NIS), retrospective school entry surveys, special area and population surveys, Clinical Assessment Software Application (CASA) surveys of clinics and private practices, and reports from managed care plans on coverage for children in their care. The NIS and retrospective kindergarten surveys estimate the coverage of the population in a given *geographical area*. In contrast, the CASA and managed care assessments estimate coverage levels for *particular entities* responsible for the children's care (health care providers in the former case and managed care plans in the latter).

Differences in the way immunization coverage is measured in various settings—differences in samples, antigens, and time periods, for example—inhibit comparisons across managed care plans, clinics, and private physicians' offices. While some differences may be unavoidable, opportunities for greater comparability may be achieved through technical assistance and program leadership. Understanding the nature and origins of the differences is important if remedies to improve the current situation are to be formulated. A brief description of the measurement strategy for each of the major sources follows.

National Immunization Survey. The NIS is a national telephone survey of households and providers that is used to estimate vaccination coverage levels for children aged 19 to 35 months (information provided by CDC). NIS studies include a two-phase design: (1) self-reports by respondents, obtained by dialing random telephone numbers, and (2) provider record checks that yield independent information on the dates of immunization for a smaller number of children identified through the household survey.

The survey is conducted in 78 Immunization Action Plan (IAP) areas, consisting of the 50 states, the District of Columbia, and 27 other large metropolitan areas. Data collection involves quarterly surveys in each of the 78 IAP areas, combined to provide annualized estimates at acceptable levels of precision. The survey asks about coverage for nine antigens[1] and reports up-to-date status for a variety of combinations. Respondents are selected at random from telephone banks within the IAP areas using complex, multistage sampling techniques, including adjustment weights for the telephone bias, so the sample approximates the population in the IAP area as closely as possible.

The NIS is the primary source of both national and statewide estimates of coverage, including estimates by poverty and ethnic status. CDC relies on NIS data to monitor state progress in achieving childhood immunization objectives, to compare coverage rates across states, and to award incentive funds to CDC grantees on the basis of their immunization of certain percentages of preschool children.

Although the NIS provides reliable baseline data for the nation as a whole, the survey methodology is not designed to identify children in need of more timely immunization. For example (General Accounting Office [GAO], 1996):

• Although the NIS includes an adjustment weight for households that do not have telephones, there is wide variation among states and metropolitan areas in the percentages of such households with children under age 2 (ranging from 2 to 25 percent across the 50 states and 28 urban areas sampled by the NIS).

• NIS respondents, as a group, differ in some respects from the populations represented by census and vital statistics estimates. Mothers with more than 12 years of education are slightly overrepresented, and in some areas, NIS respondents are more likely to report household incomes exceeding $50,000 and less likely to report incomes below $10,000.

• The sample size of the NIS is not large enough to provide subgroup statistics for each state or urban area. For example, one household survey of central and southeast Seattle found an immunization coverage rate of 57 percent, in contrast to the 79 percent reported by the NIS for the King County area incorporating Seattle (GAO, 1996:20).

• The absence of robust subgroup statistics within state or urban areas prevents states from linking changes in coverage rates reported by the NIS to specific programs. The NIS data are therefore not useful to states for diagnosing problems in their ongoing activities, targeting their efforts, or designing interventions (GAO, 1996:19).

Retrospective School Entry Surveys. Retrospective surveys (involving the review of school records to determine when immunizations were obtained relative to the child's second birthday) are the most common form of local-level coverage survey. CDC provides guidelines for conducting these surveys, which involve collecting coverage data from school health records in 35 randomly selected schools for a sample of children. These studies are the least expensive and easiest to perform of the assessments reviewed here, but their data lag the period of performance by 3 to 4 years; thus, for example, they offer little help in monitoring the effects of recent immunization efforts (Orenstein et al., 1999).[2]

Coverage levels reported in the NIS are often higher than those in retrospective school entry surveys. Several factors help explain this difference:

• The most important factor is that the NIS combines data from personal immunization records (and recall) with provider data, and coverage rates are often higher when immunizations from multiple sources are used.
• The NIS is a telephone survey, and children in families with telephones have higher coverage than those without (although, as noted, an adjustment factor is calculated and applied to account for this difference).
• Another major difference between the NIS and all other forms of assessment is the criteria for selection. The NIS uses children aged 19 to 35 months and calculates coverage at the time of the survey. Children who are 35 months old at the time of the survey have had 12 extra months in which to become up to date, while those assessed at 19 months have had 6 months less.

Special Area and Population Surveys. Determining local coverage levels in small geographic units (such as a metropolitan area, county, or census tract) or among specific populations (such as Medicaid families) requires special data analyses that have sufficient sensitivity to detect signs of change or disruption among vulnerable groups. These analyses are sometimes supported by state Section 317 grant awards. In addition, a few health departments (New York City, Detroit, San Diego, and rural Colorado) have participated in a Community Health Network demonstration study to determine whether collaboration with academic health centers or managed care organizations would influence and improve vaccination coverage within the entire population in the designated region (A. Bauer, CDC, personal communication, May 21, 1999).

As noted above, immunization coverage studies within small geographic areas or among specific populations (including low-income workers, Medicaid or Medicare participants who are served by managed care organizations, public housing residents, and migrant farmworkers) can provide important data on variations in coverage patterns that require attention through state and national health finance and health care policies and practices. Local immunization surveys provide intelligence needed to manage the community health system effectively, target needy groups, and ensure accountability within the public and private health care sectors. However, significant barriers challenge such efforts to track vulnerable groups:

- Surveys of baseline coverage for Medicaid populations, including the coverage rates for families served by managed care organizations, are not consistently available, nor can results be compared across survey designs.
- The difficulty of gaining routine access to households of very poor families, due in part to the high rates of mobility among such families, poses significant methodological barriers to data collection efforts.
- Special population studies are commonly funded for limited periods of time through research or state grant awards supported directly by CDC. These special area studies are inconsistent and often difficult to compare because they use different standards of coverage, different age groups, and different survey methods.

CASA Surveys. CASA is CDC-developed software and associated procedures for assessing coverage levels for a clinic or practice. The sample for 2-year-olds consists of children aged 24 to 35 months; coverage is calculated at the 24-month mark. Charts for children are included in the sample if there is a record of at least one medical or immunization visit; a chart can be excluded from the sample under certain stringent conditions.[3] Providers sometimes complain that the inclusion criteria are overly broad.[4] They report that parents often fail to notify their provider when they move, and when this happens, the chart does not bear a "moved or gone elsewhere" notation. Further, providers in birthing hospitals say patients may come to the hospital's outpatient clinic for the first or second visit after birth (especially if insurance is not in place for the child) and then move to a neighborhood health center or private provider.

Reports from Managed Care Plans. Managed care plans use immunization coverage as an indicator of quality, and the National Committee for Quality Assurance's (NCQA) Health Plan Employer Data and Information Set (HEDIS) 3.0 measures include immunization rates as an accountability and performance measure for managed care plans (information provided by the National Committee for Quality Assurance). HEDIS measures of immunization coverage are available for preschool children, adolescents, and adults, and are based on claims or encounter data as well as random samples validated by chart review. While useful in monitoring overall coverage patterns, HEDIS measures have several limitations:

• The sample consists of only those children who turned 2 in the reporting year who were continuously enrolled for 12 months prior to their second birthday (including members who had no more than one break in enrollment of up to 45 days during the reporting year).

• Since many managed care plans report annual disenrollment rates of 35 to 40 percent, children in the HEDIS sample may represent an atypically stable group whose rates are higher than those of all participants enrolled in the managed care plans.

• HEDIS measures for a given plan do not indicate whether the immunization was covered within the plan or was provided elsewhere.

• HEDIS measures often do not report the timing of the first immunization or the time of completion of a series.

No national surveys describe the levels of immunization coverage among individuals enrolled in U.S. private health plans during the period 1990–1998. A few organizations (such as the Employee Benefits Research Institute and the Health Research and Educational Trust, formerly sponsored by KPMG Peat Marwick) study coverage patterns for private industry to determine whether coverage levels vary by type of plan, but these studies cannot demonstrate where certain groups or regions might be vulnerable to reduced immunization protection or disease outbreaks.

Estimating the immunization status of a plan's participants within any given time period is extremely difficult in the absence of reliable performance measures. Health plans are not required to provide consistent data on a regular basis, and individual plans use a variety of different measures, discouraging comparisons across different payor sources. Moreover, immunization coverage rates may be considered private or proprietary information since they are often viewed as an important measure of quality for a given health plan.

Some business organizations have used immunization performance criteria to set penalties and incentives in purchasing negotiations. A study conducted by the Pacific Business Group on Health in 1996, for example, monitored the performance of 13 of California's largest health maintenance organizations (HMOs) that had agreed to penalties (placing a specified percentage of their premiums at risk) in return for not meeting quality-of-care goals (Schauffler et al., 1999). The authors reported that 8 of the 13 plans missed their targets for childhood immunizations, falling short by 3–12 percent. Five of the plans exceeded their targets (by an average of 9.3 percent) within a range of 2–19 percent. Some HMOs excuse low performance with claims that plan participants receive immunization services outside the network of HMO providers, in settings such as county health departments or community clinics, and data on this utilization may not be reported back routinely to the plans or recorded in patients' medical records (Schauffler et al., 1999). Many monitoring groups, however, including the Pacific Business Group on Health, hold participating plans responsible for tracking use of services, both within and outside the plan.

While some of the differences between the CASA and HEDIS criteria for inclusion are technical, the fundamental question is not. At the heart of the difference is the issue of when a provider or health plan takes responsibility for a child and when that provider or plan should be held accountable for the child's health care, including immunization coverage. The HEDIS criteria often exclude a large segment of the population— possibly too large a segment. It does not make sense to hold a plan accountable for the services delivered to a child who has just joined, but since most children have had encounters with the health care system before joining a given plan, the criteria may be too generous. It may make more sense to hold a plan accountable for seeing that a child's previous immunizations are included in his or her record and catching up with the remaining immunizations. On the other hand, the CASA criteria may be too inclusive. Providers have complained that they are being held accountable for children they do not see as "theirs," that parents may come to a given provider only once for any number of reasons. Some health departments address these issues by reporting on all children selected using the CASA criteria, and then providing additional reports for children who have been followed longer.[5] More attention is necessary to the issue of when providers should be held accountable for children who have visited them and how that accountability should be reflected in sample selection for coverage assessments.

Role of Registries in Documenting Coverage Levels

Recognizing that the assessment and documentation of immunization status are complicated by the movements of individuals, health care providers, and health finance systems, several states, local communities, and private health plans have initiated electronic registries to monitor immunization rates within a community or health plan. Immunization registries are "confidential, computerized information systems that contain information about immunizations and children" (National Vaccine Advisory Committee [NVAC], 1999b:2). They have also been described as "automated systems that manage immunization information" (Horne et al., forthcoming:3) and as "a computerized database that gathers immunization information on all children (with preschool children commonly a high priority) in a population defined by a specific geographic area, health maintenance organization (HMO), enrollment, etc." (Wood et al., 1999:233).[6]

Most efforts to develop immunization registries in this country have focused on infants and preschool children. Some managed care companies and HMOs, however, have developed and maintain information systems that they use to monitor their effectiveness and efficiency in providing both childhood and adult immunizations to their enrolled populations.

Registry development began in 1974 when Delaware created VacAttack, a community-based registry built to collect childhood immunization data from all pediatric and family practice providers in the state (Ortega et al., 1997). In the 1980s, several large HMOs started to develop immunization registries (Wood et al., 1999). For example, Group Health Cooperative of Puget Sound created a computer-based data record for all immunizations administered to its 350,000 enrollees in the late 1980s. HMOs continued to build registries in the 1990s. In 1991, CDC collaborated with several large West Coast HMOs in the Vaccine Safety Datalink project, which established both immunization registries and systems for tracking adverse reaction events (Davis et al., 1997; Wood et al., 1999).

In 1991, the Robert Wood Johnson Foundation (RWJF) launched the All Kids Count national childhood immunization registry initiative in response to both the measles outbreak of the late 1980s and the low immunization rates of preschool children in the United States (Watson et al., 1997). These computerized information systems were designed to perform three functions: (1) to provide a computerized database for use by providers in monitoring the immunization status of individual children; (2) to identify children due or overdue for immunizations and notify their parents/guardians of the need to obtain vaccinations; and (3) to provide information for use in identifying underserved populations, targeting resources to these pockets of need, and evaluating outreach program efforts. Between 1992 and 1997, RWJF collaborated with five other private foundations to partially fund 24 registry projects. In 1998, RWJF established the All Kids Count II project by allocating additional funds to 16 of the most advanced developing registries to help them become fully operational by January 1, 2000 (Watson et al., 1997; Wood et al., 1999; Horne et al., forthcoming).

To address the lack of consistency among different registry systems, the All Kids Count initiative developed a 20-item list of ideal components for registries (RWJF, 1996).[7] The CDC National Immunization Program (NIP), in conjunction with its state and local grantees, subsequently developed a list of 12 attributes that define the minimum necessary elements of an operational registry (information provided by CDC).

The registry effort received additional support in 1993, when as part of the Childhood Immunization Initiative, President Clinton offered a challenge to create "a nationwide system of state- and community-based information systems" (Kilbourne, 1998; NVAC, 1999b). In response, the NIP assembled a task force to undertake an initiative on immunization registries, guided by an NVAC work group (NVAC, 1999b). Through public meetings and focus groups, the work group determined that registries in the United States should be a "nationwide mosaic of interoperable systems" as opposed to a federally based information system (Kilbourne, 1998:10).

The development or implementation of registries is a required condition for CDC's state and local immunization grant awards. According to a 1999 CDC survey, 92 percent (59 of 64) of federal immunization grantees (states, cities, and territories) had met this requirement. Only a small number of these registries meet the fully functional standards set by NVAC or RWJF, however (information provided by CDC; NVAC, 1999b; Wood et al., 1999). Currently 34 states and the District of Columbia have operational registries that can import or export data from a central point (J. Harrison, CDC, personal communication, 1999). There are 9 states in which 75 percent or more of the children under age 6 are included in the state's immunization registry. Another 5 have registries that include 50 to 74 percent of children (see Figure 4-1).[8]

A separate measure of registry implementation is provider participation. As of January 2000, 24 states had enrolled a majority (50 percent or more) of public providers in their registries. Yet recruiting private providers has been a major barrier to registry development.[9] Only 11 state registries have over 50 percent enrollment of private providers. It is important to note that provider enrollment does not ensure provider participation.[10] For example, although Michigan has 71 percent of all providers enrolled in its state registry, only 34 percent of enrolled providers are actually submitting data (see Figure 4-2).

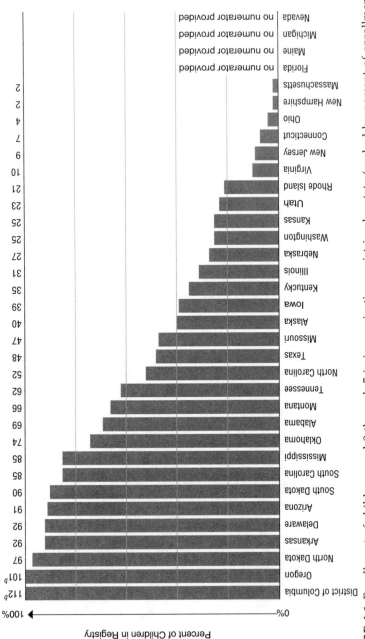

FIGURE 4-1 Enrollment of children aged 0 through 5 in immunization registries, by state (ranked by percent of enrollment[a]). [a]Enrollment is defined as children having at least two doses of vaccine recommended by the Advisory Committee on Immunization Practices and recorded in an immunization registry's database. [b]More than 100% because of duplicate records. SOURCE: CDC, 1999h.

Role of Immunization Registries in Improving Coverage Levels. Immunization registries serve multiple purposes beyond the surveillance and assessment of current coverage rates (DeFriese et al., 1999). They can facilitate service delivery, consolidate scattered records, and simplify the assessment of need for vaccine for both private and public providers. As long as significant numbers of at-risk groups are enrolled, registries can also be used to identify pockets of need in areas where immunization coverage lags behind the current high national and/or state levels. If used appropriately, fully operational registries can be an efficient means of identifying children who require intensive services and may stimulate service responses to ensure their full immunization.

In addition to improving immunization coverage for the currently recommended immunization schedule, registries can be used to monitor and ensure the full implementation of newly recommended vaccines and vaccine schedules. Just as a series completion rate for children in the registry catchment area can be assessed, uptake of specific antigens, including those newly introduced, can be monitored and changes made in implementation strategies on the basis of populations identified as being in need. The current immunization schedule is sufficiently complex to benefit from computerized monitoring, and, as noted earlier, greater complexity is anticipated in the future.

Anecdotal reports (Fairbrother et al., 1997) indicate that immunization monitoring can also improve the identification of children who require other preventive care services (such as lead screening). It is conceivable that investments in immunization registries could benefit these programs, although the scale of this potential impact is not known. The costs and benefits of immunization registries for adult populations (particularly those over age 65) are similarly uncertain.

Barriers to Registry Development and Implementation. Barriers to registry development and implementation fall into four categories: (1) technical and operational issues, (2) privacy and confidentiality, (3) provider participation, and (4) resource requirements (NVAC, 1999b; Linkins and Feikema, 1998; Kilbourne, 1998).

Difficulties have been experienced in sharing information among community-based registries because of variations in the architecture of computer systems, including different software, hardware, data entry mechanisms, and networking resources (NVAC, 1999b). Differences also exist in the methods used to receive or send registry data and in linkages to other computer systems. CDC has encouraged its state and local grantees to endorse standard algorithms to facilitate the transfer of information between systems (NVAC, 1999b; Wood et al., 1999). Duplicate records,

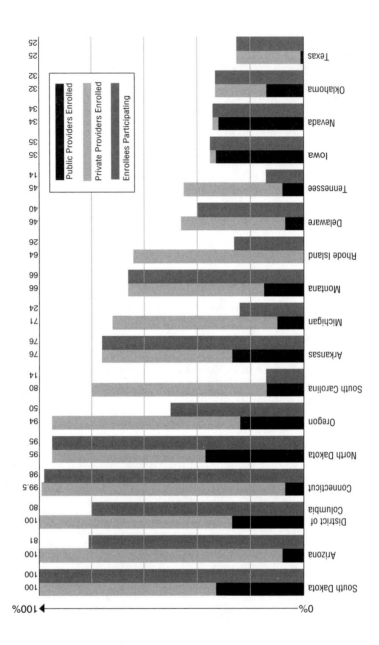

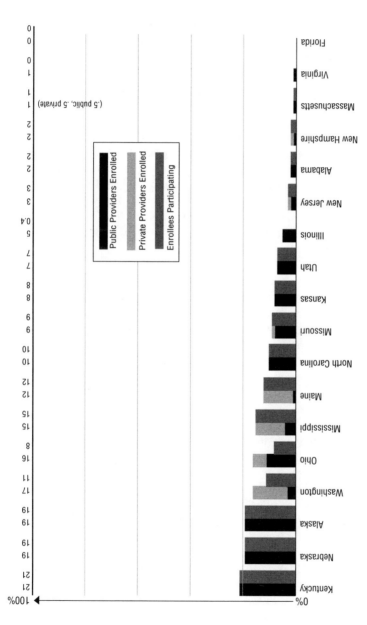

FIGURE 4-2 Provider enrollment[a] and participation[b] in immunization registries, by state (ranked by percent of provider enrollment). [a]Enrollment is defined as providers who have authorized access to the registry (e.g. written agreement, passwords, rights, and responsibilities defined). [b]Participation is defined as providers who have submitted data to (or accessed data from) the immunization registry in the last 6 months. SOURCE: CDC, 1999h.

transcription errors, and missing data are also a problem (NVAC, 1999b; Wilton and Pennisi, 1994).

Studies have shown that barriers to private provider participation in immunization registries include personnel time required to submit and obtain data; costs of technology and other necessary resources; liability for errors; and concerns about data accuracy, confidentiality, access, and security (Bordley et al., 1997; NVAC, 1999b; Wood et al., 1999). An Oregon study revealed that doctors are willing to spend only about "three extra seconds per patient" to participate in an immunization registry (Zablocki, 1996).

In addition to financial resources, immunization registries require a large investment in personnel. Staff are needed to design the system, develop community support, procure technological resources, connect providers to the system, train office personnel, enter and retrieve immunization data, maintain the system, and respond to any problems that might arise. A recent study of costs among a sample of All Kids Count projects showed that personnel time was more costly than computer time (Slifkin et al., 1999).

Finding 4-2. A successful immunization system must be able to monitor vaccine coverage rates in targeted areas where populations are at risk of disease outbreaks. When communities are successful in achieving high coverage rates, the task of identifying vulnerable populations becomes more difficult and expensive, especially if unprotected groups are dispersed across multiple service systems or are concentrated in hard-to-reach geographic regions (such as remote areas or households without telephones).

Finding 4-3. The shift in service delivery for low-income children from a small cadre of public health providers and community-based clinics to a larger and more diverse network of health plans and private providers has increased coverage rates, but has also created more complexity in assuring service delivery and monitoring immunization coverage. The transition in service settings has also complicated the information management and administration of populationwide services within public health agencies. Data from disparate sources must be combined; health plans must incorporate outreach and patient reminder–recall systems, measure immunization coverage, assess provider practices, and conduct record audits; and public health agencies must formulate oversight policies that can guide health care finance and delivery systems within the public sector.

Finding 4-4. Although each community may express immunization data collection and service strategies differently, a core surveillance effort is essential in three key areas—infectious disease patterns, immunization coverage levels (especially within high-risk groups), and adverse events from vaccines within the general population—to maintain the integrity and reliability of the national immunization system. Adequate datasets in each area are necessary to allow for comparisons within and between states and to monitor trends over time, especially among vulnerable populations. Compromising the quality of data within critical areas can lead to blind spots and uncertainties that erode health care policy and practice and waste resources in both public and private settings.

Finding 4-5. Precise and consistent measures and small-area studies are necessary to monitor coverage assessments in targeted areas and to establish performance benchmarks for different health care plans. A consistent, national standard for measuring coverage levels among diverse populations and multiple health care settings does not currently exist. The result is uncertainty in comparing rates across private and public health care plans or geographic areas. Performance standards, benchmarks, and information databases that establish consistent and comparable communitywide indicators for immunization levels among children, adolescents, and adults represent important opportunities for quality-of-care initiatives, but such efforts are in the early stages of development. They should be viewed as complements to, rather than replacements for, traditional public health surveillance and assessment efforts.

Finding 4-6. Some efforts are under way to improve immunization assessments as a measure of quality of health care delivery, but no single governmental agency is responsible for collecting datasets from multiple sources (e.g., NIS, Medicaid, and SCHIP) to ensure that relevant data are made available to state health officials. In addition, the methodology used in some assessments (such as HEDIS measures) may be inadequate to determine the true depth of coverage within hard-to-reach or mobile groups.

Finding 4-7. Several states and localities have made considerable progress in implementing registries that improve the measurement of immunization levels. Those operational systems that are in place offer a number of advantages, such as the assurance of data availability in case of disaster, reductions in the cost of record verification among providers at the point of service for a given patient, and elimination of the variations that can occur in parent/patient-carried health records. Once fully operational, registries may allow communities to target their outreach and other interventions more successfully, as well as to achieve significant savings in other surveillance programs. With the increasing importance of population-based approaches to health system planning and evaluation, immunization registries offer one of the most useful instruments for assessing the population-specific effectiveness of health and medical care programs.

Finding 4-8. The registries of most states have not achieved a level of performance that allows them to serve as effective sentinels for gaps in coverage. A number of barriers need to be addressed if registries are to be fully implemented. Broad variability, the lack of consistent technical standards, problems with access to and the operational capability of software to support registry operations, and the need to respond to the requirements of multiple jurisdictions constitute major challenges that must be resolved to improve registry performance. Making registries fully operational will entail considerable costs, as well as efforts to resolve key concerns about privacy, liability, and confidentiality.

Finding 4-9. Data gaps and unreliable measures can lead to under-estimation of coverage levels and risk of disease for vulnerable populations. These uncertainties could eventually lead to blind spots within the national immunization system that would create pressure points in policy and practice and erode the quality and integrity of the enterprise. The experience with measles outbreaks in 1989–1991 and more recent disease reports suggest that during periods of complacency, low levels of immunization coverage among vulnerable groups may remain undetected and unaddressed, and can erupt into infectious disease outbreaks (NVAC, 1991).

Monitoring Vaccine Safety

As a biological product, vaccines may cause unintended side effects, some of which can be serious. Concerns about quality, safety, and reliability can be expected to grow as use of vaccines expands, particularly as the threat of infectious disease diminishes and as knowledge of the possible long-term health consequences of vaccine use increases. The potential for adverse events argues for the need to sustain both reliable monitoring systems and sources of expertise that can investigate anecdotal and clinical reports. The ability to distinguish between causal relationships and coincidence should adverse events occur requires an evidentiary base, as well as risk assessment judgments that can guide health care and public policy decisions during periods of uncertainty. Extensive media coverage of claims about possible adverse events associated with vaccine use before research information is available to guide health professionals, policy makers, and the public prompts skepticism and even alarm that can lead to reduced vaccine use in the absence of scientific consensus.

Recent Safety Concerns. When safety claims emerge, organizations responsible for formulating recommendations that guide the use of vaccines must determine whether the reported evidence warrants the suspension or removal of a vaccine, further study, or no action. Three recent incidents—involving concerns about the safety of rotavirus vaccine, the use of thimerosal, and the reported connections between measles, mumps, and rubella (MMR) vaccine and the onset of autism—illustrate the range of issues and responses that arise in vaccine safety discussions.

In July 1999, the Advisory Committee on Immunization Practices (ACIP) and the American Academy of Pediatrics (AAP) recommended that physicians temporarily suspend administration of rotavirus vaccine. This recommendation emerged after CDC had investigated reports of several cases of intussusception (an intestinal disorder that sometimes requires surgical intervention) during the first few days after the vaccine's ingestion (CDC, 1999i). CDC is conducting an ongoing case-control study of the vaccine and expects to report results in 2000 (AAP, 1999a). In the interim, the rotavirus vaccine has been removed from the ACIP recommended schedule.

Also in July 1999, AAP issued a joint statement with the U.S. Public Health Service (PHS) alerting physicians and the public to concern about thimerosal, a mercury-containing preservative used in some vaccines to prevent bacterial contamination. Mercury can be toxic to children, depending on the form used, route of entry, dose, and age of exposure. AAP and PHS have recommended that government agencies work rapidly to diminish children's exposure to mercury from all sources, including vaccines (AAP, 1999b). Although future research findings may lead to changes in the vaccine schedule or the use of selected products, the thimerosal warning has not modified current ACIP recommendations in the absence of alternative products.

More recently, a series of stories in the media have suggested the possibility of a connection between autism and vaccines, especially the MMR vaccine. Unlike the rotavirus and thimerosal cases, in which the weight of clinical evidence attracted the attention of medical organizations, safety concerns about possible links between vaccines and autism have emerged primarily from preliminary research findings that have drawn public and political attention. Since the MMR vaccine is administered at the same time that symptoms of autism may become apparent, some parents have concluded that the vaccine is responsible for the syndrome. Two congressional hearings on vaccine safety (U.S. House of Representatives, 1999b, 2000) provided an opportunity for testimony that attracted media coverage and further stimulated public fears about vaccine safety, even though little is known about the biological origins of autism. Further research has been recommended on this subject, but the scientific groups responsible for vaccine recommendations have also urged the continued use of the MMR vaccine in the absence of research or clinical evidence that would establish a convincing connection between vaccine use and the emergence of this disorder.

Vaccine safety concerns related to other disorders (e.g., childhood diabetes and multiple sclerosis) have also drawn large amounts of media attention. When claims are made about possible links between specific health and behavioral disorders and vaccine use, extensive efforts are required to determine the strength of the evidentiary base that supports each claim. Future additions to the vaccine schedule may contribute to concerns about vaccine safety, increase the likelihood of adverse events, and necessitate more resources for surveillance and for such efforts to investigate claims of health risks at both the national and local levels.

Federal Role. Before vaccines reach the market, private manufacturers implement rigorous measures designed to ensure the safety of their products. Vaccine manufacturers are required to document and report in the clinical trials literature any adverse health effects that are detected prior to the approval and licensing of a new vaccine product. Once a vaccine is in widespread use, health providers that administer vaccines and vaccine manufacturers are expected to report any adverse effects to DHHS.

There are two federal programs related to vaccine safety: the Vaccine Adverse Events Reporting System (VAERS) and the National Vaccine Injury Compensation Program (VICP). Following the passage of the National Childhood Injury Act of 1986 (P.L. 99-66), DHHS established VAERS to accept all reports of suspected adverse events among all age groups after the administration of any U.S. licensed vaccine in the public or private sector. Operated jointly by the Food and Drug Administration and CDC, VAERS was created primarily to serve as a signaling system for adverse events not detected during premarket testing (Food and Drug Administration, 1998).

VAERS currently receives 800–1,000 reports each month. About 85 percent of the reports concern relatively minor adverse events, such as swelling at the injection site and ordinary fevers. The remaining 15 percent involve serious side effects, such as high fever, seizure, life-threatening illness, or death. Upon analysis of VAERS reports, the Food and Drug Administration has the authority to recall a vaccine if it represents a risk to the American public. Only three batches of vaccine have been recalled during the last 10 years (Food and Drug Administration, 1999).

The National Childhood Injury Act of 1986 also established VICP, which became effective on October 1, 1988, as Subtitle 2 of Title XXI of the Public Health Service Act. VICP is a federal no-fault system designed to compensate individuals, or families of individuals, who have been injured by childhood vaccines, whether administered in the private or public sector. The program is a critical component of the national immunization strategy since it authorizes compensation for those with specified injuries while also allowing the manufacture of recommended childhood vaccines to continue.

DHHS, the U.S. Department of Justice, and the U.S. Court of Federal Claims administer a collaborative process for determining qualification for compensation. VICP covers adverse events caused by the following vaccines: diphtheria, pertussis, tetanus (DTP, DTaP, DT, TT, or TD); MMR or any of its components; polio (oral poliovirus vaccine [OPV] or inactivated poliovirus vaccine [IPV]), whether administered individually or in combination; hepatitis B; *Haemophilus influenzae* type b; varicella, and rotavirus (Health Resources and Services Administration [HRSA], 2000a).

As of February 8, 2000, 5,763 VICP petitions had been filed, and 5,079 had been adjudicated (see Table 4-1). Most (74 percent) of the petitions involved vaccines administered prior to October 1, 1988. From fiscal year

TABLE 4-1 Vaccine Injury Compensation Program Petitions Filed, Adjudications, and Awards

Fiscal Year	Petitions Filed	Adjudications Dismissed	Compensable Adjudications	Awards (in millions of dollars)
1988	24	NA	NA	NA
1989	148	12	9	NA
1990	3,248	34	98	71.9
1991	962	446	142	79.6
1992	189	488	166	97.6
1993	140	589	125	125.4
1994	107	446	162	107.0
1995	180	575	160	108.4
1996	84	409	161	103.1
1997	104	197	190	118.6
1998	120	181	145	135.1
1999	411	143	97	101.7
2000[a]	46	45	58	55.1
Totals	5,763	3,565	1,514	$1,103.5

NOTE: NA = not applicable.

[a]Through February 8, 2000.

SOURCE: Health Resources Services Administration, 2000b.

(FY) 1989 to February 2000, 1,514 petitions were found to be compensable, while 3,565 were dismissed.[11]

The funding source for VICP awards depends on the date of vaccination. For vaccine administered prior to October 1, 1988, awards are financed by federal tax dollars allocated by Congress at $110 million per year. For vaccines administered on or after October 1, 1988, awards are paid from the Vaccine Injury Compensation Trust Fund, financed by an excise tax on vaccine purchases (HRSA, 2000c). In 1997, a flat-tax rate of $0.75 per antigen was introduced for all covered vaccines.

The average FY 1999 pre-1988 injury award was $855,474 (58 cases), for a total of $51.7 million. The average FY 1999 post-1988 injury award was $1,433,319 (33 cases), for a total of $50 million. Adjudication under VICP led to payments totaling $101.7 million in FY 1999 and approximately $1.1 billion in the 1990s (see Table 4-1) (HRSA, 2000b).

Finding 4-10. Vaccine safety concerns can be expected to acquire greater importance as the incidence of infectious disease diminishes and more vaccines are approved for general use. Data monitoring and reliable reporting systems need to be in place so that public health agencies can respond appropriately to concerns and uncertainties of the public and health providers about the need for vaccines during times when disease outbreaks are not apparent. Recent experiences with substantiated and unsubstantiated reports of adverse effects associated with vaccines suggest that the media have difficulty providing reliable information on this subject, especially during periods of scientific uncertainty. The demand for informed expertise can quickly overwhelm routine assessment and data collection efforts, especially if public health officials are expected to respond to antivaccine literature and anecdotal accounts as well as clinical reports.

EFFORTS TO IMPROVE AND SUSTAIN HIGH VACCINE COVERAGE RATES

The Task Force on Community Preventive Services (TFCPS) has identified a set of strategies for improving and sustaining high levels of immunization coverage (Briss et al., 2000)[12]:

- Reduce cost barriers for vaccines for disadvantaged groups.
- Expand access to immunization services.
- Develop provider-based interventions to address the problem of missed opportunities in health care or social service settings that serve high-risk families.
- Increase community demand for vaccinations.

These strategies are complementary to vaccine purchase and service-delivery efforts intended to increase coverage levels within populations that require additional assistance in achieving up-to-date immunizations. Each strategy consists of several different types of interventions. TFCPS recently reviewed the available literature to determine areas of best practice (Briss et al., 2000). An abbreviated summary of the TFCPS findings is presented here to demonstrate the impact of public health infrastructure investments on immunization coverage rates.

Reducing Cost Barriers and Building Capacity

The out-of-pocket costs of immunization constitute a barrier to obtaining vaccinations for many clients (Cutts et al., 1992). Providers are more likely to refer children with less public or private insurance coverage to other sites for vaccination, and referral practices are known to have adverse effects on both the timing and rate of immunization (Bennett et al., 1994; Mainous and Hueston, 1995; Ruch-Ross and O'Connor, 1994; Taylor et al., 1997; Zimmerman et al., 1997).

Reducing out-of-pocket costs improves vaccination coverage for diverse age groups and populations in a range of settings, from individual clinics, to statewide programs, to national efforts such as the Vaccines for Children (VFC) program (Briss et al., 2000). These positive effects have been reported whether the reduced-cost intervention has been used alone or as part of a multicomponent intervention (such as client or provider reminder–recall, communitywide education, expansion of access in health care settings, and provider education). The overall median coverage difference was found to be 10 percent (range of 8 to 35 percent). On the basis of this evidence, TFCPS strongly recommended reducing out-of-pocket costs as an effective strategy to improve vaccination coverage (Briss et al., 2000).

Although poverty is commonly accepted as a significant cause of discrepancies among immunization coverage rates, low rates of immunization coverage have been reported among populations for which cost is not a barrier (Orenstein et al., 1999). In one survey of 2-year-old children of employees of a large corporation, for example, only 65 percent of the children who had medical insurance coverage for immunizations had received the 4:3:1 series (four DTP, three polio, and one MMR) (Fielding et al., 1994).[13] There were also no differences in coverage found in a study that compared private practices in states with and without universal purchase policies (Taylor et al., 1997). The families surveyed in this study, however, were well educated, of moderate to high socioeconomic status, and therefore least likely to benefit from free vaccines (Orenstein et al., 1999).

Service utilization studies within public health clinics indicate that some low-income parents use public clinics because of the reduced cost, even though they might prefer to receive immunizations from their regular private providers (Lieu et al., 1994; Santoli, 1999). Studies of the implementation of VFC have indicated that referrals to health departments decrease when free vaccines are provided to private providers, suggesting that both parents and providers take advantage of the free vaccines (Zimmerman et al., 1997). Although parents may need to pay administration fees in private-care settings that are not assessed at health department clinics, this cost is usually less than the vaccine expense. Parents may also be motivated to make use of VFC in seeking vaccine services since they do not need to take additional time from work or incur further transportation or child care expenses to visit a public clinic. VFC enables them to obtain vaccines from their usual care provider (Orenstein et al., 1999).

Research has not yet demonstrated whether reduced-cost strategies will improve immunization rates or change provider referral practices for adolescents and adults below age 65. This absence of knowledge is especially important when one is considering new finance strategies for future generations of vaccines for these age groups. In particular, although the body of research on children and older adults (above age 65) strongly suggests that reduced costs for vaccines result in positive outcomes for many age groups, the adolescent and young adult population is sufficiently distinct to merit independent study.

Expanding Access to Immunization Services

Expanding Access in Health Care Settings. Many local and state health agencies have sought to improve immunization rates by enhancing access to vaccines in health care settings, whether by extending hours or adding staff; introducing express services; or adding immunization services to hospitals, pharmacies, and nursing homes. These strategies are designed to reduce the distance from the setting to the at-risk population, increase the hours during which vaccination services are offered, deliver vaccinations in clinical settings in which they were previously not provided, or reduce administrative barriers to obtaining vaccination services within clinics (e.g., by developing a drop-in clinic or an "express lane" vaccination service) (Briss et al., 2000). Some programs for expanded access are offered through special contractual agreements with local health care providers. Others require more substantial commitments, including additional personnel that may be more difficult to sustain during hiring or salary freezes.

The TFCPS report strongly recommends expanding access to immunizations in health care settings as part of a comprehensive intervention, indicating that insufficient evidence exists to support this intervention when used alone (Briss et al., 2000). TFCPS notes that within a comprehensive intervention, expanded access can improve vaccination coverage among children and older adults in a range of contexts, but the contribution of individual components to the overall effectiveness of such comprehensive interventions cannot be determined. The TFCPS report further observes that there are several barriers to implementing expanded access, including difficulties of coordination among settings, a lack of appropriate records, difficulties in clients' recall of immunization status, high numbers of clients with contraindications to vaccination, and the lack of a relationship between vaccination programs and the primary missions of other settings.

Building capacity to serve new populations, especially adolescents and young adults, is a challenge that requires major consideration of the nature of the immunization partnership and funding patterns. New vaccines may be introduced in nontraditional settings (such as school clinics, workplace sites, and pharmacies) in which strategic oversight is required to monitor coverage levels and address safety concerns, including the potential for adverse events. The scale of investment required for public health agencies to exercise a leadership role in linking programmatic efforts, guiding the implementation of future generations of vaccines, and introducing vaccines to new populations has not been addressed.

Expanding Access in Nonmedical Settings. Numerous interventions have been designed to reach important target populations in nonmedical settings where they congregate. These interventions usually involve assessment of a child's immunization status, and the referral of underimmunized persons to appropriate providers or the provision of vaccinations on site. Four nonmedical settings have been evaluated in this regard: (1) Women, Infants, and Children (WIC) sites; (2) home visits; (3) vaccination programs in schools; and (4) child care centers.

WIC Sites. WIC is a special supplemental nutrition program for women, infants, and children, a federal grant program administered by the U.S. Department of Agriculture and implemented through state health departments and tribal organizations. The primary mission of WIC is to provide supplemental foods and nutrition education; the program can also serve as a gateway and coordinator for other health and social services, including immunizations. WIC is the single largest point of access to health-related services for low-income preschool children since it serves more than 45 percent of the U.S. birth cohort, and in some cities serves up to 80 percent of low-income infants. Participants (usually mothers with young children) commonly visit WIC sites every 2–3 months to receive nutrition services and to pick up food vouchers; more comprehensive health status evaluations are conducted every 6–12 months.

The TFCPS report recommends vaccination programs for immunization interventions in WIC settings, but observes that certain barriers may prevent implementation of this strategy. Many WIC providers believe vaccination requirements or monthly voucher pickups constitute disincentives for WIC participation. Two evaluation studies compared dropout rates between intervention and control groups. It was concluded that small differences in dropout rates do not demonstrate a causal link between vaccination interventions and WIC dropout (Hutchins et al., 1999; Birkhead et al., 1995).

Home Visits. Home visits provide face-to-face health services to clients in their homes. These services can include education, assessment of need, referral, and provision of vaccinations. Home visiting interventions can also involve telephone or mail reminders.

The TFCPS report recommends that home visits be used to improve vaccination coverage among socioeconomically disadvantaged populations. Home visit interventions, however, when applied only to improve vaccination coverage, are highly resource-intensive relative to other available options for improving coverage since they require specialized staff training and must address concerns for staff safety.

School-Based Programs. School-based programs provide opportunities for vaccination interventions that extend beyond the simple requirement of certain vaccinations for school attendance. School interventions are intended to improve delivery of vaccinations to school attendees and to improve coverage rates among children and adolescents aged 5–18. In some cases, the programs may also target preschool siblings.

School interventions generally consist of vaccination-related education of students, parents, teachers, and other school staff; provision of vaccinations or referrals; and occasionally other components, such as incentives or written consent requirements. School-based programs often involve collaborations among schools, local health departments, private hospitals, and community clinics. They provide a unique opportunity for reaching young adolescents, since approximately 90 percent of U.S. children aged 11 and 12 attend school (Kominski and Adams, 1991). School-based vaccination programs can be used to determine each student's immunization status, identify those who have missed doses, and ensure completion of vaccine series (especially for hepatitis B vaccine) among most students. However, TFCPS found there was insufficient evidence to assess the effectiveness of such programs because limited studies have been conducted to evaluate their impact.

There are several potential barriers to the implementation of school-based vaccination programs. These barriers can include difficulties in coordinating among different programs, staff training requirements, disruption of school routines, and confidentiality concerns.

Child Care Centers. Children in child care centers are at increased risk for communicable diseases. In 1995, approximately one-third of preschool children (31 percent) were cared for in such settings (information provided by Children's Health Working Group). Child care center interventions involve efforts to encourage vaccination of preschool children (younger than age 5) by assessing each child's immunization status upon entry into child care and at some point or at periodic intervals during the child's enrollment. Vaccination interventions can also include education or notification of parents, referral of underimmunized children to health care providers, and sometimes provision of vaccinations on site. TFCPS concluded that there is insufficient evidence available to assess the effectiveness of such interventions (Briss et al., 2000).

Addressing Missed Opportunities

Many researchers and health care providers used to attribute the lack of complete immunization coverage to poverty and the economic barriers that discouraged families from seeking vaccines or gaining access to a primary care provider. In the wake of the 1989–1991 measles outbreak, however, it was found that underimmunized children had substantially more access to the health care system than had previously been assumed. The 1988 National Health Interview Survey on Child Health, for example, revealed that 90 percent of children had a source of routine health care, although only 77 percent of 2-year-olds had achieved full immunization coverage (St. Peter et al., 1992). This finding was reinforced by a later analysis of the 1993 National Health Interview Survey, which demonstrated that 90 percent of underimmunized children reported having a usual source of health care (Tatande et al., 1996).

These findings caused many researchers and health professionals to rethink traditional strategies for improving vaccination coverage levels and to focus on addressing missed opportunities in health care and other public service settings (Santoli et al., 1998). Researchers recommended several new strategies aimed at encouraging providers to vaccinate both children and adults. These strategies included checking records of immunization status and implementing reminder–recall systems for public and private providers; introducing immunization services in nontraditional medical settings (e.g., emergency departments or acute care clinics); linking immunization assessment efforts with other services that involved high-risk families (e.g., Head Start, WIC clinics, and the welfare system); and encouraging health professionals to offer simultaneous immunizations during acute care appointments (Orenstein et al., 1999). Four such provider-based interventions have been evaluated in the research literature (Briss et al., 2000):

- provider reminder–recall,
- provider assessment and feedback,
- standing orders, and
- provider education.

Provider Reminder–Recall. This strategy involves alerting those who administer vaccinations that individual clients are due (reminder) or overdue (recall) for particular vaccinations. Issued before, during, or after a scheduled appointment, such notices can be provided through such means as client charts, computer records, or mail.

Provider reminder–recall has been shown to improve vaccination coverage for various age groups (adults, adolescents, and children) in a range of settings and populations (Briss et al., 2000). Positive impacts have been demonstrated whether the reminder notice was used alone or as part of a comprehensive intervention. Positive results were also associated with a range of methods (e.g., computerized or simple reminders, checklists, or flowcharts).

The TFCPS task force strongly recommends the use of reminder–recall interventions to improve vaccination coverage for all age groups. However, some studies have revealed that provider offices experience difficulty with placing reminders in charts, and some health care professionals do not use reminders when provided, suggesting that the administrative burden associated with this strategy may be a major barrier to its use (Briss et al., 2000). Lack of information about vaccination status may also inhibit use of this approach. A 1992 study indicated that fewer than 20 percent of providers operated any kind of credible reminder–recall system (Szilagyi et al., 1992). A 1999 study led to a similar finding (Darden et al., 1999).

Provider Assessment and Feedback. Many providers tend to overestimate the coverage rates of their clients. In a California study, for example, physicians estimated that about 90 percent of their patients were up to date, although record audits indicated that the actual rate was well below 70 percent (Watt et al., 1998). Assessment and feedback interventions (also called AFIX for Assessment, Feedback, Incentives, and eXchange of information) involve performing a retrospective evaluation of the performance of providers in delivering one or more vaccinations to a client population. This information is then given to providers and sometimes others (e.g., comparing performance against a goal or standard with incentives or benchmarking in a health plan). Specific interventions vary in content, intensity, and use of incentives.

Use of assessment and feedback can change provider knowledge, attitudes, and behavior, and may also stimulate additional system-level changes, such as the routine use of reminders or standing orders. TFCPS strongly recommends the use of assessment and feedback interventions, whether alone or as part of a comprehensive intervention, across a range of settings, age groups, and populations (Briss et al., 2000). At the same time, the TFCPS report notes that this intervention may constitute an administrative burden for some providers or systems, and there may also be barriers to its implementation, such as the lack of an adequate information infrastructure.

Standing Orders. Standing orders provide a protocol by which non-physician personnel prescribe or deliver vaccinations to client populations (primarily adults) without direct physician involvement at the time of the interaction. This intervention has been implemented in clinics, hospitals, and nursing homes. Standing orders are designed to improve delivery of immunizations by reducing both barriers to vaccination (such as the requirement for a physical examination) and missed opportunities (resulting from a lack of physician personnel).

TFCPS concluded that there is insufficient evidence to assess the effectiveness of standing orders in improving vaccination coverage in children (Briss et al., 2000). No studies have evaluated the effectiveness of standing orders in improving vaccination among adolescents or increasing delivery of hepatitis B or tetanus vaccinations. In contrast, TFCPS strongly recommends the use of standing orders for both influenza and pneumococcal vaccinations for adults in such settings as hospitals, clinics, and nursing homes (Briss et al., 2000). Again, however, the TFCPS report notes that the use of standing orders may be difficult. The strategy requires effective interprofessional communication and the sharing of responsibility for the associated administrative burden among busy providers and systems, especially in pediatric clinics.

Provider Education. Increasing the knowledge or changing the attitudes of providers regarding vaccination can lead to improvements in immunization coverage if providers act on this information in a positive manner. Provider education can lead to additional vaccinations; change provider–

client interactions to increase client acceptance of vaccinations; or motivate providers to implement other system-level changes, such as reminder–recall systems or standing orders.

Given the paucity of studies of this intervention, limitations in their design and conduct, and small effect sizes, TFCPS concluded that there is insufficient evidence for assessing the effectiveness of provider education interventions. The TFCPS report suggests that this approach be used only in conjunction with other interventions until better information becomes available (Briss et al., 2000).

Improving Awareness and Documentation of Immunization Status

Strategies to promote community and client awareness and documentation of individual immunization status have been proposed in the expectation that such efforts will stimulate requests for immunization services during interactions with health care providers. Three such strategies have been formulated:

- Increasing community demand for vaccinations through various educational and reminder interventions
- Establishing requirements or incentives for immunization
- Enhancing awareness of immunization status through devices such as client-held medical records

Increasing Community Demand for Vaccinations. Three specific strategies are commonly used to increase community demand: client reminder–recall systems, comprehensive interventions that include education, and communitywide or clinic-based education-only interventions.

Client Reminder–Recall Systems. Reminders and recalls inform clients when vaccinations are due or overdue. They differ in content and timing and are provided in various forms, including telephone, letter, or postcard. Client reminders can be either general or specific (i.e., certain vaccinations are due on a specific date).

Client reminder–recall interventions have proven effective whether used alone or as part of a comprehensive intervention. TFCPS therefore strongly recommends the use of these interventions for both children and adults, in a range of settings and populations, and at different levels of scale (Briss et al., 2000). Barriers to implementation include lack of datasets and the administrative burden on providers or systems.

Comprehensive Interventions That Include Education. Comprehensive interventions focused on clients address health concerns and barriers to vaccination in an integrated way. They make community members aware of vaccination services, highlight the utility and relevance of these services, and provide information that can help clients take advantage of the services. The interventions may incorporate a variety of associated strategies to improve vaccination, including client and/or provider reminders, provider education, expanded hours or access in clinical settings, lowering of out-of-pocket costs, client-held vaccination records, and WIC interventions.

Having reviewed the relevant research, TFCPS strongly recommends the use of comprehensive interventions that include education for children and adults in communitywide and clinic-based settings in a range of contexts (Briss et al., 2000). Barriers to the implementation of this intervention include the difficulties involved in coordinating strategies among various programs and administrative systems.

Communitywide or Clinic-Based Education Only. Education-only programs provide information to most or all of a target population in a geographic (communitywide) or institutional (medical or public health clinic-based) setting. The information may be provided to clients only, providers only, or both. Educational materials can take the form of brochures (including mail), videotape, posters, vaccine information statements (standardized statements often used to obtain consent for vaccination), and announcements in the media (radio, newspapers, and television). The goal of educational interventions is to increase client acceptance of and demand for vaccinations.

A limited evidentiary base exists for this intervention. TFCPS therefore concluded that there was insufficient evidence regarding the effectiveness of either communitywide or clinic-based education-only interventions (Briss et al., 2000).

Establishing Requirements and Incentives. States or local governments may develop specific requirements or incentives to ensure immunization coverage.

Vaccination Requirements for Child Care, School, and College Attendance. During the 1970s and 1980s, all 50 states adopted immunization requirements for entry to elementary school, and more than 95 percent of children are now appropriately vaccinated with recommended doses of vaccine upon entering school. The required immunization schedule varies from state to state. More recently, immunization requirements have been adopted for child care and college attendance. Enforcement levels for the latter vary greatly among the states.

Having reviewed the relevant body of evidence, TFCPS recommends vaccination requirements for child care, school, and college attendance among all relevant populations (Briss et al., 2000). TFCPS found that the extent to which specific legal characteristics or intensity of enforcement influenced the effectiveness of state requirements could not be determined.

Client or Family Incentives. Many immunization programs offer positive incentives (e.g., baby toys, money, or discount coupons) to motivate their clients to seek vaccinations for themselves or their children. Incentives can also be negative (penalties that can lead to the client's exclusion from a program). After reviewing the relevant literature, TFCPS concluded that insufficient evidence exists to assess the effectiveness of client incentives in improving vaccination coverage, and observed further that the potential for coercion represents a potential barrier to their implementation.

Enhancing Awareness of Immunization Status. Client-held (also called hand-held) medical records are provided to members of a target population or their families to indicate which vaccinations have been received. The records can improve a client's awareness of vaccinations needed or due and can be used to assess immunization status in medical and other settings. Many state and local health departments and providers have encouraged use of client-held medical records to improve coverage rates by increasing clients' knowledge about vaccinations and/or reducing missed opportunities in health care settings.

Based on the small number of studies of this strategy, limitations in study designs, and variations in the interventions and research findings, TFCPS concluded that insufficient evidence exists to assess the effectiveness of client-held medical records in improving vaccination coverage (Briss et al., 2000). Furthermore, although 80 percent of providers in one survey reported positive or very positive overall reactions to a "health diary," 17 percent also believed that such records negatively affect client flow (Dickey and Petitti, 1992).

Finding 4-11. There is sufficient evidence in the research literature to support strongly recommending the use of certain strategies to improve immunization rates across the United States, within either the general population or targeted groups. These strategies include client and provider reminder–recall; assessment and feedback for vaccination providers; multicomponent interventions that include education; lowering of out-of-pocket costs to families for vaccinations; elimination of the gap in immunization coverage rates between minority groups and the general population; expanded access to vaccinations in health care settings; and the use of standing orders to vaccinate adults in clinics, hospitals, and nursing homes. Other interventions—such as school or child care vaccination requirements, home visits to promote vaccinations, and vaccination programs in WIC settings—can be recommended when they are well matched to particular needs and capabilities. In other cases, additional work is necessary to determine whether a specific intervention has the potential to increase coverage levels and to be implemented successfully within different communities. Support and leadership are required from local public health agencies to test the effectiveness of and to implement promising interventions within a given community. Nationwide programs are not the best approach; instead states and local communities need to experiment with multiple strategies. Interventions designed to enhance the use of reminder–recall and assessment and feedback efforts in the private sector are likely to be highly effective. There is also a need for extensive and ongoing collaboration among local public health agencies, private health plans, and public and private health care providers to monitor and improve coverage levels.

Finding 4-12. Data on baseline and current immunization coverage levels are essential for determining the reliability or effectiveness of a selected intervention. Disruptions in data collection and assessment efforts impede the evaluation of intervention strategies and inhibit the determination of best practices.

Finding 4-13. It is unlikely that private health care plans will allocate adequate resources for populationwide services or community activities that promote the health of at-risk or hard-to-reach populations under current contractual arrangements.

SUMMING UP

The continued presence of many vaccine-preventable diseases throughout the world requires a persistent effort within each U.S. state to monitor disease reports and be prepared to respond swiftly to disease outbreaks. Similarly, surveillance and assessment of immunization coverage rates are still required so that discrepancies can be identified and resolved by reducing barriers or creating appropriate incentives within the health care system. Interventions such as assessment and feedback for public and private health care providers and client reminder–recall have been shown to improve immunization rates, and their implementation in a broad range of communities deserves full support. In areas where evidence of impact is uncertain, multiple strategies are necessary until certain approaches have achieved a significant enough impact to warrant their implementation across multiple populations. Policy linkages are also needed to strengthen system performance and to bridge gaps between the health care finance and health care delivery systems. System-level interventions can improve immunization coverage rates when they benefit key target audiences, but such interventions can be difficult to achieve when their implementation requires changes in professional behavior or organizational practices.

Ongoing developments within the science of vaccines, changes in the organization of the U.S. health care system, and movements within the population at large all place extraordinary demands on the public health infrastructure for immunization (see Chapter 2). These demands, in turn, have generated two key forces: (1) a persistent national need for the best available expertise, technology, tools, and leadership to complement state efforts to fulfill important public health functions, and (2) a strong desire to maintain flexibility in services and policies at the state and local levels to ensure responsiveness to immediate situations and state-driven priorities. These twin forces shape the infrastructure for immunization nationwide.

Finding 4-14. The immunization infrastructure within each state needs to have the capacity to perform a set of critical surveillance, disease control, safety oversight, and immunization improvement strategies to sustain current coverage rates. Reductions in this capacity will contribute to a weakening of vaccination levels and possible disease outbreaks.

Chapter 5 considers the various forms of local, state, and federal investments in each of the three roles discussed in this chapter. Recognizing that variations in organizational style can affect the level of resources required, we examine how some states have spent federal funds to support stand-alone as well as integrated services. Determining the level of resources necessary to sustain a viable and flexible infrastructure and how such investments should be allocated across state and national budgets is essential to ensure a viable, flexible, and stable national immunization system in the future. The particular roles and contributions of the National Immunization Program and Section 317 funds are considered in this context.

ENDNOTES

1. Diphtheria, tetanus, and pertussis (DTP) vaccine; poliovirus vaccine; measles, mumps, and rubella (MMR) vaccine; *Haemophilus influenzae* type b vaccine; and hepatitis B vaccine.

2. Up-to-date coverage is calculated for children at the 24-month mark. However, the retrospective nature of this survey results in a 3-year lag time in the data reported. Thus, for

example, data collected in fall 2000 on 5-year-old kindergarten entrants reflect coverage 3 years ago, when these children were age 2 (information provided by CDC).

3. Such conditions include the following: the records were transferred to another provider; the chart indicates that the child has moved or gone elsewhere; a mailed reminder card was returned without another local forwarding address; and the chart indicates that the parent says the child is seeing another provider, or that a home or telephone visit revealed the child was seeing another provider.

4. Examples cited are based on personal communication with providers in the New York inner-city area.

5. The New York City Department of Health provides such separate reports.

6. What constitutes a "fully functional registry" has been discussed and debated. Both NVAC and Wood et al. (1999:232) define a fully functional registry as one that tracks more than 95 percent of children under age 2 in the specified catchment area and provides an electronic immunization record that is accessible to providers. The Robert Wood Johnson Foundation (RWJF) considers a fully functional registry as one that includes all children in a given catchment area, with information about all doses of all vaccines delivered by all providers (NVAC, 1999b:16).

7. The items were derived from a conceptual definition prepared by the Cecil G. Sheps Center for Health Services Research at the University of North Carolina at Chapel Hill, which served as the national evaluation office for the All Kids Count initiative. RWJF also established a national program office for the initiative at the Task Force for Child Survival at the Carter Center in Atlanta, Georgia.

8. Duplicate records are included in these statistics, causing some states to show more than 100 percent of their children enrolled in the state registry.

9. The CDC survey defined public providers as "facilities operated partially or wholly with public funds (e.g., county public health clinics, community/migrant health centers, Indian Health Services, etc.) and/or the individual practitioners providing immunizations in such facilities." Private providers are defined as "health care facilities or practices operated solely with private funds and/or the individual practitioners providing immunizations in such facilities."

10. For the purposes of the CDC survey, enrollment was defined as "providers who have authorized access to the registry (e.g., written agreement, passwords, rights and responsibilities defined)" (information provided by CDC). Participation entails actually having submitted data to a registry in the last 6 months.

11. The percentage breakdown of vaccines claimed to cause adverse events is as follows:

DTP/P/DTP-Hib	71.7%
MMR or components	14.5%
IPV or OPV	10.0%
Tetanus/Td/DT	1.9%
New vaccines	0.5%
Other*	1.5%

*Vaccine not covered under VICP or unspecified vaccine (www.hrsa.dhhs.gov/bhpr/vicp/ABDVIC.htm and www.hrsa.dhhs.gov/bhpr/vicp/qanda.htm).

12. The TFCPS report includes only three strategies (increasing community demand for vaccination, enhancing access to vaccination services, and implementing provider-based interventions). Reducing out-of-pocket costs is described in the report as one of six interventions under the strategy of enhancing access to vaccination services. Given the importance of finance approaches in the present study, out-of-pocket cost intervention is categorized as a fourth strategy in this discussion.

13. It is possible that immunization records for these children were not available, contributing to a lower reporting rate than actually was the case.

5

Immunization Finance Policies and Practices

This chapter examines the finance policies and practices that enable the performance of the five roles of the national immunization system discussed in Chapters 2 through 4. Recognizing that immunization is the shared responsibility of the private and public sectors, including federal, state, and local governments, we consider how roles and responsibilities for immunization are distributed across different levels of government. We give particular attention to how current policies and practices establish the set of arrangements used to manage the community health system, target needy groups, ensure accountability within the public and private health care sectors, and allocate costs for these efforts. Our emphasis in this chapter is on children, since childhood immunization initiatives have been a major area of emphasis within the Section 317 program and the exclusive focus of the Vaccines for Children (VFC) effort. Although the federal government has established national goals to improve the rate of coverage for adult immunization among different age groups and special populations, financial resources to support this effort have been extremely limited and remain largely undocumented at the federal and state levels.

When public health clinics served as the primary point of service for delivering immunizations directly to disadvantaged populations, they had self-contained programs that performed multiple functions, including the purchase and administration of vaccines, the measurement of infectious disease patterns, the analysis of vaccine coverage rates and safety concerns, the development of programs to improve immunization coverage, and the performance of immunization policy and leadership roles within their communities. The public clinics were able to draw on patient revenues for specific services to help finance multiple types of public health activities.

The emphasis on providing vaccines as a fundamental part of primary health care in the private sector and the creation of the VFC program separated these roles. Vaccine purchase and service-delivery responsibilities were shifted largely to the private sector (although many public clinics continue to immunize children under Medicaid contracts and other service arrangements to meet the needs of children in local communities who do not qualify for federal assistance). Public health agencies were expected to sustain their traditional prevention and measurement efforts, while also assuming new responsibilities for administering the VFC program by enrolling private providers and monitoring a much larger set of immunization records. The policy role of public health agencies was thus expanded to include encouragement and oversight of private-sector performance in meeting national immunization goals; however, the VFC program did not provide the additional administrative resources that would enable the exercise of these functions at the local level.

This redefinition of roles and responsibilities occurred during a time when federal resources for state immunization infrastructure efforts were diminishing, and greater reliance was being placed on the states and the private sector to meet national health needs. States took on new responsibilities for the health care of infants and children through programs such as the State Children's Health Insurance Program (SCHIP), for example, which provided greater opportunity to work with managed care organizations in providing primary health care services (including immunizations) for Medicaid families.

These transitions and shifts in roles and responsibilities have resulted in ambiguity with regard to leadership, measurement, and finance responsibilities for the national immunization system. Resolving this ambiguity will require careful consideration of the level of oversight and resources necessary to ensure that the private and public health sectors can each contribute effectively in addressing national immunization needs. The new system of private-sector responsibility for clients who were once served by public health clinics is still evolving, and an array of issues is emerging that requires careful consideration before judgments are made about the successes or limitations of this new approach. In this context, the following sections review in turn the immunization roles and responsibilities and associated finance policies and practices of the private sector, local health departments, the states, and the federal government.

PRIVATE-SECTOR ROLES AND RESPONSIBILITIES

As noted earlier, most children receive their immunization services today from a private health care provider. Although the federal and state governments purchase more than half of the childhood vaccines distributed in the United States, private-sector health plans play an equally important role in determining how immunizations are delivered and influence how the costs of vaccine purchase, vaccine administration, and record keeping are distributed across the different levels of the immunization system. Three important concerns deserve attention in considering the roles and responsibilities of the private sector within this system: (1) whether immunization is a covered benefit within primary care health plans offered in the private sector, (2) whether private health plans monitor the immunization coverage levels of their members to determine whether their rates are up to date, and (3) whether private health plans are prepared to take action to improve coverage rates if disparities are found within their membership or their members' communities.

Immunization as a Covered Benefit

Most but not all private health plans include immunizations, but health plans and insurers do not cover all immunizations fully as a covered benefit. Private plans are more likely to cover immunizations for infants and children than for adults.[1] A preliminary draft of the Healthy People 2010 report included a goal of increasing to 90 percent the number of 2-year-old children who receive vaccinations as part of comprehensive primary care (baseline: 66 percent in 1996), which would constitute a 50 percent improvement over the year 2000 objectives (Department of Health and Human Services [DHHS], 1998). To achieve this goal, immunizations must be covered within primary care health plans. But even though earlier health objectives (DHHS, 1999) included a proposal to have all private plans cover immunizations fully as a basic benefit (Objective 20.15), many plans do not do so.[2]

Coverage of adult vaccines as a benefit within private health plans is highly variable and remains largely undocumented. The Healthy People 2010 objectives include increasing the level of coverage to 90 percent for annual influenza vaccinations (baseline: 63 percent in 1997) and for one-time pneumococcal vaccinations (baseline: 43 percent in 1997) for non-institutionalized adults aged 65 and older (DHHS, 2000). The 2010 objectives also propose increasing the level of coverage to 60 percent for annual influenza vaccinations (baseline: 25 percent in 1997) and for one-time pneumococcal vaccinations (baseline: 11 percent in 1997) for noninstitutionalized high-risk adults aged 18 to 64. However, no initiative has been announced within the federal or state governments that would advocate mandatory coverage of these vaccines within private health plans.

The National Vaccine Advisory Committee (NVAC) has recommended that the private health sector assume greater responsibility for improving and sustaining high levels of immunization coverage. For example, NVAC concluded in 1999 that the nation's immunization system is incomplete and cannot ensure the timely vaccination of the 11,000 U.S. infants born each day with a schedule that incorporates newly recommended vaccines (NVAC, 1999a). NVAC offered 15 recommendations for improving the immunization delivery system in both the public and private health sectors, including efforts to expand the scope of immunization coverage in private health plans (NVAC, 1999a). Among these recommendations were the following:

• All health insurance plans, including Employee Retirement Income Security Act (ERISA) self-insured plans, should offer first-dollar coverage for childhood vaccines recommended in the harmonized immunization schedule (NVAC, 1999a).[3]

• Managed care organizations and managed Medicaid plans should ensure complete immunization of their members based on the harmonized schedule. These efforts should include the use of effective strategies to improve and maintain immunization coverage rates, such as reminder and/or recall systems, practice-based coverage assessments, and provider incentives and education (see Chapter 4).

• All immunization providers, public and private, should assess the immunization coverage levels within their practices annually with assistance from state and local health departments, professional associations, and managed care organizations and other insurers.

One source of continuing uncertainty within both private and public health plans is the changing nature of the recommended immunization schedule (see Chapter 2). The federal government does not set universal immunization standards for the entire population. National recommendations are developed through collaboration among governmental bodies (e.g., the Advisory Committee on Immunization Practices [ACIP]) and professional advisory organizations (e.g., the Committee on Infectious Diseases of the American Academy of Pediatrics [AAP]), whose recommendations influence the scope of coverage benefits within federal programs such as Medicaid/Early and Periodic Screening, Diagnosis, and Treatment (EPSDT), SCHIP, and VFC. These same recommendations are considered by private health plans and state health agencies, which issue guidelines and enact requirements for their own populations, including immunization standards for school entry, day care licensing, and insurance coverage. As a result, immunization coverage requirements are not mandatory, and benefits vary by state and by health plan (see Appendix G).

Difficulties in Achieving Immunization Coverage Goals

In negotiating Medicaid or SCHIP contracts with private health care plans, many states have included immunization rates as key performance measures. Recent legislation, such as the Balanced Budget Act of 1997, has required health maintenance organizations (HMOs) that provide services for public beneficiaries to develop internal quality assurance processes that can be reviewed externally to assess contractor performance in meeting certain goals. To assist this effort, the Health Care Financing Administration (HCFA) has undertaken several quality-of-care activities, including a quality improvement system for managed care (known as QISMC). These initiatives are designed to help the states comply with their legal requirements to develop and implement quality assessment and improvement strategies. Public health officials have technical skills and expertise that can support these initiatives, but financial resources to support collaborative efforts involving HCFA, CDC, and state officials are not readily available within each state.

State health finance agencies can hold providers accountable for outcomes and performance in areas such as quality of care and basic benefits coverage through health contract negotiations as well as the use of incentives or penalties. State officials have indicated, however, that they often avoid adding such requirements to Medicaid health plans because doing so would make the plans unduly burdensome, and could discourage private providers or managed care organizations from participating in Medicaid at all or enrolling hard-to-reach participants. Similarly, private health plans with Medicaid or SCHIP contracts may incur additional costs in the use of evidence-based prevention strategies, such as recall and/or reminder systems, immunization registries, practice-based coverage assessments, and provider education.

In theory, physicians within a managed care system will offer preventive services (including immunization) that reduce the probability of costly illnesses. In the ideal world, managed care's emphasis on population-based health outcomes, analysis of small-area variations, data tools, provider profiling and accountability, coverage of prevention services, and benchmarking should promote the achievement of high immunization coverage rates for enrolled populations (Mullen, 1999). In practice, however, frequent changes occur in the mix of clients, providers, and health plans. Half of those enrolled in managed care plans do not remain for longer than 3 years. The transience of hard-to-reach patients contributes to a diffusion of responsibility, since providers are not obligated to check on or improve the immunization status of clients who visit their offices only once.

At present, little compelling evidence has emerged that managed care plans do any better or worse than fee-for-service systems in improving the immunization status of their members (Fairbrother et al., 1996). More important, variations in measurement and the movement of covered populations make it difficult to compare plan performance in improving immunization rates. The exclusion of providers that serve predominantly low-income clients or hard-to-reach groups from enrollment or assessment measures can contribute to positive measures of immunization coverage that suggest good performance. Such exclusionary practices are difficult to detect, especially in the absence of small-area population-based assessments that have sufficient sensitivity to reveal disparities in coverage rates and service utilization patterns among vulnerable groups. The lack of national or state-level trend data for Medicaid and other disadvantaged populations within private health plans (whether capitated managed care organizations or fee-for-service) also makes it difficult to follow immunization coverage rates within high-risk groups. States and local communities thus rely on special population-based studies to monitor coverage rates and to determine whether private plans within their areas are providing immunizations as expected (see Box 5-1). These special studies are generally financed by state public health agencies or CDC; both types of studies are commonly supported by the Section 317 program.

Inconsistencies in the measurement of immunization status within high-risk populations inhibit efforts to monitor community health, as well as the impact of private health plans on client and community outcomes. The absence of reliable data confounds attempts to hold plans accountable for the quality of their performance in improving the health status of their most vulnerable participants.

Several factors make it difficult to monitor service-delivery patterns within the private sector:

• Large numbers of uninsured and Medicaid families shift between public health clinics and private health plans (often as a result of monthly eligibility determinations), and the scattering of immunization records becomes a significant problem in establishing accountability requirements within multiple health plans. In California, for example, 40 percent of children lose Medicaid each year (Kuttner, 1999; Fairbrother, 2000; Fairbrother, 1999).

• Most health plans do not provide separate reimbursements to service providers for immunizations that are included in capitation payments for primary care or well-baby services for infants and children.

BOX 5-1
Small-Area Analysis for Detroit and Newark

Detroit, Michigan, and Newark, New Jersey, are cities with high poverty rates and large minority populations. Detroit residents in particular have problems with access to primary care. The immunization coverage rates of both cities are among the lowest for municipalities in the country and are well below the rates in the rest of their respective states. Detroit's rate for the 4:3:1 series for 2-year-olds in 1998 was 71.6 percent, while the rate for the rest of Michigan was 80.0 percent; Newark's rate in the same year was 66.3 percent, while that for the rest of New Jersey was 85.9 percent.

In Detroit, a multiyear CDC grant funds the university-based Child Health Network Immunization Project (CHNIP), providing $1.5 million for each of 5 years for innovations in practices designed to improve immunization coverage and for evaluation of these practices. The Detroit Medical Center at Wayne State University initially undertook neighborhood-specific door-to-door surveys to determine local health care resources and access to primary care providers. These surveys represented an effort to identify neighborhoods in which children were most at risk for underimmunization, and thus the most appropriate targets for CHNIP's outreach and facilitation services. This neighborhood-based assessment was conducted independently of the city's health department, which has neither the technical nor financial resources needed to conduct this type of study.

The Newark health department likewise has not conducted any small-area surveys of immunization coverage or access to primary care in recent years. It has, however, applied to the State of New Jersey for Public Health Priority Funds—state-appropriated monies that must be used for state-identified priorities—to conduct a study of immunization coverage rates within selected neighborhoods. City health officials and leaders appreciate the value of small-area analysis of immunization coverage rates in identifying pockets of need and targeting resources and special interventions accordingly. They frequently lack the resources needed to conduct such special studies and interventions as a routine function, however, and thus depend for this purpose on state and federal initiatives and resources.

• Immunizations for adolescents and adults may generate bills, but such data often are not available in a form that would allow comparisons of service patterns across health plans or regions.

• Although some plans may incur costs for developing and maintaining medical records data, the costs of compiling (or searching) immunization information are not recorded separately. As noted earlier, such compilation can be labor-intensive if records are scattered across multiple health settings.

Improving Performance and Implementing Prevention Methods

Managed care organizations based in large group practices (such as Kaiser Permanente and the Henry Ford Health System) have developed comprehensive medical record databases (often in electronic form) that provide information on a patient's health history, including immunizations. Such databases create provider performance profiles and, on occasion, may generate reminder–recall notices for immunization updates. Managed care organizations that serve Medicaid and other low-income populations (e.g., those served by SCHIP) expanded rapidly in the 1990s. These plans have less fully developed central patient information systems and contend with disenrollments of around 4 percent per month, often the result of monthly eligibility determinations (Kuttner, 1999; Fairbrother 2000; Fairbrother 1999). Thus, the potential for enrollment-based data systems to improve immunization coverage levels for Medicaid and SCHIP enrollees has not yet been realized.

Furthermore, given competition among various care networks and cost-containment practices of Medicaid managed care providers, data sharing efforts or performance assessment measures will be difficult to implement in the absence of a broader strategic approach that can provide either stability for clients (e.g., 1- or 2-year eligibility periods for services such as Medicaid or SCHIP); stability in the vaccine schedule; or financial incentives for providers so they can commit administrative resources to promoting high immunization coverage rates, the addition of new vaccines, and efforts to cover hard-to-reach populations. Restructuring financial incentives and payment methods for small inner-city practices in particular so they can implement quality improvement and preventive approaches (such as reminder–recall systems) would help mitigate personal and systemic barriers to care for families that already have access to a medical home and a primary care provider.

In ensuring that significant disparities in access to vaccines and coverage do not emerge within vulnerable groups, state public health agencies will need to assume leadership and coordination roles in the assessment, documentation, and improvement of immunization rates in the private sector. Other IOM reports (1988 and 1997) have described in detail the information gathering and analytical functions associated with these roles. Since the delivery of immunization services has shifted from the public to the private sector over the past decade, careful attention will need to be focused on ways to gather and compare data on immunization status, vaccine coverage benefits, and service-delivery costs from both public and private health insurance plans. Key concerns include the following:

• What is the appropriate measure of coverage of a given population? (the whole population? all of those enrolled with a selected group of providers? those enrolled for a certain length of time with certain providers?)

• How do we know we have accurate data on selected groups within a given population? What sample size and population characteristics are the appropriate selection criteria?

• What level of vaccine coverage is an acceptable measure of immunization coverage within a given population?

• What constitutes a reasonable effort to determine and improve coverage levels within specific population groups?

In addition to the assessment of immunization coverage levels, public health agencies are consistently encouraged to exercise leadership in working with private providers to adopt model strategies (such as routine audits and reminder–recall systems) to maintain high rates of coverage. A recent NVAC report, for example, urges indemnity health and self-insured plans to cover immunization benefits for their members, and recommends that all Medicaid-enrolled providers who immunize children participate in the VFC program (NVAC, 1999a). Despite this encouragement, a national consensus about the implications of not meeting certain performance standards does not yet exist. Who is to be held responsible if a large percentage of Medicaid clients do not acquire immunizations in a timely manner? Who is obligated to ensure that high-risk adults are encouraged to receive influenza and pneumococcal vaccines?

How to finance such assessment, assurance, and leadership roles lies at the crux of the present study. It is clearly in the national interest to have a strong public health system in place nationwide that can provide reliable data and indicators, and support public and private health care providers and local communities in improving their immunization performance. At the same time, private health plans and providers need to share the burden of incorporating prevention efforts into their practices and programs (see Box 5-2). A shared partnership, responsive to local needs and resources, can integrate public health activities within the complex maze of state health finance and health insurance initiatives to improve the health status of vulnerable groups.

Finding 5-1. Child and adult immunization coverage requirements are not mandatory, and benefits vary by state and by health plan. Disparities in covered benefits between public and private health plans and within the private sector make it difficult both to assess immunization levels and to fix responsibility for addressing coverage gaps on a population-wide basis.

BOX 5-2
Rochester Private–Public Partnership Approach

One example of a coordinated, strategic private–public partnership approach has been demonstrated in Rochester, New York, with favorable results. Szylagyi (1999) prepared a randomized sample of 30,000 charts from Rochester's 80 pediatric provider practices, and reported 1993 coverage rates as follows: 55 percent in the inner city, 65 percent in the remaining urban areas, and 75 percent in the suburbs. The study tested the impact of an intervention consisting of a tiered reminder–recall–outreach intervention, with outreach (the most expensive approach) targeted to the most hard-to-reach portion (5–10 percent) of the study population. The results of the tiered intervention included a 20 percent increase in immunization coverage and an 11 percent increase in preventive service visits, which had the spillover effect of increasing anemia screening (by 12 percent) and lead screening (8 percent). The same intervention was implemented countywide, and a follow-up survey in 1996 showed significant increases in coverage. The greatest improvements were for inner-city children, whose rates increased from 55 percent in 1993 to 75 percent in 1996. These interventions have been financed by a unique collaboration between the county and state health departments that has allowed county health officials to pool money from several categorical programs. As more clients seek immunizations within their medical homes among private providers, other sources of revenue are able to finance some of the costs of the immunization program.

Finding 5-2. Responsibility for ensuring the immunization status of selected communities or at-risk groups is currently diffused among multiple parties, including clients themselves, health care providers, health plans, health finance agencies, and public health agencies. Although the assessment of immunization coverage rates within local communities remains a fundamental responsibility of public health agencies, few local or state agencies have sufficient resources to conduct independent studies, and most must rely on data provided by others.

Finding 5-3. Needy populations are increasingly receiving care within the private health sector as Medicaid and SCHIP contract with health plans to provide benefits, including immunizations. However, the absence of reliable indicators of this shift to privately managed care has made it more difficult to monitor immunization coverage levels for the total population as well as vulnerable groups. Both private and public health care providers must be held accountable to a consistent set of measures that can be used to assess and compare their performance in adequately immunizing public program beneficiaries.

Finding 5-4. Collaborative efforts with private health plans and local providers can improve the quality of data available to support assessment studies. However, state health agencies must provide the leadership, technical expertise, and independence that are essential to the integrity of assessment efforts.

Finding 5-5. The private sector plays a significant role in offering immunization benefits and has the capability to implement prevention practices that would improve and sustain immunization coverage rates among vulnerable groups. To exercise this capability, however, the private sector requires assistance and oversight so that accurate immunization coverage rates can be established, and the causes of coverage disparities can be monitored.

Finding 5-6. If immunization assessment is to be enhanced within private provider offices, the private health sector must make behavioral changes that require more than the infusion of federal or state funds. Such efforts must involve partnerships with national, state, and local professional groups and private health plans so that common strategies can be developed and implemented at the local level. States require incentives as well as financial assistance if these public–private partnerships are to be implemented at the local level to improve the quality of local immunization services and sustain high rates of immunization coverage among vulnerable populations.

LOCAL HEALTH DEPARTMENT ROLES AND RESPONSIBILITIES

More than 3,000 public health agencies across the United States provide a broad array of programs and services staffed by technical, administrative, and support personnel within county, metropolitan, and statewide jurisdictions. As noted in an earlier IOM report, the jurisdictions and authority of local health departments overlap, and their service responsibilities and fiscal capabilities are heterogeneous (IOM, 1988). Significant variation exists in their funding sources, ranging from completely state supported to funded exclusively at the local level.

Many states rely on a county system to deliver public health services, and in recent years, many local governments have dealt directly with the federal government to obtain financial assistance in meeting the needs of vulnerable populations. The importance of using federal funds to support local initiatives is reflected in the administration of the Section 317 program within CDC. In addition to the state and other political jurisdiction grants awarded by the National Immunization Program, five metropolitan regions are eligible to receive federal immunization grants (Houston and San Antonio, Texas; New York City, New York; Chicago, Illinois; and Philadelphia, Pennsylvania).[4]

The basic responsibility for public health is at the state level, but states differ in the ways in which they administer local public health programs. Some states rely entirely on state employees for local services. Others delegate their responsibilities to county or local health departments that must rely upon local revenues to supplement state resources. In some metropolitan areas, local health departments are larger than the entire public health staff of smaller or more rural states. Some states have highly centralized data collection efforts used to monitor disease outbreaks and vaccination coverage status, while others have only the results of scattered studies within local health departments that can afford to conduct them. Similarly, some states use their own or federal funds to support programs such as Women, Infants, and Children (WIC) linkages or outreach efforts to improve local coverage levels, while such initiatives are supported entirely with local funds in a limited number of jurisdictions.

Infrastructure Investments and Immunization Programs

Prior to the expansion of the Section 317 program in the early 1990s, most local health departments served primarily as providers of immunizations. Only a handful of state agencies were actively involved in data collection, coverage assessment, or partnership initiatives. With the increase in Section 317 funding in the early 1990s and legislative changes that allowed the federal government to support direct services within the states, funds became available for local immunization programs, extensive experimentation with new measurement efforts, and the formation of new public and private partnerships.

According to an informal survey conducted by the National Association of City and County Health Officials (NACCHO), in the early 1990s local health departments used Section 317 funds to develop new immunization programs in such areas as increased assessment, outreach, performance measurement, program linkages, and information management (NACCHO, 1999). Staff time and clinic hours devoted to immunization activities increased in urban areas, and health clinics were established in rural areas and isolated communities to improve access to immunization services. Evening, weekend, and satellite clinics, specialty clinics (hepatitis B and school-based clinics), and partnerships with other organizations such as WIC and Head Start were developed to target hard-to-reach populations. Local health departments also used federal funds to send staff to health fairs, strengthen advertising and public information campaigns, and improve tracking and recall systems used to survey at-risk populations. Incentive programs for patients were established, and staff training was enhanced to keep all providers up to date on changing vaccines and schedules. More localities had the time and support necessary to become involved in the development of regional immunization registries.

These investments in broader outreach, access, and educational efforts had contributed to a significant increase in immunization coverage rates by the latter part of the decade. National childhood immunization rates increased from 74.2 to 79.2 percent for the 4:3:1:3 series between 1995 (surveying children born between February 1992 and May 1994) and 1998 (surveying children born between February 1995 and May 1997) (information provided by CDC) (see Table 1-2 in Chapter 1). Research has indicated that certain types of programs, especially in such areas as provider record audits, reminder–recall systems, and WIC linkages (see Chapter 4), contributed to the increased coverage rates reported during the past decade.

Impact of Program Cutbacks and Budget Reductions

When federal appropriations for infrastructure grants began to decline in 1996, local budgets for immunization services were substantially reduced, and in some cases eliminated entirely (programs were eliminated, for example, in Duvall County, Florida; Zanesville-Muskingum County, Ohio; Noble County, Ohio; Dakota County, Minnesota; and Hennepin County, Minnesota). In some cases, local governments used local tax dollars to subsidize immunization program activities; in other cases, money was redirected from flexible funding sources or cut from programs and services such as environmental health, home health visits, and WIC clinics (NACCHO, 1999). But few local jurisdictions had sufficient resources to support technical personnel or broad initiatives, and project cutbacks became routine.

Many cities and counties experienced up to a 50 percent reduction in immunization infrastructure funding relative to the original grant funds in the early 1990s (NACCHO, 1999). The decrease in federal funding affected each of the six roles of the immunization system with the exception of vaccine purchase, since the new VFC and SCHIP programs covered the latter costs. For example (NACCHO, 1999):

• Cutbacks occurred in direct clinical services, resulting in reductions in clinic hours and staff, the closing of entire clinics in some areas, elimination of physician training, and reductions in update notices for private providers.
• Resources for computer upgrading and maintenance were reduced, slowing the use of electronic records and automated tracking.

• Community assessment activities were discontinued, diminishing the tracking of immunization coverage levels.

• Local health departments decreased programs designed to improve immunization coverage rates among hard-to-reach populations, such as home visits and outreach activities.

• Partnerships with organizations such as WIC and Head Start were discontinued because of the lack of staff time to assist with outreach.

• Health departments' capabilities to conduct community education were reduced, and local agencies had fewer resources to assist with regional immunization registries.

In addition, the reduction or elimination of many local program coordinator positions resulted in a loss of leadership that disrupted communication and assistance from state health departments. The resulting delays in obtaining information from state health departments have made it more difficult for local health departments to remain informed about changes in vaccine schedules and to address professional and public concerns in a timely manner. Record and recall systems became increasingly fragmented, and today many health departments no longer conduct full immunization audits of local providers.

In some areas, local health officials responding to the NACCHO survey reported frustration and sometimes resentment with regard to the impact of the federal cutbacks on programmatic efforts. One Western state noted: "As a result of the efforts staff supported through the immunization program, we have been able to raise our immunization rates from 56 percent to almost 90 percent. It seems tragic that funding should be cut when we are finally beginning to see some success" (NACCHO, 1999:1). Similarly, according to a Midwestern state, "It seems ironic that while immunization rates have risen slowly, we know that the last 25–30 percent will be the most difficult to reach, and now funds are cut" (NACCHO, 1999:1).

Cuts in local programs not only reduced public health services, but also decreased the emphasis placed on the importance of adhering to immunization schedules within the private sector. One health official in a Western state reported: "The greatest impact is the loss of sufficient infrastructure to sustain highly effective systems change and to sustain necessary community assessment activities that not only track coverage outcomes, but also served as a source of community opinions and knowledge, attitudes and behaviors" (NACCHO, 1999:2).

Finding 5-6. Local health departments have the capability to play important roles in working with public- and private-sector providers to assess and improve immunization coverage rates. However, they require state and federal assistance to perform these roles.

Finding 5-7. Reductions in federal assistance grants to the states have decreased and sometimes eliminated important local infrastructure efforts in areas related to data collection, technical assistance, immunization assessment, and community outreach.

STATE ROLES AND RESPONSIBILITIES

States have important responsibilities for public health services in general and immunization in particular (IOM, 1994b; IOM, 1988). In particular, they:

• Adopt policies and practices that influence vaccine coverage and the delivery of immunization services within local jurisdictions (including the adoption of universal purchase policies in 15 states).
• Create and enforce state mandates for the inclusion of immunization benefits in private health insurance plans.
• Establish immunization requirements for day care and school entry, as well as long-term health care facilities.
• Set Medicaid and SCHIP eligibility criteria and provider reimbursement levels within federal requirements, negotiate managed care terms and contracts within the limits of federal mandates, and determine the scope of services to be included in the benefits package above the federal minimum.
• Distribute publicly purchased vaccines and administer immunizations as part of their responsibility for direct health care for indigent populations.
• Contract with health plans for state and county employees, set health guidelines for their welfare clients (such as immunization requirements), and provide public health services for the general public.
• Have historically borne the burden of disease surveillance; containment (initially through the use of quarantines); vaccine safety oversight; and health records management in the areas of infectious disease and, more recently, immunization coverage.

Despite this array of activities, state immunization infrastructure efforts are poorly described in the research literature. States do not track routine expenditures for assessment, assurance, or regulatory activities. The common practice is simply to divide costs between vaccine purchase budgets and program operations as general categories.

Infrastructure Investments and Immunization Programs

Immunization infrastructure encompasses the direct labor, administration, supplies, facilities and equipment, training, and overhead costs related to each state's overall program. Every state immunization program is concerned with vaccine purchase and service delivery, but variations exist in the scope of the population that is served and the settings in which services are delivered. In most states, the core mission and basic purpose of the state program are focused solely on children, ensuring that they receive the immunizations recommended by ACIP (Freed et al., 1999). At the same time, the state survey and eight case studies prepared for the present IOM study demonstrated significant variation in state activities that reflect differences in levels of need, resources, and local practices (see Appendixes D and E).

Section 317 Infrastructure Support. The vast majority of infrastructure support for immunization within the states comes through Section 317 grant awards administered by CDC. Following the 1989–1990 measles outbreaks, federal and state officials expressed alarm about the adequacy of existing immunization delivery systems and identified strategies designed to improve immunization coverage rates among vulnerable populations.

In the midst of turbulent health care reform and the expanded reliance on private managed care plans to deliver public health benefits to individuals eligible for federal assistance, the increased budget for Section 317 (1992–1994) and the creation of the VFC program (1994) enabled states to do more to improve immunization coverage levels. In the high-funding years of the Section 317 program, states used their grant awards primarily to expand local services (33 of 50 states) and outreach and education (33 of 50 states) (see Table 5-1). About one-third of the states developed new partnerships with WIC clinics (13 of 50 states) or initiated state or regional registries with encouragement from CDC (16 of 50 states). A few states used their federal grants to improve statewide assessment efforts (7 states), expand vaccination campaigns in general or specialized areas (5 states), or add state staff to assist with coordination and policy development (8 states). In addition to the national studies supported by CDC, 11 states conducted their own immunization coverage surveys during 1995–1997, using methods that included annual birth certificate studies, retrospective school surveys, cluster surveys, and registries (see Box 5-3).

Beyond operating their own programs, many states used their Section 317 funds to monitor and help improve immunization rates within the private sector. These efforts, such as the use of Clinic Assessment Software Application (CASA) audits[5] and general management of the VFC program, represent important features of the new roles of public health agencies in assessing and ensuring the quality of private health care services financed through public funds. Yet such efforts are often the most difficult to document because they do not constitute a defined "program" in many public health agencies. The ability of health agencies to

TABLE 5-1 Main Uses of Section 317 Infrastructure Grant Funds in High-Funding Years (1994–1996)[a]

State	Outreach and Education[b]	Assessment	WIC Linkage[c]	Registry[d]	Addition of State Staff	Local Service-Delivery Expansion[e]	Expanded Vaccination Campaigns[f]
AL	✓		✓		✓	✓	
AK	✓					✓	
AZ	No specific information; used for activities focused on meeting immunization goals for 2-year-olds					✓	✓
AR							
CA	✓					✓	
CO	✓					✓	
CT	✓	✓		✓			
DE	✓	✓	✓		✓	✓	
DC	✓	✓	✓			✓	
FL	✓					✓	
GA							✓
HI							
ID	✓	✓					
IL	✓		✓		✓	✓	
IN	✓		✓			✓	
IA						✓	
KS	✓		✓	✓		✓	
KY				✓			
LA	✓						
ME	No information						
MD	✓	✓	✓	✓		✓	
MA	✓	✓	✓			✓	
MI	✓					✓	
MN						✓	
MS	✓				✓	✓	
MO				✓		✓	✓
MT	✓						✓
NE	✓		✓			✓	

NV	✓		✓		✓	
NH	✓		✓		✓	
NJ	✓	✓				
NM	No information					
NY	No information	✓			✓	
NC	✓		✓		✓	
ND	✓					
OH	✓		✓	✓		
OK	✓					
OR	No specific information; passed on to LHDs and CMHCs for immunization activities					
PA	✓					
RI	No information					
SC	✓	✓	✓		✓	
SD	✓	✓	✓		✓	
TN	✓	✓	✓		✓	
TX	✓	✓	✓			
UT	✓					
VT	✓					
VA	✓		✓	✓	✓	
WA	✓	✓			✓	
WV	✓	✓			✓	
WI	✓		✓		✓	
WY					✓	

[a]Not a comprehensive (or mutually exclusive) list of state activities, but rather the activities they chose to highlight.

[b]Outreach and education includes such activities as work with coalitions, media campaigns, and provider education.

[c]WIC = Special Supplemental Nutrition Program for Women, Infants, and Children.

[d] Registry activities include software development and purchase of hardware and other equipment.

[e]Local service-delivery expansion includes contracts with local health departments (LHDs), community and migrant health centers (CMHCs), and other partners to extend clinic hours, offer weekend clinics, add nursing staff, and so on.

[f]Expanded vaccination campaigns include adult and adolescent campaigns, as well as campaigns focused on specific vaccines (e.g., hepatitis B).

SOURCE: Freed et al., 1999.

BOX 5-3
Sample of State and Local Immunization Coverage Surveys*

Birth Certificate Survey
    Georgia
    Mississippi
    Tennessee
    Florida
    Oregon

Retrospective School Survey
    California (this year)
    Minnesota (performed once "a few years ago")
    New York (annual)
    Kansas

Cluster Survey
    Washington (performed for several counties 2 or 3 years ago)

Registry-Based Survey
    South Carolina

Child Health Network
    New York City (cluster survey)
    Detroit (cluster survey)
    Colorado
    San Diego (random digit dialed survey)

*Surveys supported by state or local funds. Full range of surveys is not known.

SOURCE: A. Bauer, CDC, personal communication, May 21, 1999.

support management and oversight roles is challenged by programmatic restrictions within federal programs such as VFC, Medicaid, and SCHIP and the absence of general funds at the federal or state level (apart from the Section 317 grants) that can support monitoring and assessment functions. Health agencies realized that they were expected to assume new responsibilities that were difficult to justify and were unable to obtain the necessary resources to exercise this role.

States initially had broad discretion in the use of federal funds, although CDC provided guidance each year to emphasize certain program objectives and priorities. In 1998, CDC announced a set of required activities under 18 program components to guide state programs and to provide a basis for comparison of state efforts (information provided by CDC) (see

Figure 1-5 in Chapter 1). The 18 program components, called "core functions," are currently used by CDC to track federal and state allocations for immunization activities (information provided by CDC).

Other Federal Support. In addition to categorical grants from federal immunization programs, some states receive funding for immunization-related activities (including vaccine purchase, infrastructure support, or both) through other federal programs (Freed et al., 1999). This type of federal support is very limited, however, and is often focused on a particular program or one-time support, rather than general and ongoing infrastructure support. For example:

- Four states receive Medicaid matching funds to support registry or outreach activities.
- Ten states report using Maternal and Child Health (MCH/Title V) block grant funds to support immunization efforts.
- Four states draw on Public Health Service (PHS) block grant funds for immunization programs.
- A small number of states draw on other funding sources, including WIC (2 states), Temporary Assistance for Needy Families (TANF) (1 state), and other state/federal grants (4 states).

In a few cases, federal programs require states to carry out certain functions without federal financial support. The VFC program, for example, restricts its expenditures primarily to the purchase and distribution of vaccines. Although some funds are available to coordinate provider enrollment, the VFC program does not support the administration of vaccine products, the recruitment or training of VFC providers, or the records management of immunization coverage levels. By necessity, state public health agencies support VFC administration with other funds, and routinely draw on their Section 317 grants for this purpose.

State-Level Funding. CDC first requested estimates of state-level contributions for immunization programs in the proposals for fiscal year (FY) 2000 grants. Self-reports by the states indicated that they expected to provide $109 million for vaccine purchase and $231 million for program operations to support immunization efforts in the year 2000. This figure includes funds provided by other federal agencies that are used within the state for immunization programs, along with state-level revenues and private resources. The state-level contributions are not evenly distributed: half the states (25) directly fund infrastructure support, and 4 of these states have such funding as a substantial portion (more than 40 percent) of their infrastructure budget (Freed et al., 1999) (see Figure 5-1). A few states

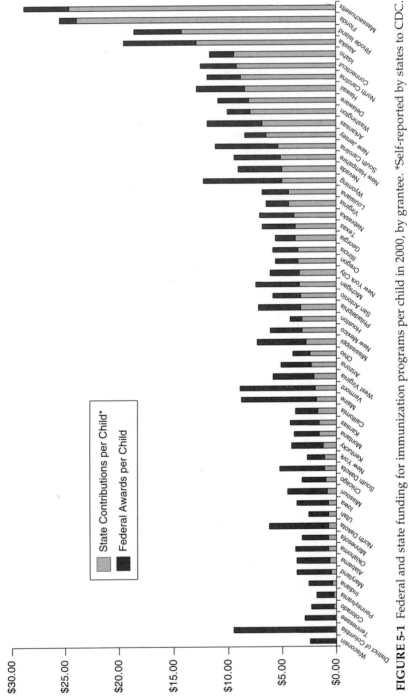

FIGURE 5-1 Federal and state funding for immunization programs per child in 2000, by grantee. *Self-reported by states to CDC. NOTE: May not include all appropriated and in-kind contributions. SOURCE: Information provided by CDC.

provide support for specific initiatives. For example, 15 states have direct or in-kind state funding for registry development (although the size and length of such funding vary).

Twenty-one states do not fund immunization infrastructure, and four recently redirected state funds from vaccine purchase to infrastructure support. More common across states is indirect support of the immunization program through intergovernmental transfers, involving other state or federal programs or services. In addition, many states provide in-kind contributions in the form of assistance from school nurses and secretaries, who conduct school-based assessments of children's immunization status, and from local health departments (e.g., facilities and overhead, and locally funded staff who perform multiple duties, including the delivery of immunizations) (Freed et al., 1999). Five states mentioned the contributions of volunteers in conducting various immunization activities.

State Finance Practices

State vaccine purchase grants from CDC remained relatively stable during the 1990s (close to about $130 million per year in the period 1996–1999; see Table 5-2). Although the VFC program assumed responsibility for distributing large quantities of vaccine directly to providers that immunized disadvantaged children, changes in the vaccine schedule and initial uncertainties about the reliability of the VFC program caused state health officials to stockpile surplus vaccines. Reliance on federal funds for vaccine purchase also allowed some states to use their own revenues for other, more risky investments in community assistance and registry programs. In one year (1995), a significant decrease in state vaccine expenses created a surplus of $60 million in the Section 317 vaccine purchase awards, which CDC transferred to state operations/infrastructure support with congressional approval (information provided by CDC).[6]

Several factors within each state influence levels of public health investment and administrative systems, including demographics (such as population size and urban/rural distribution), per capita wealth, tax revenues, the size of the uninsured populations, and health care traditions (Marquis and Long, 1997). Finance practices may also be affected by the organizational structure of state health programs. For example, in states such as Maryland and Texas, where Medicaid is located administratively or fiscally within the department of health, state agencies used vaccine purchase savings from the implementation of VFC to increase provider reimbursement fees, or to purchase additional vaccine for school health programs or other groups not covered by VFC. In states where Medicaid is not housed within the department of health, VFC savings were commonly not captured within the immunization program, and sometimes

TABLE 5-2 Annual Awards and Expenditures of Section 317 Direct Assistance (DA) Vaccine Purchase Funds (in millions of dollars)

Year	New Funds	Re-awarded Funds[a]	Total Award	Expenditures	Percentage of Total Award Expended[b]
1990	149.0	0.0	149.0	106.3	71%
1991	112.9	37.5	150.3	102.5	68%
1992	156.2	26.8	183.1	121.6	66%
1993	171.2	43.9	215.1	156.2	77%
1994	136.2	86.3	222.5	171.9	61%
1995[c]	83.1	74.3	157.4	96.3	59%
1996	133.3	11.0	144.2	111.2	77%
1997	124.0	34.7	158.7	128.4	81%
1998[d]	108.2	34.9	143.1	135.6	95%
1999	128.0	8.0	136.0	NA	NA

NOTE: CDC notes that 1990 was the first year in which grants were administered centrally, instead of by regional offices. There is limited background information with which to substantiate these amounts, and as a result their accuracy is questionable. In 1994, an additional $30,672,686 in appropriated vaccine purchase funds was paid directly to the Department of the Treasury for floor stock excise taxes on behalf of all the grantees when the Vaccine Compensation Act was reauthorized.

[a]Funds awarded in previous years but not obligated.
[b]Based on year-end unobligated balances for 1990–1997 reported to CDC as of April 1, 1999.
[c]$53 million rescinded from unobligated balances in fiscal year 1996 (comprising funds from 1993, 1994, and 1995).
[d]CDC estimates for expenditures and percentage of 1998 award expended.

SOURCE: Information provided by CDC.

were not protected within the general health budget at all (Freed et al., 1999).

An additional finance issue involves differences in federal and state fiscal years. Legislatures in many states appropriate federal funds, so that expenditures cannot be made until the legislature has approved them. State legislatures do not meet every year in every state. State purchasing and hiring procedures are legal controls of major importance that can delay action in response to federal initiatives. The processes for the preparation and approval of capital budgets and general expenditure budget processes are often separate in many states and involve lengthy and detailed procedures.

States also differ in the extent to which they respond to unmet needs; CDC has reported more than a five-fold variation across states in the proportion of the population served by health department–operated clinics. Fifteen states have adopted universal purchase policies (see Chapter 3); the remainder contribute a relatively small amount of state funds (i.e., less than 30 percent of total public vaccine purchase in the state) or nothing at all to supply vaccines to disadvantaged adults and children.

In 1994, an earlier IOM committee warned state and federal officials that "current approaches to immunizing children are not sufficient to reach the 1996 target of 90 percent coverage" (IOM, 1994b:26). This prediction was borne out: the overall immunization rate for preschool children (aged 19 to 35 months) increased to just 79.2 percent in 1998 (information provided by CDC). The committee's report states: "To guide the development of new programs and the allocation of funding and other resources, states must have comprehensive information on children's unmet needs for immunizations and on the factors that keep them from receiving those immunizations" (IOM, 1994b:26). Recognizing that state needs will vary, the report continues:

> No single plan will lead to comprehensive immunization coverage in every state. Common themes may exist, but each state must find a solution that takes into account the specific immunization needs of its children and how its providers and organizational resources can be used to meet those needs. The committee is persuaded that solutions will require state collaboration with local health departments, private providers, state and local chapters of providers' professional organizations, community groups, and others. States should be exploring how to strengthen primary care to meet not only children's immunization needs but also their other important health care requirements. (IOM, 1994b:27)

In addressing the finance requirements for this enhanced set of efforts, the report notes: "States are expected to apply CDC funds previously spent on vaccine purchase to improving the infrastructure for delivering immunization services" (IOM, 1994b:22).

The present committee's analysis of budgetary trends, conducted 5 years after that earlier IOM study, suggests that this expectation has not been realized. In many respects, state immunization programs received mixed messages during the 1990s about the delivery of immunization services. On the one hand, the Childhood Immunization Initiative and the early increases in Section 317 funding encouraged the states to rely on their public health clinics to improve access to immunizations by increasing hours of service, availability of walk-in appointments, mobile service units, immunization fairs, and other activities. Many states directed Section 317 infrastructure funds to these areas by supporting additional staff and equipment (Freed et al., 1999).

At the same time that states were encouraged to use their public clinics to expand access and foster outreach, however, the VFC program and Medicaid reforms created a counteremphasis by promoting immunizations for children in their private medical homes and encouraging greater reliance on managed care organizations to serve populations that once relied on public health clinics. In the majority of states, VFC has made strides in this area, assisted by the increasing penetration of managed care plans, the proliferation of Medicaid managed care plans, and the implementation of SCHIP. Of the 46 states that reported this information in response to the survey conducted for the present study, 40 had experienced decreases in the proportion of children receiving vaccines in the public sector, and some of these decreases were substantial (Freed et al., 1999).

Still, the need for public-sector immunization services has not disappeared. As discussed earlier, most children receive their services from private providers, but the trend toward private-sector immunization delivery is uneven (see Table 5-3). Indeed, the number of doses of vaccine provided in the public sector did not decrease appreciably during the 1990s even though the overall numbers of clients were reduced, a fact that can be attributed to the increase in the number of recommended doses for newborns and adolescents (Freed et al., 1999). Residual needs for vaccine remain in most public clinics, reflecting the realities of serving vulnerable children and adults who have urgent needs and are unable to take advantage of other health care resources. Furthermore, the clientele of public health clinics has changed; the current clientele requires more effort to maintain and improve immunization status because they are often more transient, more socially isolated within their community, and more likely to have contact with multiple health care providers in the public and private sectors.

Furthermore, recent trends in poverty measures suggest that the needs of those who depend on public programs may become more complex. While the overall proportion of children living below the poverty line has declined somewhat during recent years, the number of children in extreme poverty may be increasing (Center on Budget and Policy Priorities, 1999). These trends suggest that although fewer children may be eligible for federal and state assistance programs, those who are eligible may face more barriers, and require greater assistance, than was previously the norm. Anecdotal reports from clinical sites have confirmed this observation (Szilagyi, 1999).

State health officers in various regions of the United States have reported that managed care providers sometimes refer their patients to public clinics for vaccine services because such immunizations can then be provided without cost to the managed care plan (and the plan's assess-

TABLE 5-3 Estimated Vaccination Coverage with 4:3:1:3[a] Series Among Children 19–35 Months of Age by Provider Type, Census Division, and State—United States, National Immunization Survey (NIS), 1998[b]

Division/State	NIS Population Size[c]	Vaccinated by Public Provider (%)	Vaccinated by Private Provider (%)	Vaccinated by Mixed Providers (%)	Vaccinated by Other Provider (%)
National	5,634,624	16.9	54.6	7.9	20.5
East North Central	893,232	18.0	51.3	9.5	21.2
Illinois	265,220	17.6	51.7	7.2	23.5
Indiana	120,294	22.0	44.6	13.6	19.8
Michigan	192,317	21.2	46.9	13.1	18.8
Ohio	216,883	16.0	58.1	6.1	19.8
Wisconsin	98,518	12.2	52.0	11.4	24.4
East South Central	324,385	31.9	38.7	10.7	18.7
Alabama	88,454	24.3	45.0	11.3	19.4
Kentucky	74,893	32.2	40.9	10.7	16.2
Mississippi	58,458	49.3	20.6	8.1	22.0
Tennessee	102,580	28.2	42.1	11.7	18.1
Middle Atlantic	758,284	7.7	65.9	4.2	22.2
New Jersey	168,721	5.7	66.3	7.0	21.0
New York	376,586	8.9	65.6	2.0	23.5
Pennsylvania	212,976	7.0	66.1	5.8	21.0
Mountain	369,444	21.6	46.1	10.4	21.9
Arizona	105,862	17.3	50.1	4.7	27.9
Colorado	77,203	17.1	52.4	8.9	21.6
Idaho	26,666	28.2	47.9	14.5	9.3
Montana	15,582	25.6	42.1	13.0	19.2
New Mexico	39,573	19.4	38.1	14.0	28.5
Nevada	40,496	33.3	40.9	12.5	13.2
Utah	55,177	24.2	39.1	16.2	20.4
Wyoming	8,886	23.7	48.2	13.4	14.6
New England	249,411	7.2	72.1	2.4	18.2
Connecticut	64,926	4.6	77.0	2.0	16.4
Massachusetts	113,833	7.1	72.0	2.0	18.9
Maine	21,136	7.5	68.2	1.9	22.4
New Hampshire	21,355	7.5	68.4	5.7	18.3
Rhode Island	18,183	18.2	67.2	1.1	13.5
Vermont	9,976	5.4	66.8	6.3	21.5
Pacific	1,014,554	11.6	56.2	7.5	24.7
Alaska	14,136	32.1	30.8	10.6	26.4
California	793,466	11.1	56.8	7.2	24.9
Hawaii	26,902	6.2	61.7	4.9	27.2
Oregon	64,318	18.0	50.5	9.9	21.7
Washington	115,732	10.1	57.3	8.3	24.4
South Atlantic	984,856	17.0	58.2	8.1	16.6
District of Columbia	10,816	14.5	58.9	3.1	23.5
Delaware	13,865	6.4	63.5	2.5	27.6

continued

TABLE 5-3 Continued

Division/State	NIS Population Size[c]	Vaccinated by Public Provider (%)	Vaccinated by Private Provider (%)	Vaccinated by Mixed Providers (%)	Vaccinated by Other Provider (%)
Florida	288,797	15.5	61.8	7.9	14.7
Georgia	165,386	24.3	52.2	9.4	14.2
Maryland	111,625	5.3	73.1	1.6	20.0
North Carolina	151,281	17.4	51.5	11.9	19.2
South Carolina	75,919	34.5	36.3	12.8	16.4
Virginia	138,479	12.7	64.5	6.3	16.5
West Virginia	28,687	15.5	59.2	10.1	15.2
West North Central	363,354	19.5	52.4	8.1	20.1
Iowa	52,688	21.8	48.1	12.4	17.8
Kansas	53,968	30.4	42.1	10.3	17.3
Minnesota	94,025	6.6	65.6	4.1	23.7
Missouri	104,231	25.9	49.6	8.6	15.9
North Dakota	10,748	29.0	34.8	11.6	24.6
Nebraska	32,466	11.4	53.7	6.2	28.7
South Dakota	15,228	18.5	50.8	8.9	21.8
West South Central	677,104	25.9	45.9	9.7	18.5
Arkansas	51,925	49.3	22.1	11.7	16.9
Louisiana	89,357	32.6	42.7	10.5	14.2
Oklahoma	66,406	30.7	36.2	10.3	22.8
Texas	469,416	21.4	50.4	9.2	19.0

[a]4:3:1:3 = Four or more doses of diphtheria, tetanus, and pertussis vaccine; three or more doses of poliovirus vaccine; one or more doses of a measles-containing vaccine; and three or more doses of *Hemophilus influenzae* type b vaccine.
[b]Children in this survey period were born between February 1995 and May 1997.
[c]Weighted estimates.

SOURCE: CDC, 1999e.

ment measures will count the immunization status of the patient regardless of service-delivery setting). These reports have stimulated advisory notices by the HCFA and CDC warning that patterns of deliberate referral are subject to penalties (Richardson, 1999; Richardson and Orenstein, 1999).

Impact of State Program Cutbacks and Budget Reductions

Federal budget cutbacks in the Section 317 program during FY 1996, 1997, 1998, and 1999 were significant (see Figure 5-2). In some cases, grantees saw their infrastructure support budgets reduced by one-third

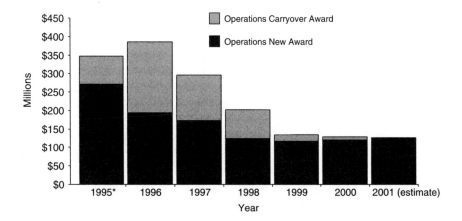

FIGURE 5-2 Section 317 grant operations funding history, 1995–2001 (dollars in millions). *In 1995, CDC transferred funds not needed for vaccine purchase to state operations. SOURCE: Information provided by CDC.

each year. As was the case with local health departments, discussed earlier, these reductions caused states to cut back many immunization efforts, including assessment, outreach, performance monitoring, program linkages, and information management (see Table 5-4).[7] Two of the most common activities initiated with the original increases in Section 317 funding—outreach and education efforts and expanded service delivery— were also the most common targets of cuts (Freed et al., 1999). For example:

• Almost all state program managers made substantial cuts in contracts with local health departments, even though they viewed local outreach activities as critical and effective.

• Half the states reduced staffing within the immunization program by cutting staff, consolidating positions, or leaving vacancies unfilled. Eight states transferred full-time equivalents (FTEs) or activities to other programs.

• Several states expressed concern that they do not have the workforce capacity required to investigate disease outbreaks, to work with providers, and to continue registry development. Officials in one state pointed out that it does little good to identify children who are behind on their immunizations if there is no outreach component for follow-up and subsequent vaccination.

TABLE 5-4 State Responses to Section 317 Funding Cuts[a]

State	Activities Eliminated or Reduced							Other/Notes
	Outreach and Education[b]	Assessment and Surveillance	WIC Linkage	Registry[c]	State Staff[d]	Local Service-Delivery Expansion[e]	Expanded Vaccination Campaigns[f]	
AL								No cuts because of increasing amounts of incentive funds.
AK	✓		✓	✓				
AZ	✓		✓	✓	✓	✓	✓	State provided funds for registry, transferred full time equivalents (FTEs) to other program.
AR			✓		✓			No major cuts; VFC infrastructure funds increased.
CA	✓				✓	✓		
CO	✓				✓	✓		
CT	✓		✓		✓			State provided funds to build back up. VFC infrastructure funds increased.
DE					✓			
DC			✓	✓	✓			
FL	✓					✓		
GA		✓			✓			
HI		✓			✓			
ID	✓	✓		✓	✓	✓	✓	Changed or increased responsibilities per FTE.
IL	✓			✓	✓	✓	✓	
IN	✓			✓	✓	✓		
IA	✓		✓	✓	✓	✓		
KS	✓							
KY								Not much impact yet.
LA	✓		✓			✓		
ME					✓			
MD	✓	✓				✓		No information available.

State	Notes
MA	Shifted some FTEs from federal to state funds. State provided funds for registry. VFC infrastructure funds increased; some contracts forward funded.
MI	
MN	
MS	Redirected some state vaccine purchase funds to registry.
MO	
MT	Received block grant funds; moved FTEs to other programs.
NE	
NV	
NH	
NJ	
NM	
NY	Redirected some state vaccine purchase funds; not much impact yet.
NC	
ND	
OH	Moved FTEs to other program.
OK	
OR	Received other funding sources.
PA	
RI	
SC	Shared costs with other programs.
SD	
TN	Shared costs with other programs at local level.
TX	
UT	Redirected some state vaccine purchase funds to support local health departments (LHDs). Shifted costs to other programs.
VT	
VA	

continued

TABLE 5-4 Continued

State	Activities Eliminated or Reduced							Other/Notes
	Outreach and Education[b]	Assessment and Surveillance	WIC Linkage	Registry[c]	State Staff[d]	Local Service Delivery[e]	Expanded Vaccination Campaigns[f]	
WA	✓					✓		VFC infrastructure funds increased.
WV						✓		LHDs lobbied for state funds.
WI			✓	✓				Changed universal policy (i.e., no longer covers insured children).
WY		✓	✓					

NOTE: WIC = Special Supplemental Nutrition Program for Women, Infants, and Children. VFC = Vaccines for Children. FTE = full-time equivalent. LHD = local health department.

[a]Not a comprehensive (or mutually exclusive) list of state responses, but rather those they chose to highlight.
[b]Outreach and education includes such activities as work with coalitions, media campaigns, and provider education.
[c]Registry activities include software development and purchase of hardware and other equipment.
[d]State staff includes staff cuts as well as vacancies that were not filled.
[e]Local service-delivery expansion includes contracts with LHDs, community and migrant health centers, and other partners to extend clinic hours, offer weekend clinics, add nursing staff, and so on.
[f]Expanded vaccination campaigns include adult and adolescent campaigns, as well as campaigns focused on specific vaccines (e.g., hepatitis B).

SOURCE: Freed et al., 1999.

• Many states have discontinued funding for local organizations engaged in immunization outreach activities. States have reported that doing so has damaged their credibility as partners with local agencies (such as WIC clinics and community centers).

State Efforts to Adjust to Budget Declines

As federal assistance declined, many states attempted to secure from other sources, public and private, funding that would preserve essential services and alleviate the impact of the reductions. Such alternative sources included other federal funding, redirection of state vaccine purchase funds to infrastructure support, and additional state funding, among others. Only 11 states were able to replace federal funds for vaccine purchase with funds provided by their health departments and/or state legislatures. Success in procuring funds for infrastructure is generally limited to support for new vaccines, a specific immunization initiative (e.g., providing hepatitis A vaccine in Texas' border counties), or registry development (Freed et al., 1999:22). In cases where state legislatures did support infrastructure (about 25 states), funds were sometimes appropriated directly to the local health departments. Half of the state agencies are looking for other funding sources, primarily from the state budget.

In some cases, private sources were identified to support educational or outreach efforts within the state agencies. For example, vaccine manufacturers in 31 states supported educational activities (especially provider education) and information dissemination. Statewide and/or local immunization coalitions in 19 states became significant contributors to immunization efforts, particularly outreach activities. Insurers or managed care organizations provided support in 7 states for registry efforts, vaccine purchase, or outreach and education. Most of the states obtained partial funding from other direct or indirect funding sources, including All Kids Count grants for statewide registries (12 states), county- or city-level registry efforts (11 states), and philanthropic assistance from other groups.[8]

Yet even with additional funding sources, as of the end of the decade almost all state immunization programs had obtained few good answers to their serious financial questions. According to one state source:

> It's a never-ending situation around here with new vaccines and all the funding issues. Immunization program managers around the country are being stretched beyond their limits. At some point, either things are going to have to be broken down differently or . . . I don't know what the answer is. All of these things are important, but we're just not able to do it all. At what point do you just say enough is enough? (Freed et al., 1999:23).

*Finding 5-8. States have devised various approaches and made invest-
ments in vaccine purchase and program operations, but the level of
investment is unevenly distributed across the states. Expenditures for
infrastructure efforts are poorly documented, and the financial base for
these efforts is not stable. State variability in caring for indigent populations has impeded the development of a national consensus about what
level of care, what age groups, and what types of public health assessment, assurance, and leadership responsibilities are adequate to support
a national immunization system.*

*Finding 5-9. Many states have attempted to maintain direct service
efforts to meet residual needs, especially among young children, while
also expanding their public health assessment, assurance, and policy
development roles in monitoring and responding to trends within the
private health sector. These enhanced efforts were undertaken without
additional resources during a period when federal budgets for infrastructure support declined.*

*Finding 5-10. The loss of federal funds in Section 317 infrastructure
grants has diminished state and local activities in such areas as immunization services, outreach, educational programs, data surveillance and
measurement, and technical assistance. These reductions have impaired
the ability of state health agencies to carry out effective assessment,
assurance, and policy development roles. States now have less flexibility
to initiate comprehensive efforts in response to new vaccines, to serve
new age groups (such as adults) or selected populations, or to detect and
respond quickly to sudden disease outbreaks. Their ability to meet the
immunization needs of underserved communities and to encourage the
uptake of new vaccines among the general population has declined.*

*Finding 5-11. Changes in the roles of the public- and private-sector
health care system in delivering immunizations have generated uncertainty about the appropriate balance of responsibilities among public
and private agencies, and between federal and state programs, in bringing expertise and resources to bear on immunization coverage concerns
within local communities. This uncertainty has been exacerbated by the
instability of and reductions in the funding stream for state immunization infrastructure.*

*Finding 5-12. The growing complexity of the vaccine schedule has
increased the states' burden of record assessment in routine procedures.
Assessment studies are often reduced or eliminated when more pressing
needs arise, such as vaccine purchase or service-delivery requirements.*

States with large areas of concentrated poverty or populations that lack immunization as a result of underinsurance may require additional federal resources to coordinate data collection efforts, to conduct targeted assessments, and to synthesize the collection of records that are scattered across diverse health care settings.

Finding 5-13. States had provided more than $300 million to support immunization efforts as of midsummer 1999. While half the states (25) directly support infrastructure, only 4 states fund a substantial portion of their infrastructure budget (i.e., more than 40 percent). Twenty-one states currently provide no direct state support for immunization infrastructure. Four states receive such funding only by drawing on vaccine purchase funds provided by their legislatures.

Finding 5-14. Some states have identified other finance sources to support immunization services, and new private-sector sources may eventually emerge that can contribute to state programs. However, these other sources are limited in scope and are restricted to particular initiatives, such as the development of registries, education for providers, or community partnership efforts.

FEDERAL ROLES AND RESPONSIBILITIES

The National Immunization Program (NIP) within CDC is the primary agency concerned with federal policy and practices in support of state immunization efforts. NIP works with many different agencies and organizations, including other divisions within CDC, HCFA, NVAC, the Health Resources and Services Administration, and the Interagency Committee on Immunization (Rosenbaum et al., 1992; Fine, 1999; Association of Maternal and Child Health Professionals, 1999). In addition, the Departments of Agriculture, Education, and Housing and Urban Development all participate in the development and implementation of federal immunization policies and programs (Kelley et al., 1993). As one report observes: "The diversity of agencies involved is indicative of the importance of immunization to the overall well-being of children and the complexity of providing this service" (Kelley et al., 1993:1).

Although public health is commonly viewed as a primary function of the states, federal interventions have occurred frequently, beginning with the creation of public health hospitals in port cities in 1798 (DHHS, 2000). The federal government has exercised two separate but often overlapping roles in addressing immunization:

- *State assistance*—The federal government has consistently sought to supplement and support state efforts through policy coordination, technical assistance, and data collection. Federal grant awards also offer assistance to help states improve their ability to meet the needs of underserved populations, including the uninsured and urban poor, rural residents, immigrants and migrant workers, the elderly, and infants and children. As discussed earlier, federal immunization grants to the states expanded to include infrastructure support in the early 1990s, allowing the states to use federal funds to hire personnel and contractors for specific purposes such as outreach, data collection, and program development.

• *Federal initiatives*—In addition to state assistance, the federal government has undertaken special initiatives to expedite the introduction of new vaccines or technologies into the health care system; to reduce inequities in access to immunization services; and, more recently, to address concerns about the safety and quality of vaccines. These initiatives require close collaboration with the states to ensure that federal funds are distributed according to the priorities of the federal program, rather than simply augmenting state revenues for public health.

The combination of state assistance and federal initiatives has evolved through a series of special programs and policies (see Appendix B). The result is a patchwork quilt of policy guidance that places particular emphasis on certain issues while omitting others. By using their Section 317 grant awards, states were able to stitch this quilt together in a cohesive manner that responded to local needs and circumstances. As funds were reduced, states were forced to balance responding to local conditions while also complying with federal mandates.

Infrastructure Investments and Immunization Programs

Federal investments in immunization programs in the 1990s had two basic objectives: (1) improving immunization coverage rates and sustaining high rates among hard-to-reach populations using a variety of evidence-based prevention and linkage strategies, and (2) integrating immunization services within comprehensive primary care plans and medical homes in the private health care sector. Congress has formulated specific guidance for the development of the national immunization program in a few additional areas as well:

• In the initial buildup of the Section 317 infrastructure grants, Congress clearly intended that federal funds be used to improve access within high-risk communities by extending clinic hours and hiring staff to administer immunizations (U.S. House of Representatives, 1991; U.S. Senate, 1993, 1994).

- Congress has directed CDC to help states target pockets of need so that federal funds can be focused on disadvantaged communities (U.S. House of Representatives, 1989; U.S. Senate, 1992, 1995, 1998).
- Congress has supported the use of incentive grants to reward states that achieve high rates of immunization coverage (U.S. Senate, 1993, 1994, 1995, 1998).
- Congress has guided the development of vaccine safety concerns through the creation of a federal injury compensation plan financed by a special excise tax on vaccine sales.
- Congress has urged CDC to provide leadership in improving adult immunization coverage rates (U.S. House of Representatives, 1992).
- Congress has urged CDC to develop the worldwide polio eradication program, drawing on carryover funds in the state infrastructure grants to support the program's early development (U.S. House of Representatives, 1996).

Congress has not addressed the issues of state data collection or the assurance and assessment roles of public health agencies in the oversight of private-sector performance, which now represent significant aspects of immunization infrastructure. These latter areas raise fundamental concerns about the extent to which federal agencies should support and guide state practice through financial assistance and other incentives, including penalties and reporting requirements. These areas also reveal challenges that emerge when federal and state agencies attempt to guide or change professional practices within the private health care sector. Recently, legislation has been introduced that seeks to require comprehensive health insurance coverage for childhood immunization.[9] But such initiatives must address the complex regulatory structure for group and individual health insurance coverage within the private sector and face the traditional political resistance to federal mandates for the private health insurance system.

Federal Finance Practices

As discussed earlier, significant increases in the federal immunization grant awards to the states occurred in the early 1990s, followed by rapid decreases in the latter part of the decade (see Figures 1-2 and 1-3 in Chapter 1). In 1990 and 1991, infrastructure grants (called Financial Assistance [FA] grants) and state expenditures were about one-fourth the level of those for vaccine purchase (called Direct Assistance [DA] grants) (see Tables 5-2 and 5-5). At mid-decade, FA levels increased substantially, rising to twice the levels for DA. New money for FA grant awards increased more than seven-fold from a total of $37 million awarded for 1990

TABLE 5-5 Annual Awards and Expenditures of Section 317 Financial Assistance (FA) Immunization Program Funds (in millions of dollars)

Year	New Funds	Re-awarded Funds[a]	Total Award	Expenditures	Percentage of Total Award Expended[b]
1990	36.9	0.0	36.9	25.8	70%
1991	37.0	6.3	43.3	32.2	74%
1992	92.3	5.9	98.2	43.0	44%
1993	98.2	42.2	140.4	81.8	58%
1994	227.6	27.3	254.9	135.4	53%
1995	261.4	75.2	336.6	195.4	58%
1996	179.7	191.4	371.1	247.7	67%
1997	158.6	121.7	280.4	241.1	86%
1998[c]	115.9	77.8	193.7	179.5	93%
1999[d]	110.6	17.8	128.4	128.4	NA[e]

[a]Funds awarded in previous years but not obligated.
[b]Based on year-end unobligated balances for 1990–1997 reported to CDC as of December 21, 1998.
[c]CDC estimates for 1998 expenditures and percentage of 1998 award expended.
[d]Projected amounts for 1999.
[e]Not available.

SOURCE: Information provided by CDC.

to $261 million for 1995. By the end of the decade, newly awarded FA grants had declined to $116 million for 1998 and $111 million for 1999 (more than a 50 percent decrease). In FY 1999, expenditures for DA and FA were roughly comparable. Four factors affected the buildup and subsequent cutbacks in the Section 317 state infrastructure grants:

• Implementation of a pockets-of-need strategy.
• Use of incentive grants to improve immunization rates within the states.
• The existence of significant carryover in the early years of the state infrastructure grant awards.
• Initiation of the global polio eradication program.

Pockets of Need. Since numerous studies have demonstrated that low socioeconomic status is strongly associated with low immunization rates, CDC employed a strategy throughout the 1990s designed to enhance efforts to identify and provide vaccination interventions to underserved populations, particularly within large urban areas. In 1991, NIP identified

23 urban areas (in addition to 5 urban grantees) as targets for new Immunization Action Plans.[10] For each of the 28 target areas, an average immunization coverage rate was calculated with National Immunization Survey (NIS) data, and traditional public health providers and nontraditional community partners were encouraged to collaborate in program planning and implementation.

Several years later, the FY 1996 Senate Appropriations Committee (U.S. Senate, 1995) directed CDC to develop a strategy that would identify pockets of underimmunized children and help the states target resources to raise immunization coverage in these areas. Although NIP designated 11 major urban areas as pockets of need that would receive intensive follow-up and technical assistance, additional financial resources to support these efforts were not forthcoming in the state grant awards.[11] In 1997, CDC instructed all grantees to place additional emphasis on identifying geographic subdivisions at high risk for underimmunization, measuring immunization coverage in these areas, and implementing measures designed to achieve high coverage among vulnerable groups.

CDC recommended three strategies for intensifying efforts to improve coverage rates in pockets-of-need areas: linkages between WIC and immunization services; Assessment, Feedback, Incentives, and eXchange of information (AFIX) interventions; and reminder–recall systems. State and local grantees were expected to implement these key strategies fully and to report progress in using them along with other initiatives, such as immunization registries, in areas identified as pockets of need.

The 1997 annual progress reports submitted to CDC included data provided by 58 grantees (information provided by CDC).[12] About three-quarters of the respondents collected information on the key strategies recommended by CDC (WIC linkage, 79.3 percent; reminder–recall, 60.3 percent; and AFIX, 67.2 percent). However, only 11 grantees (19 percent) monitored the number of target WIC sites implementing high-risk protocols for immunization, an important strategy promoted by CDC as part of routine program management.[13]

In their progress reports, significant numbers of grantees indicated that they had redirected personnel (67.2 percent) or funds (55.2 percent) to work on pockets-of-need issues. The effects of these redirected efforts are not known, however. Neither CDC nor the state grantees have attempted to measure changes in coverage levels in the pockets of need against specific interventions. The prohibitive costs of small-area surveys are commonly cited as a major obstacle to such analysis.

In 1999 NVAC once again called on CDC and state and local immunization programs to focus resources on underimmunized populations. Immunization programs were encouraged to collaborate with WIC to assess each enrolled child's immunization status, and state immunization leaders were urged to participate in negotiating the state's contracts for Medicaid managed care (NVAC, 1999a).

Despite these mandates, state and local immunization programs have few resources to dedicate to program coordination and leadership initiatives. As noted earlier, collaborative and partnership efforts were often the first activities to be reduced within the states when budget cutbacks occurred. The elimination of staff positions within the states, as described earlier, also resulted in multiple task assignments for remaining personnel that reduced their ability to take on new roles. While states have received additional federal assistance in the forms of SCHIP funds and VFC, the application of these resources to state immunization program needs has been constrained by the strict eligibility guidelines and limits to spending for program administration (including the costs of setting up outreach and record-keeping systems) (see Figure 5-3). These guidelines and restrictions leave little margin for collaborative program development in areas of mutual interest and common goals.

Use of Incentive Grants. In an effort to improve state performance in reaching national immunization goals, the Senate Appropriations Committee instructed CDC in 1993 (for FY 1994) to set aside approximately $32 million annually from the state infrastructure awards for incentive grants (U.S. Senate, 1993). These funds are distributed to the grantees according to their levels of immunization coverage, as reported by the NIS. Once the size of the base award has been determined for each state in response to its original request, states with higher coverage rates receive "bonus" awards from the incentive funds to reward their achievement.

In the mid-1990s, when infrastructure grants amounted to more than $300 million annually, incentive grants constituted less than 10 percent of that total. In recent years, as the total funding for infrastructure grants has diminished, the $33 million set-aside has become an increasing source of concern. Incentive grants now represent about 24 percent of the total grant awards, and grantees with low immunization coverage rates have indicated that they are being "punished" by lower total awards when they require additional assistance to meet urgent local needs.

The Carryover Problem. As noted earlier, in the aftermath of the rapid and unplanned buildup of state infrastructure grants in the early 1990s, significant amounts of carryover emerged within the state immunization budgets (see Table 5-5 and Figure 5-2). Although the states had acquired extensive experience over several decades in working with federal agencies to purchase vaccines, the large increases in infrastructure support were targeted to areas that required new personnel and new efforts (such as outreach, record assessment, performance measures, and the develop-

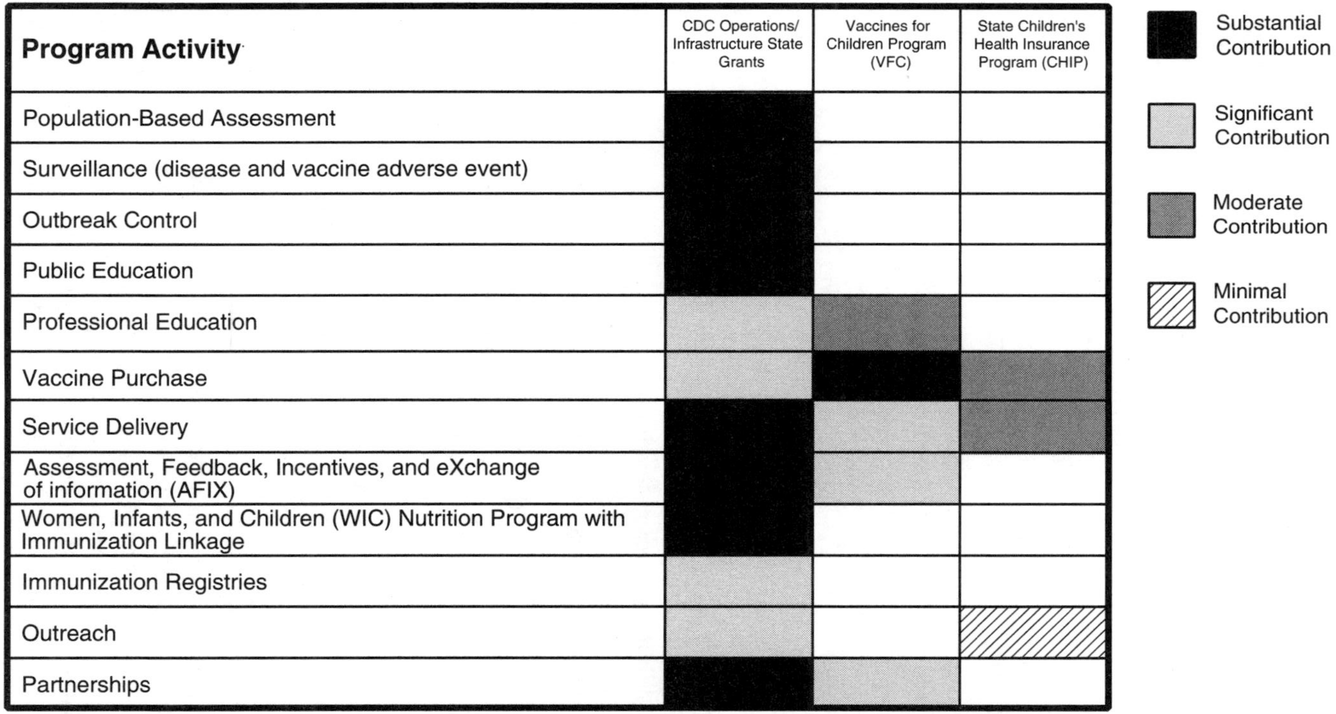

FIGURE 5-3 Immunization activities by funding source. SOURCE: Information provided by CDC.

ment of immunization registries). Moreover, the increases occurred swiftly without adequate lead time to plan for how the funds would be used within existing state administrative and management systems.[14]

Although increases in Section 317 funding for infrastructure support in the early 1990s were viewed as a tremendous opportunity, states reported serious administrative impediments to reaping the full benefit of those funds (Freed et al., 1999). For example:

• Many states had difficulty in predicting the level of funding for any given year. This made it problematic to create accurate budgets for the immunization program, engage in strategic planning, or hire full-time permanent staff.

• Funds were awarded late in the fiscal year, often as a result of delays in congressional approval of federal health budgets. In some cases, multiple allocations were made within a given year.

• The federal grant requirements obligated the states to spend their funds before the end of the fiscal year.

• Statewide internal restrictions in some cases affected hiring, budgeting, or spending. Some state legislatures must allocate or approve all state agency spending, including federal grants, especially if personnel appointments are involved. States were unable to abolish personnel positions once the funding decreased; the result was administrative obligations that inhibited program development.

Two overall problems resulted from these circumstances: (1) states did not have adequate time to assess their needs and use federal funds effectively, and (2) states with cumbersome internal procedures for budgeting, spending, or hiring were unable to obligate their funds expeditiously (Freed et al., 1999). Some legislatures meet every other year, creating further delays. Both problems contributed to the buildup of carryover or unexpended funds that had been obligated by the federal government to the states, which Congress eventually viewed as excessive (U.S. Senate, 1995). The delay in expenditures during the startup period led Congress to reduce the state infrastructure grant funds in the period FY 1996–1998.[15] These reductions resulted from mid-decade pressures to reduce the size of federal discretionary programs in general, making it more difficult to sustain ongoing efforts while also starting up new initiatives, such as the polio eradication program. The decreases are commonly viewed by state officials as "punishment for factors beyond their control" (Freed et al., 1999:16). Many state officials also noted that the curtailment of Section 317 carryover funds occurred precisely at the point when they believed they had made significant strides in the organization of immunization delivery, outreach, and other activities.

When Section 317 grant awards were reduced, state expenditure rates gradually increased, demonstrating the states' growing capacity to use federal funds for immunization services. The states' needs eventually became greater than the resources available to them. Expenditure rates of the infrastructure grants during 1997 and 1998 were in the range of 86 percent and 96 percent, respectively, and total carryover of funds is currently estimated at less than $10 million for 1998 Section 317 FA awards. CDC and state officials now report that the current level of federal funds for Section 317 infrastructure support (requested at $117 million for FY 2000) is no longer sufficient to support their efforts (Thompson, 1998).

Global Polio Eradication Initiative. Reasoning that the health and economic benefits of polio eradication would be perpetual and that extra funds would be needed for a few years only to achieve this goal, CDC launched a global polio eradication initiative in 1996, with congressional support. The initiative involved an extensive partnership (including funding and technical support) with Rotary International, the United Nations Foundation, the United Nations International Children's Emergency Fund (UNICEF), the World Health Organization, and governments of other industrialized countries.

In the period FY 1996–1998, when budget cutbacks were common throughout DHHS, CDC received explicit guidance from both the House of Representatives and the Senate to fund the new initiative for polio eradication (as well as measles elimination) at the expense of state vaccine purchase and infrastructure development funds (U.S. House of Representatives, 1996). Recognizing that prior increases had occurred in the state infrastructure grants, and disturbed by reports of large amounts of unspent state funds from prior years, the Congress expressed strong support for the global polio eradication program and encouraged CDC to expand the effort using available resources—by reducing the state infrastructure grant awards. This decision to cut the base of the state infrastructure program to support the global polio eradication effort plays an important role in explaining the shortfall now being experienced by the states.

Impact of Budget Reductions

Reductions in state infrastructure grants have affected each of the six key roles of the national immunization system. For example:

- *Infectious disease prevention and control*—At present, the NIP does not have a separate pool of funds within the Section 317 grant program to support the purchase of vaccines for outbreak control (information provided by CDC). Funds are likewise not available within the Section 317 program to support the training needs for outbreak control recommended by NVAC (1999a); such support may be provided by a new bioterrorism initiative financed elsewhere within CDC.

• *Surveillance and monitoring*—During the 1990s, CDC maintained support for the NIS (see Chapter 4). CDC also encouraged the development of immunization registries as a key component of the future immunization surveillance system. Between 1994 and 1999, CDC allocated a total of $178.4 million in Section 317 funds within the state infrastructure awards to support immunization registries, but the size of these awards has declined in recent years (see Box 5-4) (A. Bauer, CDC, personal communication, May 21, 1999). Cutbacks in federal grants have caused several states to reduce their own surveillance and monitoring efforts, as discussed earlier. These reduced efforts represent critical omissions in the development of important baseline and benchmark coverage measures in certain key areas, such as the immunization status of Medicaid or VFC-eligible clients. The cutbacks also diminished the states' abilities to expand surveillance for diseases such as varicella that are now vaccine-preventable while maintaining current surveillance efforts for traditional vaccine-preventable diseases. Furthermore, in areas where states are designated for special immunization initiatives (such as the ACIP recommendation that 11 states universally vaccinate children against hepatitis A), additional funds are not available to help these states with program implementation or enhanced surveillance. In such cases, states are given further program responsibilities by federal agencies without additional federal funding.

BOX 5-4
Total Section 317 Funds Awarded to Support Registries as of July 1, 1999 (in millions of dollars)*

1994	$ 6.6
1995	50.9
1996	42.5
1997	35.1
1998	23.8
1999	22.2

*Data sources varied by source and by year (for 1994, 1995, and 1999, grantees provided data; for 1996–1998, CDC coded data from grant awards).

SOURCE: Information provided by CDC.

• *Assessment and technical assistance*—State immunization officials have been strongly encouraged to exercise leadership and technical assistance in a variety of areas, including the immunization of adults, the negotiation of Medicaid managed care contracts, the coordination and regulation of private insurance and VFC benefits, the auditing of private-sector immunization records, and the integration of datasets from multiple sites (NVAC, 1999a). Reductions in federal grants have severely constrained the states' ability to exercise their current roles, much less assume enhanced responsibilities for monitoring private-sector performance, ensuring vaccine safety, and encouraging the immunization of adults. The cutbacks have also occurred at a time when negotiations regarding the distribution of government-financed vaccines have become more complex; an example is questions that have emerged about the use of VFC for clients who are covered by private (non-Medicaid) SCHIP plans. In most states, public health immunization efforts and public health insurance plans (such as Medicaid and SCHIP) are administered in separate agencies and even separate departments. Opportunities for coordination and integrated efforts are often limited. For example, state immunization programs may have technical expertise that is relevant to contract specifications for the purchase of managed care services for state beneficiaries. But those who are involved in negotiating Medicaid or SCHIP contracts may be unaware of or reluctant to involve other state employees in developing benchmark and performance standards for their contractors.

• *Programs to improve immunization coverage rates*—The reductions in federal grants have had significant effects on interventions such as outreach, provider education, and service delivery, as described earlier. Efforts such as WIC linkages, reminder–recall systems, and record audit procedures, all of which have been found to be highly effective in improving immunization rates in disadvantaged communities, have been reduced routinely as a result of federal cuts that decrease resources for state and local programs.

Changes in Program Composition

Total appropriations for the Section 317 program declined by only about 5 percent in the latter part of the 1990s (decreasing from $464 million in FY 1995 to $448 million in FY 1999). Significant shifts occurred within the major components of the program during this time (see Table 5-6); for example, the program operations category (the portion of the program that is administered directly by CDC) expanded, while the state infrastructure grants were reduced. During FY 1995–1999, the program operations category increased from $104 million (23 percent of the

TABLE 5-6 Composition of CDC Immunization Appropriations, 1995–1999, Amounts and Shares (fiscal years; dollars in thousands)

Type	1995	1996	1997	1998	1999
Grants					
DA[a]: Vaccine purchase	151,893	139,393	139,393	119,393	139,629
State operations	23,800	23,800	23,800	23,800	23,467
Parent/patient notification	2,900	2,900	2,900	2,900	2,859
Surveillance and response	5,100	5,100	5,100	5,100	5,029
Infrastructure	108,400	108,400	88,400	42,400	41,806
Program-based incentives	33,000	33,000	33,000	33,000	32,537
Assessment activities	3,500	3,500	3,500	3,500	3,451
Immunization information systems	8,232	8,232	8,232	0	0
Adult/adolescent vaccination	0	0	0	0	0
Adult immunization	0	0	0	0	0
Other grants	22,552	23,576	23,361	30,741	30,311
Subtotal, Section 317 grants	359,377	347,901	327,686	260,834	279,089
Program operations					
Prevention activities	38,660	37,917	37,825	37,825	38,439
Polio technical assistance	5,727	11,227	19,277	19,277	30,874
Polio vaccine	4,116	16,000	28,000	28,000	35,565
Measles technical assistance	0	0	0	0	7,944
Measles vaccine	0	0	0	0	7,944
Adult adolescent vaccination	0	0	0	0	0
Vaccine R&D[b]/A&E[c]/lab support	24,130	23,146	23,146	23,146	22,525
Vaccine safety	4,451	4,451	4,451	4,451	4,389
National Immunization Survey	16,000	16,000	16,000	16,000	12,472
Immunization information systems	1,029	1,004	1,004	1,004	0
Information/education	4,244	4,244	4,244	4,244	4,185
Interagency group research	6,000	6,000	6,000	6,000	5,916
Subtotal, program operations	104,357	119,989	139,947	139,897	170,253
Administrative rescission	0	0	0	0	–1,394
Total, Section 317 program	463,734	467,890	467,633	400,731	447,948

[a]Direct Assistance.
[b]Research and development.
[c]Assessment and evaluation.

SOURCE: Information provided by CDC.

total NIP budget in FY 1995) to $170 million (38 percent of the total budget in FY 1999). In the same period, the grants portion of the budget (which includes state infrastructure and vaccine purchase grants, research support, and congressionally mandated studies) decreased by 20 percent (from $359 million or 77 percent of the total in FY 1995 to $279 million or 62 percent of the total in FY 1999).

The committee finds these compositional shifts troubling because they suggest an unintended reorientation of the Section 317 program that diminishes the state assistance role while expanding the federal presence. Although international polio eradication efforts are important, federal support for such efforts should not come at the expense of state immunization grant awards. It may have been reasonable during a period of national budget reductions to start up the polio eradication initiative with carryover funds from the state grants program. This finance strategy has long-term consequences, however, that require attention and merit remedial action.

Furthermore, cuts have occurred in the infrastructure grants during a time when VFC vaccine purchase funds have increased. The greater reliance on VFC and the private sector has allowed states to reduce their service-delivery role in the public health sector, but important functions remain and new roles have been added, all of which need to be supported.

Finding 5-15. Infrastructure support in the state immunization grants program lacks a strategic vision that can guide federal and state investments. Congress has not made infrastructure support within the states a priority for the national immunization program.

Finding 5-16. The federal government has traditionally assisted the states in supporting such areas as outreach and clinical services. A new emphasis is required, however, in areas that involve assurance, access, and policy development as result of the shift in the delivery of immunization services to the private sector. Administrative and staff support is needed in these areas so that local public health agencies can provide leadership and technical assistance in monitoring key indicators of quality of care and disparities in immunization coverage rates within their communities.

Finding 5-17. New federal funds for state infrastructure grants were reduced from $261 million annually (1995) to $111 million annually (1999) during a time when the health care system and immunization schedules were becoming more complicated. Resources are not available to help local communities adapt to new vaccines; monitor trends that can influence immunization rates; or implement new initiatives in the areas of assessing private-sector performance, improving coverage of adult vaccines, and conducting vaccine safety education programs.

Finding 5-18. Programs such as VFC, Medicaid, and SCHIP have administrative resources that can help states monitor vaccine coverage rates among public and private health providers. However, no coordi-

nated strategy currently exists for encouraging states to draw on these resources in building their immunization programs.

Finding 5-19. Although the federal government has traditionally supported the concept of partnership with the states to achieve national immunization goals, extensive ambiguity exists regarding the scope and forms of infrastructure that are adequate to meet national objectives while also responding to local needs. Some infrastructure services (such as providing immunizations within school health clinics or other community settings) can be undertaken by state and local health departments alone. Others require federal–state collaboration to help local agencies do more with limited resources (such as extending clinic hours). Interventions that are focused on systemic change, such as addressing missed opportunities for immunization assessment and referrals within WIC and Head Start programs, require interagency and community partnerships at the federal, state, and local levels. In implementing these interventions to serve vulnerable families, public health officials must interact with other agencies and offer resources so that high priority is given to the immunization effort.

SUMMING UP

During the past decade, the federal government assumed increasing responsibility for the immunization of vulnerable populations. The development of new vaccines, their increased costs, and the appearance of new diseases requiring immunization to protect the population have changed the nature of immunization from a niche to an increasingly integral component of the health care universe. At the same time, global travel and increased social mobility have multiplied the probabilities of dangerous infections affecting large populations throughout the United States.

As the federal government aggressively assumed a major role in the financing of vaccines, the gap between financing and delivery of primary care health services (including immunizations) expanded for large numbers of children within the United States. Many children who previously did not have access to vaccines or were immunized in public health clinics now receive vaccines in their medical homes in the private sector. Older adults (above age 65) have access to vaccines in the private sector through plans that are financed with Medicare funds. While the expanded role of the private sector in serving disadvantaged populations has served important public health objectives by increasing coverage rates, significant questions remain about the adequacy of existing services, as well as the capability of private providers and health plans to offer timely and routine vaccinations. In addition to the use of VFC funds, many communities rely on the Section 317 program for vaccines to meet residual needs among adults and children.

Recent reductions in federal grants for immunization infrastructure and shifts in the Medicaid provider base within the states have reduced the resources available to support immunization programs at the same time that the roles and responsibilities of state and local health agencies have expanded and diversified. The assurance and assessment mission and role of state health agencies require them to take on responsibilities for monitoring and improving provider behavior in the private sector, collecting and evaluating data on immunization trends within private health plans and special populations, adding new vaccines and age groups to the immunization schedule, addressing growing concerns about vaccine safety, and developing regional immunization registries and other sources of surveillance data. Although a few states have supplemented essential activities by drawing on other federal sources, shifting state budget allocations, or developing new sources of revenue (such as tobacco settlement funds), the demand on state public health agencies continues to exceed their current capacity.

Policy reforms within the private health care sector (such as the trend toward managed care, the inclusion of immunization services in private insurance benefits, and first-dollar coverage requirements for immunization services) have fostered a climate that encourages greater use of performance standards and assessment of immunization status within private practice. Yet access to reliable and timely data that accurately describe the immunization status of at-risk populations served by private plans remains elusive and uneven. Preventive services (including access to vaccines) in primary care health plans are fragmentary and unpredictable in both quality and scope. As part of their mission, public health leaders and programs bear responsibility for encouraging private providers to incorporate evidence-based strategies and new vaccines into routine primary care services, participating in regional registries, monitoring and improving immunization coverage rates in the public and private health sectors, and addressing concerns about vaccine safety.

Local and state governments have demonstrated both interest and ability with regard to developing immunization programs and services that have positive populationwide benefits, but few states have the resources needed to sustain infrastructure programs on their own. Efforts to increase and sustain coverage levels require diversified approaches, including community outreach and linkage programs, as well as systemic interventions, such as provider assessment and feedback systems and reminder–recall services.

It takes time to put new management and administrative services in place, particularly when consensus must be developed about how clients, providers, payers, and health departments should collaborate to ensure that immunizations are provided as part of appropriate health care (IOM, 1994b). State efforts to foster public awareness of the importance of immunization coverage are particularly challenged in the current environment with the addition of new vaccines to the childhood immunization schedule, the addition of new population groups (adolescents and adults) to the immunization system, public concerns about vaccine safety, and diminished public perception of the importance of timely immunization coverage in the absence of disease outbreaks (Orenstein et al., 1999).

Recent cuts in Section 317 state grant awards have reduced the ability of the states to carry out their traditional surveillance and outreach responsibilities or improve their oversight roles. Although state and local health programs have been urged to assume new leadership and oversight roles (such as strengthening coordination with new health finance practices, monitoring immunization status within private health care plans, and developing registry initiatives), it is unlikely that such efforts can be undertaken on a national scale without federal funding committed to their support.

As new vaccines are recommended in the next few decades, health plans, health care providers, and the public will need to confront the problem of recognizing, accepting, and applying these recommendations in routine medical care. Public health interventions at both the provider and community levels are necessary to sustain quality health care services and reduce disparities in coverage that result from barriers to access or attitudes and behavior. In the absence of such interventions:

• Efforts to track the immunization status of individuals who move across public and private health care plans will become increasingly difficult.

• Delays may occur in the integration of new vaccines into routine medical care.

• Further improvements in immunization coverage rates may be reduced, and significant disparities will probably occur in levels of vaccine coverage. The most severe effects are likely to be felt by those who are hard to reach and often most vulnerable to vaccine-preventable disease.

• States may be unable to develop appropriate immunization benchmarks, impeding their efforts to use appropriate performance measures in purchasing vaccines and health care services for disadvantaged populations and monitoring quality of care within public and private health plans.

• National and local data systems designed to monitor vaccine coverage status and disease outbreaks may become unreliable.

• Sustaining public acceptance of vaccines may become more difficult as a result of decreased exposure to information on the need for immunizations, as well as the complexities involved in documenting increasing numbers of vaccines across the life span.

ENDNOTES

1. A 1997 survey of employer-sponsored health plans (Partnership for Prevention/ William Mercer Survey) indicated that 82 percent of employers' most popular health plans (i.e., the plans with the highest employee enrollment) provided immunization benefits for infants and children, while 71 percent provided coverage of immunizations for adolescents. The survey also indicated that adult vaccines are least likely to be covered: 57 percent of employers' most popular health plans included coverage for influenza vaccines, while only 41 percent covered pneumococcal vaccines.

2. Data collected by the Health Insurance Association of America (HIAA) show that between 1989 and 1992, immunization as a benefit covered by conventional insurance plans increased from 45 to 53 percent, by preferred provider organization plans increased from 62 to 65 percent, and by health maintenance organization plans decreased from 98 to 95 percent (information provided by HIAA).

3. The harmonized schedule is endorsed by the Advisory Committee on Immunization Practices (ACIP), the American Academy of Pediatrics (AAP), and the American Academy of Family Physicians (AAFP).

4. These metropolitan regions represent the remnant of a larger group of urban grantees once associated with the Section 317 program.

5. CASA is a menu-driven relational database developed by CDC as an assessment tool for immunization clinics and providers. CASA provides programmatic feedback that can highlight areas that may have lower levels of immunization coverage, identify the up-to-date immunization status of the age group served by the clinic or practice, describe antigen-specific levels, and disclose the proportion of children that has dropped out of the vaccination schedule or experienced missed opportunities. CASA can also generate reminder and recall letters and postcards for a specified facility.

6. This one-time transfer occurred in the middle of the budgetary cycle and contributed to the carryover problem in the state grants. States were not able to expend these funds expeditiously and reported them as carryover, and the vaccine transfer funds inflated the infrastructure budget for several subsequent years.

7. See, for example, a letter from the Association of State and Territorial Health Officials to DHHS Secretary Donna Shalala (Thompson, 1998): "The severe cuts (upwards of 60%) to infrastructure over the last two years have resulted in major cutbacks on the state level including: reductions in every aspect of programs, from development of materials to staffing of clinics; cancellations of contracts with WIC, private providers, community health centers, TANF, and community coalitions; severe reductions in registry development and maintenance; reductions in clinic hours and the delivery of shots; and cancellation of assessment programs, evaluation and surveillance improvements. In addition the severe cutbacks do not allow for states to plan and implement the institutionalization of vaccine delivery strategies that work...." Proposed reductions in state efforts have also been described in materials provided by CDC to NVAC (information provided by CDC).

8. Such groups included Rotary Clubs (2 states), McDonald's (2 states), United Way (1 state), and other private foundations (2 states).

9. Senator Durbin (D-IL) and Senator Reed (D-RI) introduced S.2444 in April 2000 to require such coverage through amendments to the Employee Retirement Income Security Act of 1974, the Public Health Service Act, and the Internal Revenue Code of 1986.

10. The selection criteria included coverage rates (as determined by the National Immunization Survey), population size, and the proportion of individuals from racial and ethnic minority groups residing in the core city.

11. The 11 metropolitan areas were New York City, Philadelphia, Newark, Miami, Chicago, Detroit, Dallas, San Antonio, Houston, Phoenix, and Los Angeles.

12. The grantee reports used different surrogate measures to identify pockets of need, such as proportion of minorities (25 grantees), population density (21), poverty level (19), provider/service shortage (17), proportion of single-parent households (13), educational status (less than 12 years of education or GED) (12), public assistance rates (10), and vaccine-preventable disease morbidity (9). One-fifth of the grantees also used geographic information systems computer software to identify and map pockets of need. The grantees described seven direct measures for identifying pockets of need: retrospective surveys (29), provider-based surveys (21), local immunization registries (20), cluster surveys (12), birth certificate–based surveys (11), statewide immunization registries (11), and random digit dialing surveys (6). In measuring and monitoring immunization coverage in the pockets of need, grantees reported on population-based methods, provider assessments, and the frequency of measurement. Retrospective school-based surveys were used by 50 percent of the grantees to measure and monitor coverage. Most respondents relied on public clinic assessments (51 of 58 grantees) to monitor coverage rates, although private provider assessments (36) and, more rarely, managed care plan assessments (17) were also used. Assessments were usually conducted annually (69 percent).

13. Additional strategies reported by the grantees as part of their intensive efforts in pockets-of-need areas included outreach (82.8 percent), provider education (75.9 percent), and linkage with other public assistance programs (36.2 percent). Outreach efforts included public education, community awareness campaigns, coalition building, door-to-door canvassing, use of volunteers, and involvement of community-based organizations to contact families of individuals identified as undervaccinated.

14. Between 1992 and 1995, CDC awarded nearly all carryover funds in addition to, rather than in lieu of, newly appropriated funds. This compounded the problem in grantee areas that experienced difficulty in expending their funds efficiently. CDC reports that during these years, the NIP was trying to resolve the carryover issue by encouraging states to continue to build and sustain the systems needed to raise immunization coverage levels with new funds, while using the carryover funds for one-time expenses (information provided by CDC).

15. The amount of funds available for infrastructure services within the Section 317 grants in 1997 and 1998 was less than half of what was appropriated in 1996. See Table 5-6.

6

Summary Findings, Conclusions, and Recommendations

S ix questions posed by the U.S. Senate Committee on Appropriations and CDC established the initial framework for this study:

1. What was the extent of overall spending by all sources for immunizations in the United States during the 1990s?

2. How were new federal funds spent by the states, and to what extent did states maintain their own levels of effort over the past 5 years?

3. What are current and future funding requirements for immunization activities, and how can those requirements be met through a combination of state funding, federal Section 317 immunization grant funding, and funding available through the State Children's Health Insurance Program (SCHIP)?

4. How should federal grant funds be distributed among the states?

5. How should funds be targeted within states to reach high-risk populations without diminishing levels of coverage among the overall population?

6. What should be the role and financing level for CDC's current program supporting state efforts to vaccinate adults and achieve the nation's goals for influenza and pneumococcal vaccines?[1]

In preparing answers to these questions, the committee examined the roles and responsibilities required for an effective national immunization system. We identified six key roles that this national system must perform:

193

• Assure the purchase of recommended vaccines for the total population of U.S. children and adults, with a particular emphasis on the protection of vulnerable groups.

• Assure access to such vaccines within the public sector when private health care services are not adequate to meet local needs.

• Control and prevent infectious disease.

• Conduct populationwide surveillance of immunization coverage levels, including the identification of significant disparities, gaps, and vaccine safety concerns.

• Sustain and improve immunization coverage levels within child and adult populations, especially in vulnerable communities.

• Use primary care and public health resources efficiently in achieving national immunization goals.

The last of these roles provides overarching support for the other five, and was the focus of the committee's charge. In conducting the study, we gave particular attention to the responsibilities of federal and state health agencies and the burden of effort required to support each of the above roles in an integrated manner. In this chapter, we apply the findings presented in Chapters 2 through 5 to answer the six questions under the committee's charge. We then present the overall conclusions and recommendations resulting from the study, as summarized in Box 6-1.

SIX QUESTIONS AND SIX ANSWERS

Question 1. What was the extent of overall spending by all sources for immunizations in the United States during the 1990s? (Supported by Findings 3-1 through 3-6 in Chapter 3.)

The most common sources of spending for immunization in the United States during the 1990s were federal funds, state funds, private insurance reimbursements, and other private funds (e.g., foundation support for the development of registries and local outreach efforts). The federal government was and remains the primary source of assistance for both vaccine purchases and immunization programs.

Federal funding for immunization services (including vaccine purchases, infrastructure, and other grants), estimated from congressional budgets, grew from about $500 million in 1990 to more than $1 billion in 1999, an increase that reflects the expanded federal role in purchasing vaccines for disadvantaged children (see Table 1-4 in Chapter 1). Principal federal investments include the Vaccines for Children (VFC) program, Section 317 grant awards, and Medicaid reimbursements to the states for vaccine administration services. Medicare reimbursements for adult vac-

BOX 6-1
Conclusions and Recommendations

CONCLUSIONS

Conclusion 1: The repetitive ebb and flow cycles in the distribution of public resources for immunization programs have created instability and uncertainty that are eroding the continued success of immunization activities.

Conclusion 2: Immunization policy needs to be national in scope. At the same time, the implementation of immunization policy must be flexible enough to respond to special circumstances that occur at the state and local levels.

Conclusion 3: Federal and state governments each have important roles in supporting not only vaccine purchase, but also infrastructure efforts that can achieve and sustain national immunization goals.

Conclusion 4: Private health care plans and providers have the capacity to do more in implementing immunization surveillance and preventive programs within their health practices, but such efforts require additional assistance, oversight, and incentives. At the same time, comprehensive insurance and high-quality primary care services do not replace the need for public health infrastructure.

SUMMARY RECOMMENDATIONS

Recommendation 1: The annual federal and state budgets for the purchase of childhood vaccines for public health providers appear to be adequate, but additions to the vaccine schedule are likely to increase the burden of effort within each state. Therefore, the committee recommends that CDC be required to notify Congress each year of the estimated cost impact of new vaccines that have been added to the immunization schedule so that these figures can be considered in reviewing the vaccine purchase and infrastructure budgets for the Section 317 program.

Recommendation 2: Additional funds are needed to purchase vaccines for uninsured and underinsured adult populations within the states. The committee recommends that Congress increase the annual Section 317 vaccine budget by $50 million per year to meet residual needs for high-risk adolescents and adults under age 65 who do not qualify for other federal assistance. The committee further recommends that state governments likewise increase their spending for adult vaccines by $11 million per year.

Recommendation 3: State immunization infrastructure programs require increased financial and administrative support to strengthen immunization capacity and reduce disparities in child and adult coverage rates. The committee recommends that states increase their immunization budgets by adding $100 million over current spending levels, supplemented by an annual federal budget of $200 million to support state infrastructure efforts.

Recommendation 4: Congress should improve the targeting and stability of Section 317 immunization grant awards to the states by replacing the current discretionary grant award mechanism with formula grant legislation.

Recommendation 5: CDC should initiate a dialogue with federal and state health agencies, state legislatures, state governors, and the U.S. Congress immediately so that legislative and budgetary reforms can be proposed promptly when Section 317 is up for reauthorization in FY 2002.

Recommendation 6: Federal and state agencies should develop a set of consistent and comparable immunization measures for use in monitoring the status of children and adults enrolled in private and public health plans.

cine purchases have been reported only recently (fiscal year [FY] 1998). The annual budget for the National Vaccine Injury Compensation Fund, administered by the Health Resources and Services Administration (HRSA), adds another $100 million annually to the federal budget, but these funds are reserved solely for injury compensation claims and are not available to support vaccine purchase, service-delivery, or immunization programs. Trend data are not available for other federal investments, such as routine vaccine purchases and administration for military personnel and their families or veterans, or vaccines dispensed through the Indian Health Service. These budgets are designed primarily for clinical services and do not supplement infrastructure efforts within the states. Some immunization services are supported through Title V grants, the Community/Migrant Health Centers grants, and the Public Health Service prevention block grants, but such budgets are not tracked separately, nor are they reported in annual executive and congressional summaries of federal expenditures for immunizations.

The proliferation of new federal funding sources for vaccine purchase and child health care services (including VFC and SCHIP) raises the question of whether these new programs have the capability to assume many functions previously supported by Section 317 funds. These newer programs have absorbed many of the costs of vaccine purchases and office visits previously covered by Section 317 or Medicaid. Even with the expansion of public and private health plans, however, pockets of need remain in which individuals are susceptible to vaccine-preventable diseases. In addition, the increasing number of new vaccines, the fragmentation of uncovered groups, and the shift to private health care providers have increased the complexity of the national immunization system, requiring additional infrastructure and oversight within the states. As Medicaid, SCHIP, and other new federal programs are fully implemented, they may be able to absorb greater responsibilities in areas such as provider audits, assessments, outreach, and education for underserved populations and their health care providers. At present, however, these newer federal programs are not designed to perform or finance these roles.

The total amount of state funds allocated for immunization activities in the 1990s is not available. In 1999, CDC required state immunization agencies to estimate other federal (non-Section 317) funds, state funds, and private sources scheduled to support their immunization efforts in calendar year (CY) 2000. Based on these self-reported data, CDC has estimated that state budgets allocate a total of about $340 million for immunization programs and services, which include vaccine purchase and infrastructure support (information provided by CDC). This figure includes a variety of revenue sources, including state-only spending, reallocated federal budgets, and intergovernmental transfers, including school health.

However, this estimate does not include state Medicaid matches, even though a portion of these funds is allocated for immunization services. Other sources of revenue within the states, such as funds available from some private-sector plans for provider reminder–recall systems, local governmental support for registry projects, and vaccine industry support for professional education, are more limited, and no national data exist that can be used to measure such investments over time.

State budgets for vaccine purchase and immunization programs vary widely depending on the size of the state, the state's poverty level, per capita investments in public health, and the state's ability to carry out coordinated efforts that can use internal funds and cost savings efficiently. Of the total $340 million expenditures reported by the states, including state, local, other federal, and private funding (see Figures 6-1 and 6-2), states allocated approximately $109 million for vaccine purchase (including $102 million in state revenues). The remainder ($231 million) was

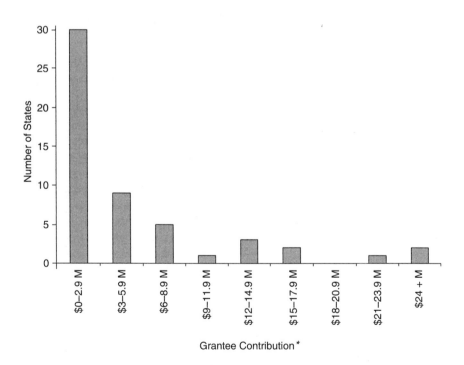

Grantee Contribution*

FIGURE 6-1 Level of grantee contribution by number of states, calendar year 2000. *May not include all appropriated and in-kind contributions. SOURCE: Information provided by CDC.

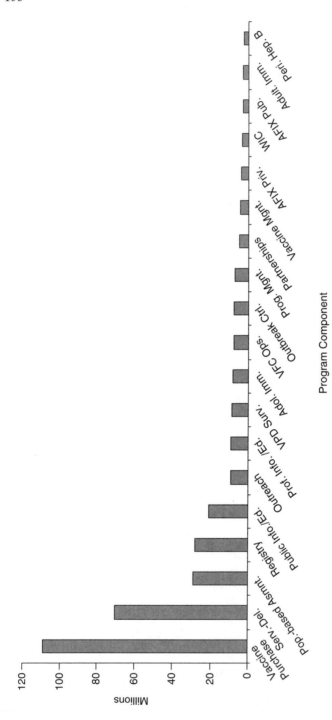

FIGURE 6-2 Level of grantee contributions by program component. SOURCE: Information provided by CDC.

allocated for infrastructure efforts and program operations (information provided by CDC).

States depend heavily on federal purchases of vaccines for all age groups, and use the Section 317 funds to serve children who are not eligible for the VFC program, to support a universal purchase policy, or to purchase selected vaccines for special programmatic needs. Ten states contribute substantially—more than 30 percent—to the total amount of publicly purchased vaccines within the state. All but two of these (Georgia and Missouri) are universal purchase states, and Georgia has expanded state purchase of vaccines for underinsured children. Twenty-four states and the District of Columbia contribute less than 10 percent to all publicly purchased vaccines, and the remaining 16 states contribute between 10 and 30 percent (information provided by CDC).

Federal grants to the states under Section 317 provide the core funding for state immunization programs, most of which is passed on to local health departments to support outreach, data collection, and program oversight efforts. The states collectively spend about twice the amount provided in federal Section 317 grants to support immunization infrastructure ($231 million in state-level budgets compared with $123 million in federal assistance grants in FY 2000), but state budgets are highly variable. Only 4 states have direct state funding for a substantial portion (i.e., more than 40 percent) of their immunization program infrastructure (Freed et al., 1999). Almost half of the states (21) provide no direct state funding for immunization program infrastructure. Eleven states have, or have had, direct state funding for registry development, although the size and length of that funding varies. Ten states fund immunization program staff, while a handful of others have small amounts of general funding. Several states devote Women, Infants, and Children (WIC), Medicaid, or Maternal and Child Health (MCH) (Title V) block grant funds to immunization-related activities, but these funds largely support specific initiatives rather than broad programmatic efforts.

In most states, local health departments provide substantial in-kind contributions, ranging from facilities and overhead to locally funded staff who perform multiple duties, including the delivery of immunizations. Major in-kind contributions come from school nurses and secretaries, who conduct school-based assessments of children's immunization status. Several states provide in-kind technical support for registry development (Freed et al., 1999).

Question 2. How were new federal funds spent by the states, and to what extent did states maintain their own levels of effort over the past 5 years? (Supported by Findings 5-8, 5-9, 5-13, 5-14, and 5-17 in Chapter 5.)

States traditionally divide their Section 317 federal immunization budgets between vaccine purchase and infrastructure or programmatic investments. Over the last 5 years, the private health care sector has assumed greater responsibility for providing immunizations to vulnerable populations (especially participants enrolled in Medicaid and SCHIP). This shift has had a profound impact on the nature of the services states are required to provide, stimulating a need for greater oversight and assessment efforts while also reducing the need, in some areas, for direct services for disadvantaged populations within public health agencies.

Vaccine Purchase. Prior to the VFC program (before FY 1995), the states routinely used Section 317 funds for vaccine purchase. In FY 1993, for example, Congress appropriated $193 million (more than 80 percent of the total Section 317 budget) for vaccine purchases by the states and $45 million for infrastructure grants (less than 20 percent of the total Section 317 budget). States were expected to gear up quickly in response to disease outbreaks, and federal funds provided them an opportunity to extend clinic hours, hire additional staff, and purchase enough vaccine to address special circumstances or short-term needs.

The implementation of VFC in the wake of the 1989–1991 measles epidemic shifted the routine purchase cost of vaccines for most Medicaid-enrolled children from state to federal funds and resulted in substantial savings to the states. The total size of these savings has not been estimated. The ways in which states used their Medicaid savings varied considerably and often depended on the state's needs and health finance organizational structure. Eight states (California, Connecticut, Idaho, Kentucky, Massachusetts, Minnesota, Nebraska, and North Carolina) used their vaccine purchase savings to increase their reimbursement fees to Medicaid providers for administration of immunizations. Some states expanded the eligibility criteria for Medicaid programs, or used the VFC savings to purchase additional vaccines for school health programs or other groups not covered by VFC, such as the underinsured (insured children whose health plans do not cover immunizations).

While total federal immunization budgets grew significantly with the creation of VFC, federal support for immunization programs within the states decreased during the past 5 years. Although states achieved cost savings with the creation of VFC, they incurred other administrative costs within the program for which they drew on other revenue streams, including Section 317 funds. In addition, states did not apply their Medicaid savings to support other immunization roles in such areas as data collection, surveillance of coverage rates, and development of preventive interventions for the general population or high-risk groups. The administrative separation of state Medicaid offices and public health agencies and the requirement that Medicaid funds be used only for Medicaid clients impeded the ability of most states to control and use revenue streams efficiently to support their multiple immunization roles. In general, the few states that housed their Medicaid program and department of health within the same agency had greater success in capturing VFC savings and applying this revenue directly to their immunization programs.

The creation of the VFC program did not eliminate the need for state-purchased vaccines. States continued to rely on Section 317 grants to meet the vaccination needs of children who did not qualify for federal assistance, which in some cases accounted for almost half of the state's total vaccine purchases. For example, a recent CDC study of 12 states[2] indicated that the proportion of total state vaccine purchases allocated to VFC ranged from 42 percent (Washington) to 87 percent (California) (CDC, 1998d). Similarly, the proportion of vaccine purchases allocated to Section 317 ranged from 5 percent (Florida) to 48 percent (Utah).

States continued to rely on Section 317 vaccine purchase funds for two reasons: (1) VFC eligibility requirements excluded many thousands of children (e.g., those enrolled in health plans that did not include immunization coverage) whom many states felt obligated to serve through a universal purchase program or an enhanced vaccine purchase policy, and (2) new vaccines (including rotavirus and varicella) were approved for children and adolescents during this period that were not automatically included within the VFC contract. As a result, Medicaid providers (which were bound by the Advisory Committee on Immunization Practices [ACIP] recommendations) were obligated to provide these vaccines, and states sought to make them available in public health clinics through their Section 317 purchases when they experienced delays in obtaining vaccines from the VFC program. In many cases, state Medicaid programs were also faced with reimbursing private providers for the private-sector purchase and administration to Medicaid clients of these very expensive vaccines.

In addition, despite the implementation of VFC throughout the United States, some states, particularly those with universal purchase programs, continue to allocate sizeable amounts of their own funds for vaccine purchase. Connecticut's vaccine purchases under the federal contract, for example, amount to half of all publicly purchased vaccine in that state (information provided by CDC). Other states, such as Alabama, Michigan, and Pennsylvania, rely primarily on federal funds for vaccine purchase.

Many states have reported that the administrative burden associated with VFC has increased considerably in the past several years, both for participating providers and for the states. This increased administrative burden raises the cost of state operations and oversight efforts, since states must provide tallies of doses administered for larger numbers of vaccines and providers, as well as estimates of VFC participants served in increasingly diverse health settings. The requirements are particularly burdensome in universal purchase programs (which were designed to reduce paperwork in determining patient or provider eligibility for state-financed vaccines). The implementation of SCHIP has added a new client base that further complicates determinations of VFC eligibility. Children who were once VFC-eligible because they were not insured now do not qualify in states that have adopted stand-alone SCHIP programs, since only Medicaid expansion programs qualify for VFC. Uncertainties about the extent to which VFC eligibility should be expanded to the entire SCHIP population have prompted requests for guidance from the Health Care Financing Administration (HCFA) (Richardson, 1999; Richardson and Orenstein, 1999), as well as legislation introduced in the Congress in September 1999 (U.S. House of Representatives, 1999a; U.S. Senate, 1999).

Infrastructure Grants. Section 317 grants to the states for infrastructure were highly unstable during the 1990s (see Figures 1-2 and 1-3 in Chapter 1). Following the 1989–1991 measles outbreak, CDC launched a national initiative designed to strengthen state immunization programs and provide resources for a broad array of direct services, outreach, and expanded access programs. The CDC budget for state infrastructure grants almost tripled between FY 1993 and 1994, growing rapidly from $45 million in new funds (FY 1993) to more than $128 million (FY 1994) (information provided by CDC). States were permitted to carry forward unobligated funds and transfer vaccine purchase funds to support infrastructure programs, further escalating the pool of funds available for state infrastructure grants in FY 1995 and 1996, even though appropriations for new awards were diminishing by this time.

Table 5-1 in Chapter 5 summarizes the principal activities to which each state directed its expanded infrastructure grants. Most commonly, states allocated their Section 317 increases to expanded service delivery, outreach and education, and development of registries. More specifically, states used this funding to improve immunization rates by, for example, undertaking collaborative efforts with groups such as WIC and Head Start to serve underimmunized clients, setting up reminder–recall systems, expanding clinic hours and locations, implementing targeted immunization campaigns for children and adolescents in pockets of need, and supporting local outreach efforts (Freed et al., 1999).

The increased Section 317 funding was viewed as a tremendous opportunity for new state efforts, especially since the creation of VFC added new responsibilities for data collection from and immunization audits of private health care providers. Yet significant barriers impeded states from reaping the full benefit of these expanded awards (Freed et al., 1999):

- Many states had difficulty predicting the level of funding for any given year, making it problematic to create accurate budgets or engage in strategic planning for the immunization program.
- The program year according to which CDC awards Section 317 grants is the calendar year. This matches no state fiscal year; most states' fiscal years (46) run from July through June, with state legislative action taking place earlier in the spring. State legislatures must thus make program and budget decisions knowing only the federal award for the first 6 months (July through December) of their upcoming fiscal year.
- Statewide hiring freezes and other administrative policies prohibited immunization programs from hiring full-time permanent staff.
- CDC grants were commonly allocated in a piecemeal way, including multiple grants within a budget cycle and the distribution of funds late in the fiscal year.
- States with cumbersome internal procedures for budgeting, spending, or hiring were unable to spend all their funds within a calendar year.
- Some state legislatures meet biennially, causing delays in accommodating additional unanticipated federal grants.
- Funds increased more quickly than states' capacity to use them, so states retained the funding as carryover until they had established the plans and personnel necessary to implement new programs reflecting their additional responsibilities.

Many states carried forward significant amounts of federal funds from one budget cycle to the next. In 1996, for example, carryover funds represented almost half of the total federal immunization funding to the states. Congress viewed the carryover funds as excessive, and over the period FY 1996–1998 reduced the base for Section 317 infrastructure funding by almost 50 percent, from $271 million in FY 1995 to $139 million in FY 1999 and 2000 (of which about $117 million is available for actual state grant awards). Most state officials have indicated that the budget reductions occurred precisely at the point at which they believed they had made significant strides in the organization of immunization delivery and other activities (Freed et al., 1999).

In response to the budget cuts, most states reduced the scale of effort of their activities, commonly reducing outreach, education efforts, and service-delivery arrangements with outside contractors. Half of the states have reported that the budget cuts affected staffing, requiring them to reduce staff, consolidate positions, or leave vacancies unfilled (Freed et al., 1999).

States have access to other direct or indirect funding sources for infrastructure, but such funds are focused primarily on specific project efforts rather than general support. Vaccine manufacturers have assisted with educational activities and information dissemination, particularly provider education, in 31 states. Statewide and/or local immunization coalitions are significant contributors to immunization efforts, particularly outreach activities, in 19 states. Twelve states have supported statewide registry development by All Kids Count grants from the Robert Wood Johnson Foundation, and another 11 states have received such grants for local registry efforts. Seven states have received support from insurers, managed care organizations, or other organizations (e.g., Rotary Clubs, McDonald's, or private foundations) for specific initiatives, such as registry efforts, vaccine purchase, or outreach and education.

These other funding sources are not sufficient to maintain a viable immunization program within each state, however, and the increasing data management and service coordination demands placed on state programs exceed their current capacity:

• Many states have discontinued funding for local organizations engaged in immunization outreach activity. Almost all program managers have reported substantial cuts in contracts with local health departments, even though they believe the most effective and critical outreach activities take place at the local level.

• The ability of states to partner with local agencies has diminished, earlier initiatives cannot be maintained, and innovative strategies cannot be implemented.

• Staff have increased responsibilities with little support or time to carry out their functions.

• Several states have expressed concern that they do not have the workforce capacity to investigate disease outbreaks, work with providers, or continue registry development.

• State officials have expressed concern that continued outreach efforts may be futile if services are not available within public health clinics to provide up-to-date vaccinations for individuals who are incompletely immunized and are not covered for such services.

Question 3: What are the current and future funding requirements for immunization activities, and how can those requirements be met through a combination of state funding, federal Section 317 immunization grant funding, and funding available through SCHIP? (Supported by Findings 2-1 through 2-4 in Chapter 2; Findings 3-2 through 3-6 in Chapter 3; and Findings 5-6, 5-7, 5-10 through 5-12, 5-15, 5-16, and 5-18 in Chapter 5.)

The funding requirements for immunization activities fall into two broad categories: vaccine purchase and infrastructure support.

Vaccine Purchase. Changes in federal and state health finance programs (including the creation of VFC and SCHIP) have improved access to vaccines for vulnerable populations within the private sector. Despite these improvements, many children continue to fall through the cracks of federal assistance programs, and new health care reforms, such as managed care, do not meet the complete immunization needs of children or adults who cycle through programs with short-term coverage arrangements. As a result, a continuing need for government-purchased vaccines remains within each state. The federal government currently spends more than $650 million annually on vaccine purchases, predominantly for childhood vaccines.[3] The states estimate that they will collectively spend an additional $109 million for vaccine purchases in 2000. This combined effort appears to be sufficient to meet the current vaccine needs of uninsured and Medicaid children, but may be inadequate if new vaccines are recommended by ACIP and if initiatives to improve adult coverage levels are launched.[4]

States are encouraged to expand their role in purchasing vaccines to meet the needs of vulnerable underinsured populations who are not eligible for programs such as VFC or SCHIP. This role can be fulfilled in one of two ways: by purchasing additional vaccines (the committee suggests an increase of $11 million) or by requiring all private insurers within the state (including Employee Retirement Income Security Act [ERISA]–preempted health plans) to provide all ACIP-recommended vaccines to their members in accordance with state immunization standards. Federal legislation would be required, however, to establish a mandate for the inclusion of childhood immunization benefits in all private insurance plans.[5]

Government expenditures for adult vaccines are currently very low (less than $4 million in federal funds in FY 2000; state estimates are not available). New vaccines are being considered for adult populations, and greater emphasis is being placed on the importance of vaccines for high-risk adults under age 65 with chronic diseases (e.g., diabetes or renal failure). Additional funds will be required to support these purchases to meet residual needs among adults who lack private or public insurance coverage. As discussed in Chapter 3, the purchase of vaccines annually for the high-risk uninsured adult population aged 18–64 requires about $19 million annually for influenza vaccine and about $24.2 million for the one-time purchase of pneumococcal vaccine. If the federal government were to absorb these combined costs, an annual increase of about $50 million in the Section 317 vaccine purchase budget would be required. Future changes to the adult immunization schedule are likely to increase these costs.

As changes occur in the vaccine schedule, the pool of federal and state funds allocated for vaccine purchase will need to expand to allow the states to continue to meet residual needs of vulnerable groups that do not have access to vaccines within private or public insurance plans. These children and adults will continue to fall through the cracks within the national immunization system unless funds are made available from programs such as Section 317 to give the states flexibility in meeting the vaccination needs of populations that cannot afford insurance, but do not qualify for federal assistance. Therefore, CDC and state health officials need to work closely and expeditiously with HCFA, state Medicaid directors, and state SCHIP program officers, as well as professional associations of health care providers, to address three objectives:

- To ensure that the states have a pool of Section 317 funds that is sufficient to meet routine vaccine needs, as well as unexpected outbreaks.
- To be certain that disparities do not emerge in public and private health plans in access to recommended vaccines.
- To develop guidelines and performance measures that will encourage providers to draw on new health finance systems (e.g., VFC and SCHIP) for vaccine coverage so that Section 317 vaccines can be reserved for residual needs.

Federal agencies (particularly CDC) also require additional resources so they can provide national and international leadership; assist in the coordination of programs among states as well as other nations; and create opportunities for the exchange of technical assistance, expertise, and experience in undertaking appropriate and adequate infrastructure efforts at the state and local levels.

Infrastructure Support. Section 317 infrastructure awards currently reflect historical patterns of expenditure and are allocated largely in response to statements of need prepared by state health agencies. Recognizing that the states spent more than 90 percent of the infrastructure grant awards distributed in 1998 and 1999, the committee believes that the demands on the states exceed their current capacity, and that their ability to respond to changes in such areas as the science of vaccines and information technology could become severely compromised. In addition, managed care contracting for Medicaid has eroded the public health infrastructure and funding base in many states so that in some areas, there is no longer a sustainable volume of personal health care demand to support the provision of public health services such as immunization. As state funds withdraw into private-sector contracts, county and local health departments have fewer resources to spend on public health services. The national immunization system is weakening, and we should not have to wait for outbreaks of vaccine-preventable disease to strengthen areas in need of support.

Current federal immunization funding for the states is significantly lower than the states' historical expenditure levels. Based on an examination of total state expenditure histories, the committee estimates that the states require a total of about $500 million in annual infrastructure funds to sustain a national immunization system that can achieve current national health goals; respond to future developments in the areas of vaccine science, information technology, and health care delivery systems; improve the sensitivity of surveillance measures so they can identify important gaps in immunization coverage levels; and extend immunization programs to the adult population. This amount was derived from two sources: it combines (1) an estimate of what is required to support the six essential roles of a viable state infrastructure program for immunization services, as outlined above, with (2) an estimate of the base level of federal funding required to direct additional resources to areas of need without reducing current levels of support for each state (known as a "hold harmless" provision).

The committee believes the annual costs for immunization infrastructure should be shared between federal and state governments. The state share is necessary because the state is the lead public health care delivery agency in the national system, because states establish immunization requirements for their residents, and because immunization efforts require state ownership and oversight. The proposed federal government share (a total of $200 million per year, representing a $74 million annual increase over current budgets) should be administered by CDC through the Section 317 state grants program. In providing their share (a total of $331 million per year, representing a $100 million annual increase over current estimates), states should be encouraged to use their own funds as well as other federal grants (e.g., Medicaid, Title V, and SCHIP). The combined increases in federal and state support are sufficient to provide resources that can stabilize existing state-level programs, respond to the needs presented by advances in the science of adolescent and adult vaccines and information technology, and address emerging concerns about vaccine safety.

Recognizing the need for a long-term strategy to build appropriate infrastructure within each state, the committee believes federal and state agencies should make a national shared commitment to the immunization partnership by investing a total of $1.5 billion in immunization infrastructure support over the first 5-year period. This figure consists of $1 billion in federal funds (approximately $200 million each year), matched by a comprehensive effort within the states to raise an annual increase of $100 million over current spending levels.

Question 4: How should federal grant funds be distributed among the states? (Supported by Findings 4-2 and 4-14 in Chapter 4 and Findings 5-12 and 5-16 in Chapter 5.)

Each state deserves some level of federal assistance, but some states require more help than others because of the characteristics of their populations. In addition, states that have more resources because of their tax base should be expected to bear a larger burden of the costs of immunization infrastructure. Finally, states that demonstrate success in increasing their immunization coverage levels should be rewarded when such increases reflect real improvements in the status of their most vulnerable populations. Since allocation by need and by achievement may run counter to each other, specific criteria will need to be developed to balance multiple goals.

For these reasons, the committee believes federal funds should be allocated to the states on a formula basis, with a state match requirement that reflects each state's capacity to bear part of the burden of infrastructure costs. A small proportion (perhaps 5 to 10 percent) of the total federal grant awards for infrastructure should also be set aside so that CDC will have discretionary funds available to respond to unexpected outbreaks, gaps in immunization coverage, or other exceptional circumstances within the states.

Four Basic Principles for a Federal Grant Formula

Allocating federal immunization grants to the states requires consideration of several factors: need, capacity, performance, and the determination of a base-level grant award. The committee offers four basic principles to illustrate the nature of each of these factors and the types of measures that should be considered in estimating their value within the proposed formula.

Principle 1: Each state requires a base grant award, regardless of population size, level of need, or match contribution. There is a strong federal interest in ensuring a stable immunization infrastructure within each state so that vaccine coverage levels can be sustained among vulnerable groups, and appropriate sentinels will be available to detect emerging trends or problems having national significance. The size of the base award should be sufficient to allow each state to perform the six roles of the immunization system discussed in this report. CDC may want to consider cost-indexing these awards, possibly through multiyear grants, to adjust for salary increases and variations in salary structures for public health employees in different regions of the United States.

Principle 2: States that have larger disadvantaged populations should receive greater amounts of federal assistance. The history of the Section 317 program demonstrates that the program is fundamentally designed so the federal government can share with the states the costs of enhancing access to immunizations for vulnerable and medically underserved populations, especially children, the elderly, and those who reside in areas of concentrated disadvantage. State needs differ according to population size, urban/rural distribution, and rate of underinsured populations. States in which 20 percent of the population is without insurance, for example, require greater investments in safety net support than those that have less than 10 percent uninsured. Determining the level of need within each state requires attention to several basic components, such as the following:

- the size of the general population (adult, adolescent, and child),
- the size of the annual birth cohort,
- the size of the uninsured population (adult, adolescent, and child),
- the size of the Medicaid (and SCHIP) population,
- the size of the immigrant population, and
- the scope and level of benefits in insurance coverage.

Principle 3: States that have a greater capacity for addressing the needs of their citizens should do more to share the costs of vaccine purchase and infrastructure development. Estimates of need, while important, are only one of the multiple concerns that require consideration in federal funding decisions. Estimates of state capacity are commonly used when determining cost-sharing formulas in other federally funded, state-administered health programs, including Medicaid, MCH grants (Title V), and SCHIP. These capacity measures reflect per capita wealth within the state and the size of the revenue base that can be raised by the state to support health programs. Such measures facilitate comparisons among states because they can help determine what each state should be expected to spend if it is to make adequate investments of its own funds in meeting critical public health needs.

A second capacity measure that is directly relevant to immunization is more difficult to determine. The capacity of the state's public health insurance system (including Medicaid and SCHIP) to cover immunizations and encourage the delivery of immunizations in each child's medical home will influence the size of residual needs, reducing or expanding the population that will seek immunization services directly from safety net health centers. States that offer generous Medicaid payments to large numbers of providers and extend client eligibility for longer periods are investing their own funds to support quality health care for disadvantaged groups and thereby encouraging the participation of private health providers in the state's Medicaid, SCHIP, and VFC programs. If the plan participants have access to adequate immunization services from their health care providers, and there are fewer administrative barriers that restrict the plan providers from offering services to vulnerable clients, the state has a stronger primary care capacity and less need for federal safety net programs to supplement its health care system.

These two measures—per capita wealth and state health care capacity—merit explicit consideration in the allocation of federal funds, including Section 317 grants. High marks for either indicator suggest that the state has the revenue to support the cost of vaccine purchase or is already investing substantially in immunization services for disadvantaged populations, reducing the demands on the public immunization infrastructure.

Principle 4: States that achieve higher levels of performance in immunization should be rewarded for those outcomes. The increasing use of performance measures in public health programs places greater importance on the selection of appropriate indicators and measures. CDC has recognized the importance of immunization performance over the past decade (with congressional guidance) by allocating a portion of the Section 317 grant awards to incentive awards based on improvements in immunization rates.

While important, statewide immunization rates can be deceiving because they often do not reveal small areas of concentrated need within the state (see Table 1-5 in Chapter 1). The size of within-state disparities is a second important measure of performance that can demonstrate how well or how poorly the state health system is doing in providing access to immunization services among hard-to-reach populations.

A third relevant performance measure is the level of immunization coverage within Medicaid and SCHIP populations. Baseline measures are especially important in determining the extent to which health finance programs can influence access to vaccines and the size of the safety net population within each state. In addition, the size of the denominator involves careful judgments about which clients should be included in performance assessment measures: all enrolled clients, all clients who make routine visits to the provider, or clients who have visited only once?

Finally, performance measures should encompass the efficiency with which the states administer federal funds. The committee did not identify any such measures in the state survey conducted for this study. Prototype research may be necessary to design and test appropriate efficiency measures for the public health environment. Relevant studies may be available in other fields (such as education) that offer insights and experience for comparative estimates of administrative efficiency in state spending patterns.

CDC should develop a set of performance criteria with these issues in mind that can be used to examine state immunization performance over a 5-year period. At the end of that time, a panel should be convened to consider whether changes in Medicaid, SCHIP, or other public or private health care plans have reduced the need for Section 317 vaccines, whether private health care plans are able to provide community-level measures of immunization coverage, and whether any other trends may influence the need for Section 317 funds within the states.

Proposal for a State Match Requirement

The committee believes the states bear responsibility for sharing the infrastructure costs of the national immunization system. The proposed formula for distributing federal funds should include a state match requirement—such as 75 federal/25 state—similar to that in place for Medicaid grants, Title V MCH grants, and block grants for the prevention and treatment of substance abuse. The committee believes a state match is desirable for several reasons.

First, the desirability of a state match requirement is based on the premise that immunization is a shared national partnership between federal and state governments. Allocating state funds for immunization infrastructure needs on a regular basis will create a line item in public health budgets that will add greater stability to the public health system and allow finance trends to be monitored over time. A state match requirement will also serve as an incentive for states that do not currently invest in infrastructure resources to commit funds to this area on a routine basis.

Second, the match requirement will stimulate greater attention to the dynamics of public- and private-sector involvement in providing immunizations to vulnerable groups and establish greater buy-in for public health efforts at the state and local levels. A match requirement will give state legislatures, state health finance agencies, and state governors' offices incentives to monitor the performance of private health care plans that operate within their borders and to determine whether plans that use state funds have the capacity to keep their clients up to date on the immunization schedule. Greater oversight of the immunization budgets of public health agencies will reveal the extent to which such budgets support safety net services to meet residual needs, as well as critical surveillance and assessment functions that benefit the general population.

Third, the state match requirement does not necessarily require new sources of funds, since many states already contribute to the support of immunization efforts. The match requirement will reveal the range of these contributions over time, and provide an opportunity for CDC to review how federal and state funds are distributed across the six roles of the immunization system discussed in this report. It is conceivable that a match requirement might prompt individual states to add their own resources or in-kind contributions to their immunization programs, or to seek such resources from outside government, since health officers will need to demonstrate a base level of grantee contribution to qualify for federal grants.

CDC has always stressed that federal funding is to be used to supplement, not supplant, each grantee's immunization effort, but a state-level contribution is not currently required for Section 317 grants. Such grants originated in a public health environment in which it was assumed that a state match requirement would delay the use of federal funds in swiftly reducing exposure to vaccine-preventable diseases for vulnerable populations. Over time, however, immunization has become a routine part of primary care services that are financed in large measure through cooperative state and federal arrangements. Additional assessment and populationwide services have also increased the costs of sustaining and improving up-to-date coverage within the U.S. population as a whole, and the federal government should not be expected to support these costs alone.

The committee considered several arguments against a state match, but did not find them compelling. Following are these arguments and the committee's response to each.

First, a matching requirement would necessitate changing the existing Section 317 legislation, and exposure of the legislation and approvals of annual budgetary contributions within the states could generate skepticism about the infrastructure grants program and create vulnerabilities in the political process. The committee believes broader exposure of the immunization grants program will strengthen federal and state collaboration. Although the legislative reform process may introduce undesirable or radical changes in the program's scope, purpose, or funding approach that could create uncertainty and confusion and disrupt programmatic efforts, at least in the short term, a state match requirement is not likely to have this effect provided the rationale for the match is sound and justified.

Second, a state match requirement might create incentives for government officials or legislators to reduce grantee contributions in areas in which the match is already exceeded. In other areas, state or local public health officials or legislators might not be able or inclined to meet a matching requirement, and federal grants could be reduced or eliminated as a result. If state contributions to public health are invested wisely, evidence should be available to demonstrate why such contributions are in the state's interest.

Third, administering a state match requirement will require additional docu-

mentation and create an administrative burden for CDC staff and state officials. It is not sound policy to introduce additional bureaucratic procedures in the public health system unless such procedures serve important goals or create new resources. State grantees will need to document their contributions to immunization infrastructure on an annual basis. This documentation will require selection criteria and finance guidelines during a start-up period, but such efforts will gradually become routine as greater familiarity is gained with the match in the budgetary cycle. Many states already have procedures for approval of match contributions, and they are accustomed to including a match in Title V and other public health grant proposals. It is doubtful that the match requirement will disrupt programmatic efforts, especially if the formula for allocation includes a base amount of federal funds for each state regardless of the size of the match contribution.

States may choose to exercise their match requirement in one of two ways: through direct or indirect support. Direct support means the states allocate their own revenues for the direct support of vaccine purchase or immunization infrastructure programs. Indirect support means the states rely on other approaches to support immunization efforts. They might use in-kind assistance in the form of contributed time from other agencies, such as the use of school nurses to monitor immunization records in the community. They might invest their own funds to provide higher fees for Medicaid and SCHIP health services and rely more heavily on these programs to cover immunizations. Indirect support might also include the oversight of private insurance plans to ensure that they provide sufficient coverage for immunization services. The direct approach involves direct payments to public health programs for immunization services, whereas the indirect approach involves greater reliance on performance assessment, incentives, and regulatory initiatives, since other agencies, including public and private health plans, are responsible for immunization services. States that cover greater numbers of children through SCHIP and serve a significant portion of their uninsured and Medicaid children with VFC through private providers may require fewer federal and state funds for Section 317 vaccine (because they receive larger amounts of federal and state funds for Medicaid and SCHIP payments). The number of children who rely on the safety net programs in these states will be smaller compared with states that use their public health infrastructure as a principal tool in serving vulnerable populations.

Determining the Appropriate Formula and Match Requirements

Although states should have flexibility in designing finance and service systems to meet their immunization needs, tracking systems should be developed that allow the states to report and compare both the scale of their investments (in direct and indirect efforts) and the outcomes achieved by using different strategies to address common goals. Interagency collaboration at both the state and federal levels may be required to support public health efforts in the field of immunization. For example, guidelines at the national level could encourage Medicaid agencies to bear the costs of administrative services (including immunization audits of provider records and registry development) as part of case management expenditures. Whatever the source, states need to be able to predict the size of their immunization budgets on a multiyear basis, rely on steady sources of income to support both vaccine purchase and infrastructure efforts, and assess the performance of those efforts according to a consistent set of measures.

A set of proxy measures focused on need, capacity, and performance should be developed that can be monitored over time. These measures can be used to guide federal grant allocation decisions and the determination of state contribution levels, as well as programmatic and reporting requirements. A small set of comparable measures will allow federal and state agencies to monitor state need, capacity, and performance without imposing unnecessary effort on the states that restricts their ability to respond to local circumstances.

The committee believes the assignment of weights to the factors of need, capacity, and performance requires careful calculations that lie beyond the scope of this report. These calculations should be informed by a democratic process that takes individual state needs into account. The calculations required include the appropriate size of the federal base grant; appropriate "hold harmless" conditions; the nature of adequate state-level contributions; an appropriate set of proxy measures that reflect need, capacity, and performance in the field of immunization; and the appropriate multiyear finance mechanism for allocating federal funds. The calculation process requires an extensive dialogue with federal and state health agencies, state legislatures, state governors, and the U.S. Congress. The committee recommends that CDC initiate this dialogue immediately so that legislative reforms can be proposed by 2002, when Section 317 is scheduled for reauthorization.

Several different types of formula factors would alter the distribution of state grant awards relative to current allocation patterns. The factors considered in making other state health grant awards are the size of the population and federal poverty level measures, which can be set at different thresholds. The inclusion of any one formula factor would cause major shifts in the current distribution of federal funds. A small number of states (commonly states with large numbers of at-risk children, such as California, Texas, New York, and Pennsylvania) frequently rank much higher in formula distributions than smaller or more rural states. It is important, therefore, to maintain stability by ensuring a base level of federal funds within each state while responding to specific state needs.

This need for stability in the national immunization system underscores the importance of increasing the size of the pool of federal funds for state infrastructure awards, as discussed under Question 3 above. CDC has estimated that the use of certain formula factors in redistributing federal awards within an annual budget of $140 or $160 million for infrastructure grants would reduce the current size of a significant number of state awards, further burdening state efforts. A annual pool of $195 million, however, would minimize the need to reduce current state awards in order to increase federal assistance to states with larger poor populations (information provided by CDC).

Question 5: How should funds be targeted within states to reach high-risk populations without diminishing levels of coverage among the over-all population? (Supported by Finding 3-6 in Chapter 3; Finding 4-11 in Chapter 4; and Findings 5-1 through 5-9, 5-12, 5-16, 5-18, and 5-19 in Chapter 5.)

The federal government's role in supporting immunization activities within each state should strike a balance between helping the states achieve important national objectives and sustaining incentives for states to use their own funds to meet the needs of their residents. Given the primacy of the role of the states in public health, the federal government's role might reasonably be restricted to certain key areas that require specific technical expertise, national data collection and analysis, and the development of benchmarks and indicators that benefit the nation as a whole. In states that do not have a sufficient revenue base to support adequate public health investments, however, the federal government has an important role to play in supplementing state funds to ensure that an adequate program is in place that can achieve national health objectives. Special considerations might include the examples that follow.

First is the size and location of the disadvantaged population within each state. Poverty remains a daunting obstacle to efforts to improve immunization coverage within any specific population. The size of a state's population that resides in poverty and the extent to which this population is distributed or clustered within the state are important factors to consider in evaluating the size of the public health infrastructure and immunization program needed within the state.

As discussed in the response to Question 4, federal immunization investments should provide greater resources for those states that have larger pockets of need. At the same time, care needs to be taken so that federal funds are not used to support basic health services that are rightfully the obligation of the state. Formula factors that might be built into the allocation of Section 317 grants might include, for example, the distribution of the state's population above and below the federal poverty level, the percentage of uninsured families, the size of the child and adolescent Medicaid populations, and the size of the high-risk adult population within the state. The application of such factors would generate new winners and losers in the distribution of federal funds, possibly creating unfair discrepancies (e.g., fewer than 10 states receiving more than 90 percent of available funds). Balance needs to be achieved in leveling the playing field among the states and ensuring that each state receives a minimal grant award that is sufficient to maintain an effective partnership with the federal government.

A second special consideration might be the marginal costs of improving immunization coverage within highly disadvantaged groups. As discussed in Chapter 4, the cost of improving coverage within the final 10 percent of a total population in any given area is thought to be significantly higher than the cost of acquiring coverage for the majority of the community. However, the scale of this difference remains uncertain. Assigning costs requires consideration of such components as outreach, case management, record maintenance, disease exposure, frequency of contacts with primary care providers, and health beliefs and knowledge that influence efforts to obtain immunization.

What is known for certain is that highly disadvantaged populations seek services more frequently from multiple providers in multiple health care settings. Such populations frequently cycle among different health plans, including public and private health care finance arrangements, and are often uninsured for lengthy periods. Their case management and record maintenance costs are greater than comparable costs for individuals who remain with the same health care provider or the same practice over a period of years, especially those who remain within one health plan during the important immunization period of the early childhood years.

Despite these barriers, research has demonstrated that certain types of programs can improve immunization coverage within highly disadvantaged groups if focused on populations that have the most to gain from those programs (see Chapter 4). It is wasteful, for example, to distribute information packages and brochures about the importance of immunization within a community where parents may be illiterate or can read only in non-English languages. Similarly, it is wasteful to improve outreach and parental education programs in communities where most parents already believe in the importance of vaccines, but mistakenly believe that their children are already up to date in their immunization status.

CDC frequently relies on technical assistance to help states direct their resources toward productive programmatic investments. However, this approach may not be sufficient in areas where states choose to distribute their own resources over a broad geographic area rather than concentrating them in areas of need where delivery systems may be weak and data collection difficult. State health agencies face difficult political obstacles when shifting public resources away from communities that have achieved high levels of coverage (sometimes with minimal state effort) so the resources can be targeted to areas where performance is poor. In such cases, the role of the federal government is to create incentives (e.g., ranking states on the basis of within-state disparities in coverage) or to provide targeted resources that enable states to do all they can to address the immunization needs of their most vulnerable citizens.

Question 6: What should be the role and financing level for CDC's current program supporting state efforts to vaccinate adults and achieve the nation's goals for influenza and pneumococcal vaccines? (Supported by Findings 3-3 and 3-5 in Chapter 3.)

Immunization coverage rates for adults are well below those achieved for childhood immunizations, although some progress in immunization was made in immunizing the adult population over age 65 during the 1990s. The Healthy People 2000 objective for influenza coverage levels was met for the noninstitutionalized elderly (individuals aged 65 and older) according to 1997 National Health Interview Survey (NHIS) data (see Table 3-6 in Chapter 3). The national average was 63 percent, up from 58 percent in 1995. According to 1997 data from the Behavioral Risk Factor Surveillance System (BRFSS), 45 states exceeded the goal of increasing influenza immunization levels to 60 percent among the elderly (CDC, 1998d). From 1995 to 1997, 48 states showed improvement in influenza vaccination rates for the elderly. The mean coverage level of states in 1997, 65.5 percent, was almost double the 1989 coverage level of 33 percent (CDC, 1998d). Nonetheless, in 1997, the percentage of adults aged 55–64 who received influenza vaccine ranged from 28.5 percent (Georgia) to 54.7 percent (Colorado), with a median of 38.2 percent. For persons aged 65–74, percentages ranged from 48.7 percent (Nevada) to 72.4 percent (Colorado), with a median of 63.6 percent. Among persons over age 75, percentages ranged from 51.7 percent (District of Columbia) to 82 percent (Arizona), with a median of 71.4 percent (Janes et al., 1999).

Pneumococcal immunization levels for the elderly are significantly lower than influenza immunization levels, even though Medicare covers the cost of this vaccine and its administration (Janes et al., 1999). The NHIS data show that only 42 percent of the noninstitutionalized elderly had ever received a pneumococcal vaccination by 1997 (see Table 3-6).

Although this was a large increase over the 34 percent coverage rate reported in 1995, the 1997 national average fell far below the Healthy People 2000 goal of 60 percent coverage, and this goal has still not been met. According to BRFSS, only 17 states had achieved immunization rates of 50 percent or greater among the elderly by 1997. Coverage in 1997 ranged from 9.5 percent (New York) to 30.7 percent (Alaska) among persons aged 55–64, with a median of 17.1 percent. For persons aged 65–74, percentages ranged from 30.1 percent (New Jersey) to 56.9 percent (Arizona), with a median of 42.6 percent. Finally, for persons over age 75, the percentages ranged from 31.4 percent (Louisiana) to 79 percent (Nevada), with a median of 53.3 percent (Janes et al., 1999).

Although differences in coverage rates among children of different ethnic groups have been significantly reduced, troublesome disparities remain in adult immunization coverage levels (see Table 3-6). According to 1997 NHIS data, elderly blacks had the lowest likelihood of receiving either influenza (45 percent) or pneumococcal (22 percent) immunizations. Elderly Hispanics had influenza and pneumococcal immunization coverage levels of 53 percent and 23 percent, respectively, as compared with coverage levels of 66 percent and 46 percent, respectively, for whites in 1997.

Noninstitutionalized high-risk adults aged 18–64 have extremely low immunization rates and may present the largest challenge to efforts to appropriately immunize adults (see Table 3-6). The 1997 NHIS data demonstrate that only 26 percent of this group had received an influenza vaccination, while only 13 percent had received a pneumococcal vaccination. Differences in coverage levels among races were not as great in the high-risk population aged 18–64 as in the population over age 65. Compared with the elderly, the high-risk group aged 18–64 had very low rates of immunization coverage. In 1997, among those with private health insurance, 29 percent of high-risk adults aged 18–64 and 63 percent of the noninstitutionalized elderly received an influenza vaccination. Among those with Medicaid, 26 percent of the high-risk population aged 18–64 received an influenza vaccination (see Table 3-6) (National Center for Health Statistics, 1997).

The 1997 NHIS also provides information on selected high-risk subgroups. Coverage rates for the noninstitutionalized elderly were higher than those for the high-risk population aged 18–64 in every subgroup. In 1997, 67 percent and 44 percent, respectively, of noninstitutionalized elderly with diabetes received influenza and pneumococcal vaccinations. In contrast, only 36 percent and 19 percent, respectively, of adults aged 18–64 with diabetes received influenza and pneumococcal vaccinations. Data on national coverage rates for adult immunizations other than influenza and pneumococcal are severely limited. According to Healthy People

2000, 67 percent of occupationally exposed workers received a hepatitis B vaccination in 1994, and 9 percent of men who had sex with men received this vaccination in 1997. NHIS data show that in 1995, 65 percent of persons aged 18–49, 54 percent of those aged 50–64, and 40 percent of those aged 65 and older had received a tetanus booster in the last 10 years (Singleton et al., forthcoming).

As with the monitoring of adult coverage levels, existing immunization finance programs tend to neglect the population aged 18–64. Adult immunizations are currently funded by a patchwork of public and private insurance that results in scattered immunization rate data, inconsistent insurance coverage among Americans, and a lack of collaborative roles and missions within the private and public health sectors.

Studies have shown that both influenza and pneumococcal vaccines are cost-effective. Yet federal funds that support adult immunization are a small fraction of the financial resources dedicated to childhood immunization. The main funding sources for adult immunization are Medicare, Section 317, and private insurance. States could spend Section 317 grants on vaccines and services for adults under age 65, but grantees have historically spent only a miniscule amount (estimated at about 2 percent) of their Section 317 funds on adult immunization. In addition, CDC did not authorize its grantees to use Section 317 funds in support of adult immunization until 1997 (information provided by CDC). Medicare has played a much larger role in adult immunization than that played by Section 317; it has covered pneumococcal vaccine since 1981 and influenza vaccine since 1993. In the future, with the dramatic rise of managed care and health maintenance organizations (HMOs) that emphasize preventive services, the committee believes adult immunizations are increasingly likely to be covered by private insurance. This trend provides an opportunity to raise awareness about the importance of immunization among health professionals who care for adults and to hold private plans and providers accountable for adult immunization performance measures.

As shown by the low coverage rates and low levels of funding, adult immunization is not a priority in the United States. Approximately 50,000 adult Americans still die each year from diseases for which both safe and effective vaccines exist, and yet as noted, only 2 percent of Section 317 funds have been dedicated to adult immunization (Poland and Miller, 2000). What is missing is a coordinated and comprehensive federal, state, and local strategy to improve adult immunization coverage levels. Health care providers are often less successful in providing age-appropriate immunizations as their clients grow from infancy through childhood to adolescence and adulthood. Immunization has not been the focus for practitioners who routinely care for adults that it has become for pediatric providers. Only rudimentary programs in state and local health departments reach out to adult populations and their health care providers regarding immunization practices. Federal and state leadership has been successful in achieving substantial coordination among the various programs devoted to specific childhood vaccine-preventable diseases. Yet the units devoted to adult vaccine-preventable diseases (e.g., influenza, pneumococcal, tetanus/diphtheria, and hepatitis B infections) typically focus on narrow goals and rarely address a comprehensive adult immunization strategy. Increased funding and coordinated programs can begin to move adult immunization beyond its current marginal status.

In the recommendations at the end of this chapter, the committee proposes a specific financing level for purchasing vaccines as part of an adult immunization program. In addition, the committee recommends that CDC develop a coordinated and comprehensive immunization effort for adults to encourage greater participation by the private and public health care sectors in achieving national goals.

CONCLUSIONS

Conclusion 1: The repetitive ebb and flow cycles in the distribution of public resources for immunization programs have created instability and uncertainty that impeded project planning at the state and local levels in the late 1990s, and delayed the public benefit of advances in the development of new vaccines for both children and adults. This instability now erodes the continued success of immunization activities.

The national immunization system that emerged in the United States in the latter half of the 20th century was created by a series of infectious disease outbreaks and governmental responses, with governmental assistance often being increased after outbreaks occurred, not to prevent them (Johnson et al., forthcoming). Substantial progress has been made in preventing and controlling disease, ensuring access to vaccines, and providing service delivery in medical homes. But three other areas require attention in renewing the national immunization partnership: improving the quality of immunization surveillance efforts and vaccine safety programs, strengthening efforts to sustain and improve immunization coverage rates, and using primary care and public health resources efficiently. The instability of funding for state immunization programs discourages the development of strategic responses designed to foster disease prevention, improve immunization coverage levels for specific populations, and ensure vaccine safety. Diminishing resources often divert attention toward protecting individual programs or interventions rather than focusing on the health and vitality of the population as a whole. The current situation is characterized by a spirit of complacency and disjointedness that creates an unstable and unpredictable environment for immunization in the midst of rapid changes in the science of vaccines and the health care system.

Conclusion 2: Immunization policy needs to be national in scope. At the same time, the implementation of immunization policy must be flexible enough to respond to special circumstances that occur at the state and local levels.

A comprehensive strategy that clarifies the roles and responsibilities of federal and state agencies as well as private-sector providers and health plans within the national immunization system is needed to sustain an important intergovernmental partnership in the midst of change and complexity. The federal presence should be adequate and stable so that state agencies can develop strategic approaches to address local needs. The state role is to ensure that appropriate systems are in place for detecting and responding to changes in immunization coverage levels and disparities in access to immunization resources. The implementation of all six immunization roles therefore requires public attention and resources at both the state and federal levels, as well as sustained commitments within the private sector.

The eligibility requirements for VFC, for example, currently discriminate against states that choose to set up stand-alone plans rather than relying on Medicaid agencies to administer their SCHIP funds. SCHIP children who are enrolled in the stand-alone plans are considered "insured" and are therefore not eligible for benefits under the VFC program, while SCHIP children in another state may continue receiving their benefits because they are still technically enrolled in Medicaid. These types of administrative distinctions disrupt the national immunization partnership and cause states to turn unnecessarily to other federal programs (e.g., Section 317) to meet their needs.

National initiatives that provide immunization coverage for larger numbers of disadvantaged families under private and public health insurance plans require state public health responsibilities to shift from direct service delivery to oversight roles concerned with assessment, assurance, and policy development. Yet certain residual immunization needs will remain that will necessitate reliable access to vaccines within the public health sector. States need flexibility and resources to adapt to these shifts, which occur unevenly across and within state borders.

Conclusion 3: Federal and state governments each have important roles in supporting not only vaccine purchase, but also infrastructure efforts that can achieve and sustain national immunization goals.

The federal government needs to work with the states to ensure that appropriate infrastructure efforts are present within each state, to distribute national resources fairly, and to build on the strengths of the private sector in meeting community health care needs where feasible. The federal government should be the senior finance partner for the national immunization system because of the central importance of vaccines in contributing to the nation's health, and because disease outbreaks in one region can threaten the health of another without respect for political borders. However, the federal role is to supplement and support state efforts, not replace them.

State legislatures and governments should be expected to sustain an immunization infrastructure that reflects each state's need, capacity, and performance. Since states are the ultimate stewards of public health policy, they are responsible for delivering services to those whose immunization needs are not met by the private sector. In maintaining coverage standards for at-risk groups, state public health agencies require a surveillance capacity that allows them to measure population-based coverage rates, assess the quality of care within public and private immunization plans, offer safety net services to meet residual needs, and improve access to immunization services within many different public and private entities. Performance monitoring, including the development of immunization registries, is important to ensure that vulnerable groups have access to adequate primary health care and that residual needs are met with public resources where necessary. Finally, state agencies are also responsible for ensuring that the public and private health care sectors work collaboratively within their jurisdiction so that public resources are used efficiently. To carry out these roles, state health agencies require a national immunization policy that provides them with adequate resources, stability, and flexibility.

Conclusion 4: Private health care plans and providers have the capacity to do more in implementing immunization surveillance and preventive programs within their health practices, but such efforts require additional assistance, oversight, and incentives. At the same time, comprehensive insurance and high-quality primary care services do not replace the need for public health infrastructure.

The committee believes health plans should not have the option of providing selective coverage for vaccines once they have been recommended for widespread use, as is currently the practice in most states. A federal mandate may be necessary to achieve this goal, particularly for ERISA-exempt plans. For example, all health plans (public and private) that offer primary care benefits for children and adults should bear the costs of integrating all vaccines recommended for widespread use into their basic health care package. Private health plans should also be expected to bear at least some of the costs of "catch-up" conditions following the licensing of new vaccines (e.g., coverage of hepatitis B vaccine for older children who were too old to have been affected by the universal recommendations). Public health agencies should not be expected to supplement public or private health insurance plans except under short-term conditions, such as responding to emergency outbreaks or reducing disparities that result from "catch-up" conditions. Coordinated efforts, such as billing practices that allow public health clinics to be reimbursed for immunizations given to individuals who are covered by private health care plans, can help reduce the burden on public health agencies. Ideally, however, immunizations should be offered routinely in each plan participant's medical home as an integrated part of primary care benefits.

Health plan providers should also be prepared to assess immunization coverage rates among their enrollees by using measures that can contribute to accurate community health profiles at the state and local levels. These efforts require independent oversight, however, to ensure that all groups are included in such assessments and that the measures used accurately reflect the immunization profile of those not currently enrolled in public and private health plans. Public health agencies can provide important measurement and audit services, such as assessment and feedback for private providers, as an investment in the quality of community health. These and other surveillance efforts should be supported by the national immunization partnership as a national health priority, with appropriate recognition of the issues of privacy and confidentiality.

SUMMARY RECOMMENDATIONS

Recommendation 1: The annual federal and state budgets for the purchase of childhood vaccines for public health providers appear to be adequate, but additions to the vaccine schedule are likely to increase the burden of effort within each state. Therefore, the committee recommends that CDC be required to notify Congress each year of the estimated cost impact of new vaccines that have been added to the immunization schedule so that these figures can be considered in reviewing the vaccine purchase and infrastructure budgets for the Section 317 program.

The committee believes the annual allocation of federal funds for the purchase of vaccines through the VFC program ($505 million for FY 2000) and the Section 317 state grant program ($162 million per year for

FY 2000) is sufficient to meet state requests for child vaccines within the immunization schedule recommended by ACIP as of January 2000.[6] But additions to the ACIP schedule will expand the burden of preventive health care costs to state and federal health agencies as well as private health plans. Such additional costs should be expected as part of the changing immunization system. Congress should anticipate such cost increases by requiring that CDC notify Congress each year of two trends: (1) the estimated cost impact of new vaccines (including administration fees) that are scheduled for consideration as additions to the recommended immunization schedule, and (2) the length of time that may be involved from the point at which such vaccines are recommended by ACIP to the establishment of a VFC contract. Federal and state vaccine purchase budgets should then be adjusted as necessary.

> **Recommendation 2: Additional funds are needed to purchase vaccines for uninsured and underinsured adult populations within the states. The committee recommends that Congress increase the annual Section 317 vaccine budget by $50 million per year to meet residual needs for high-risk adolescents and adults under age 65 who do not qualify for other federal assistance. The committee further recommends that state governments likewise increase their spending for adult vaccines by $11 million per year.**

These estimates are based on calculations of the residual vaccine needs for uninsured and underinsured at-risk populations, including adults who are younger than age 65 and suffer from chronic disease (see Box 3-3 in Chapter 3); for hepatitis B coverage among adolescents; for adults who are at risk because of sexual behavior or occupational settings; and for tetanus coverage. Both federal and state vaccine purchase budgets will require annual adjustments as vaccine costs change or new vaccines or age groups are added to the adult immunization schedule. Therefore, CDC notification of the impact of such changes should be required annually, as indicated in Recommendation 1.

The improvement of adult immunization rates will require more than increased vaccine purchases. A comprehensive and coordinated adult immunization program needs to be initiated within each state, with leadership at the national, state, and local levels, to encourage the participation of private and public health care providers in offering immunizations to adults under the guidelines established in the ACIP schedule.

> **Recommendation 3: State immunization infrastructure programs require increased financial and administrative support**

to strengthen immunization capacity and reduce disparities in child and adult coverage rates. The committee recommends that states increase their immunization budgets by adding $100 million over current spending levels, supplemented by an annual federal budget of $200 million to support state infrastructure efforts.

The committee believes state immunization programs could achieve stability and carry out their roles adequately through the adoption of a national finance strategy that involves investing a total of $1.5 billion in the first 5 years—an annual increase of $175 million over current spending levels—to support infrastructure efforts within the states. The federal budget figure is derived from three calculations: (1) annual state expenditure levels during the mid-1990s, (2) the level of spending necessary to provide additional resources to states with high levels of need without reducing current award levels for each state (known as a "hold harmless" provision), and (3) additional infrastructure requirements associated with adjusting to anticipated changes and increased complexity in the immunization schedule. The additional state contribution is necessary to reduce current disparities in state spending practices and to address future infrastructure needs in such areas as records management, development of appropriate performance measures and immunization registries, and outreach and education for adult vaccines. This increased budget could strengthen the state roles in immunization, with a special emphasis on infectious disease prevention and control, surveillance of vaccine coverage rates and safety, and programs to sustain and improve immunization coverage rates.

Different types of administrative support can be offered to the states to strengthen their immunization efforts. For example, federal reporting requirements for immunization grants should be reduced to six key areas that reflect the six fundamental roles of the national immunization system discussed in this report. In addition, grant budgetary cycles should be extended to 2 years to give states greater discretion and flexibility to plan and implement multiyear efforts in each area.

Recommendation 4: Congress should improve the targeting and stability of Section 317 immunization grant awards to the states by replacing the current discretionary grant award mechanism with formula grant legislation.

The formula should reflect a base level as well as factors related to each state's need, capacity, and performance. A state match requirement should be introduced so that federal and state agencies share the total costs of supporting the infrastructure required to operate a national immunization program and respond to the needs of disadvantaged populations.

As discussed in an earlier section of this chapter, the committee believes the states bear responsibility for sharing the infrastructure costs of the national immunization system. About half of the states currently invest in immunization programs in addition to their vaccine purchases; the remaining half do not support infrastructure costs on a routine basis.

To reduce this disparity, the proposed formula for distributing federal funds should include a state match requirement—such as 75 federal/ 25 state—similar to that in place for other federal programs, such as Medicaid grants, Title V MCH grants, and block grants for the prevention and treatment of substance abuse. The details of the match requirement and the conditions under which it would operate should be developed through a series of dialogues with state and federal officials and public health leaders to ensure that the match is fair and equitable and that it does not disrupt ongoing immunization efforts.

> **Recommendation 5: CDC should initiate a dialogue with federal and state health agencies, state legislatures, state governors, and Congress immediately so that legislative and budgetary reforms can be proposed promptly when Section 317 is up for reauthorization in FY 2002.**

The committee believes the grant formula should include weights that reflect factors of need, capacity, and performance. The calculation of these weights and the analytical process of constructing a formula must reflect special considerations that account for individual state needs and lie beyond the scope of this report. The calculations required include estimating the appropriate size of the federal base grant; determining appropriate "hold harmless" conditions; determining the nature of adequate state-level contributions; developing an appropriate set of proxy measures that reflect need, capacity, and performance in the field of immunization; and choosing the appropriate multiyear finance mechanism for the allocation of federal funds.

> **Recommendation 6: Federal and state agencies should develop a set of consistent and comparable immunization measures for use in monitoring the status of children and adults enrolled in private and public health plans.**

Immunization coverage measures are important for identifying both community health needs and performance outcomes for selected service interventions. Measurement research can guide future federal and state budgetary decisions, as well as state contribution, programmatic, and reporting requirements. A small set of comparable measures that can harmonize the Health Plan Employer Data and Information Set (HEDIS) and the National Immunization Survey, for example, will allow federal and state agencies to monitor state need, capacity, and performance without imposing unnecessarily burdensome reporting efforts on the states that would restrict their ability to use federal funds productively in responding to local circumstances (Fairbrother and Freed, forthcoming). Such measures can also facilitate efforts by state and federal health officials to assess the quality of primary care health services within private-sector health plans, so that public health agencies can direct appropriate resources to areas in which private-sector plans do not have sufficient capacity to meet health care needs. Assessments of these rates should allow state and federal governments to monitor immunization levels and identify disparities in need, capacity, and performance over time and among regions, including small geographic areas and selected health plans (e.g., Medicaid, SCHIP, and private insurance).

The use of consistent immunization measures within the public and private sectors offers a valuable opportunity to conduct research on the factors that can contribute to disparities in coverage rates within different types of health plans. Finally, immunization measures offer benefit not only for immunization efforts, but also for other national programs that require national investments in primary health care.

ENDNOTES

1. Question 6 was added by CDC during negotiation of the study contract with IOM.

2. The study was conducted as part of the CDC core functions initiative, and involved a detailed set of survey questions and site visits to the states.

3. This estimate consists of $467 million for VFC and $140 million in vaccine purchase awards for the states in FY 1999; $474 million for VFC and $159 million in vaccine purchase awards for the states is estimated for FY 2000 (information provided by CDC).

4. In February 2000, for example, ACIP recommended that a newly licensed pneumococcal conjugate vaccine be added to the early childhood schedule. The vaccine is recommended for all infants up to age 2 and all high-risk children up to age 5 (CDC, 2000d). The pneumococcal vaccine (estimated to cost $232 for a four-dose series) will add an extraordinary incremental cost to state vaccine budgets, for which resources were not allocated in either the FY 2000 or FY 2001 federal Section 317 budget (Stolberg, 2000).

5. In April 2000, Senator Durbin (D-IL) and Senator Reed (D-RI) introduced a bill to require comprehensive health insurance coverage for childhood immunization (S. 2444).

6. ACIP approval of the pneumococcal conjugate vaccine occurred after the committee had formulated its vaccine purchase recommendations and is not reflected in this calculation.

References

Agency for Healthcare Research and Quality
    1996   Medical Expenditure Panel Survey. Washington, D.C.
Altman LK
    1999   Front line in meningitis campaign: Freshmen. *New York Times*. The
                Doctor's World. (November 2).
American Academy of Family Physicians
    1999   Flu vaccine recommended for people 50 and over: American Academy
                of Family Physicians announces new guidelines. News Release (Sep-
                tember 15). [online document] www.aafp.org/news/990915d.html.
American Academy of Pediatrics
    1999a   Possible association of intussusception with rotavirus vaccination.
                Pediatrics 104(3):575.
    1999b   Thimerosal in vaccines—An interim report to clinicians. *Pediatrics*
                104(3):570–74.
    1992   Policy statement: The medical home. *Pediatrics* 90(5):774.
Annie E. Casey Foundation
    1999   *Kids Count Data Book: State Profiles of Child Well-Being*. Baltimore, MD:
                Annie E. Casey Foundation.
Anonymous
    1990   A Shot in the Arm for Vaccine Advocates. *Medicine and Health Perspec-
                tives* (July 30). Washington, D.C.: Faulkner & Gray.
Association of Maternal and Child Health Professionals
    1999   Immunization and Title V: State MCH Programs Promoting Compre-
                hensive Care Through Immunizations. (March). Washington, D.C.
Bates AS and Wolinsky FD
    1998   Personal, financial, and structural barriers to immunization in socio-
                economically disadvantaged urban children. *Pediatrics* 101(4): 591–96.

Bennett NM, Lewis B, Doniger AS, Bell K, Kouides R, LaForce FM, and Barker W

1994   A coordinated, community-wide program in Monroe County, New York, to increase influenza immunization rates in the elderly. *Archives of Internal Medicine* 154:1741–45.

Birkhead GS, LeBaron CW, Parsons P, Grabau JC, Maes E, Barr-Gale L, Fuhrman J, Bordley WC, Freed GL, Dempsey-Tanner T, and Lister ME

1997   Challenges to private provider participation in immunization registries. *American Journal of Preventive Medicine* Supplement to 13(2):66–70.

Briss PA, Zaza S, and Pappaioanou M

2000   Reviews of evidence regarding interventions to improve vaccination coverage in children, adolescents, and adults. *American Journal of Preventive Medicine* 18(1S):97–140.

Brooks S, Rosenthal J, and Hadler SC

1995   Immunization of children enrolled in the special supplemental food program for women, infants, and children (WIC): Impact of different strategies. *Journal of the American Medical Association* 274:312–16.

Bureau of the Census

1999   *Supplement to the Current Population Survey*. Washington, D.C.: U.S. Government Printing Office. (March).

Center on Budget and Policy Priorities

1999   Progress in reducing child poverty slows, study finds; children remaining poor have become somewhat poorer. News Release (December 23). [online document] www.cbpp.org/12-23-99wel.htm.

Centers for Disease Control and Prevention

2000a   Prevention and control of influenza: Recommendations of the Advisory Committee on Immunization Practices (ACIP). *Morbidity and Mortality Weekly Report* 49(RR03):1–38.

2000b   Recommended childhood immunization schedule—United States, 2000. *Morbidity and Mortality Weekly Report* 49(2):35–38, 47.

2000c   Estimated vaccination coverage with 4:3:1:3 among children 19–35 months of age by selected geographic areas—United States, National Immunization Survey, 1995–1999.

2000d   Preventing pneumococcal disease among infants and young children: Recommendations of the Advisory Committee on Immunization Practices. *Morbidity and Mortality Weekly Report* 49(RR09):1–38.

2000e   Estimated vaccination coverage with 4:3:1:3 among children 19–35 months of age by race-ethnicity of the child and census division and state—United States, National Immunization Survey, July 1998–June 1999.

2000f   Vaccination coverage in percent with individual and vaccination series among children aged 19–35 months living below the poverty level by census division and state—United States, National Immunization Survey, July 1998–June 1999.

1999a   Summary of notifiable diseases, United States 1998. *Morbidity and Mortality Weekly Report* 47(53):1–93.

1999b   Withdrawal of rotavirus vaccine recommendation. *Morbidity and Mortality Weekly Report* 48(43):1007.

1999c   Notice to readers: Recommended childhood immunization schedule–
            United States, 1999. *Morbidity and Mortality Weekly Report* 48(01):8–16.
1999d   Outbreak of West Nile-like viral encephalitis—New York, 1999.
            Morbidity and Mortality Weekly Report 48(38):845–49.
1999e   Estimated vaccination coverage with 4:3:1:3 series among children 19–
            35 months of age by provider type, by census division and state—
            United States, National Immunization Survey, 1998.
1999f   Ten great public health achievements—United States, 1900–1999.
            Morbidity and Mortality Weekly Report 48(12):241–64.
1999g   Transmission of measles among a highly vaccinated school popula-
            tion—Anchorage, Alaska, 1998. *Morbidity and Mortality Weekly Report*
            47(51 and 52):1109–11.
1999h   CDC/NIP 1999 Immunization Registry Annual Report. Self-reported
            data. [online document] www.cdc.gov/nip/registry.html.
1999i   Intussusception among recipients of rotavirus vaccine—United States,
            1998–1999. *Morbidity and Mortality Weekly Report* 28(27): 577–81.
1998a   Vaccination coverage levels for selected vaccines among children aged
            19–35 months living below poverty level and all children, by race/
            ethnicity. *Morbidity and Mortality Weekly Report* 47(44):957.
1998b   Summary of adolescent/adult immunization recommendations. (May
            17). [online document] www.cdc.gov/nip/schedule/adult/
            default.htm.
1998c   Vaccine supply policy. (April 1998). [online document] www.cdc.gov/
            nip.
1998d   Influenza and pneumococcal vaccination levels among adults aged ≥65
            years—United States, 1997. *Morbidity and Mortality Weekly Report*
            47(38):797–802.
1997   Vaccination coverage by race/ethnicity and poverty level among chil-
            dren aged 19–35 months—United States, 1996. *Morbidity and Mortality
            Weekly Report* 46(41):963–69.
1996   Prevention of hepatitis A through active or passive immunization: Rec-
            ommendations of the advisory committee on immunization practices.
            Morbidity and Mortality Weekly Report 45(RR15):1–30.
1995   Notice to readers: Licensure of varicella virus vaccine, live. *Morbidity
            and Mortality Weekly Report* 44(13):264.
1991   Current trends: measles—United States, 1990. *Morbidity and Mortality
            Weekly Report* 40(22):369–72.
Cochi SL, Broome CV, and Hightower AW
1985   Immunization of U.S. children with *Haemophilus influenzae* type b
            polysaccharide vaccine: A cost-effectiveness model of strategy assess-
            ment. *Journal of the American Medical Association* 253(4):521–29.
Copeland C and Pierron B
1998   Implications of ERISA for health benefits and the number of self-funded
            EI plans. *EBRI Issue Brief* (193):1–26.
Cutts FT, Orenstein WA, and Bernier RH
1992   Causes of low preschool immunization coverage in the United States.
            Annual Review of Public Health 13:385–98.

Darden PM, Taylor JA, and Brooks DA
 1999   Polio Immunization Practices of Pediatricians. Paper presented before the Pediatric Academic Societies meeting, San Diego, California.
Davis, RL
 2000   Vaccine extraimmunization—Too much of a good thing? *Journal of the American Medical Association* 283(10):1339–40.
Davis RL, Black S, Vadheim C, Shinefield H, Baker B, Pearson D, and Chen R
 1997   Immunization tracking systems: Experience of the CDC Vaccine Safety Datalink sites. *HMO Practice* 11(1):13–17.
DeFriese GH, Freeman V, and Miller S
 1999   Immunization Registries. Background paper prepared for the Institute of Medicine Committee on Immunization Finance Policies and Practices. Washington, D.C.
Department of Health and Human Services
 2000   *Healthy People 2010* (Conference Edition, in two volumes). Washington, D.C. (January).
 1999   *Healthy People 2000 Review, 1998–1999.* Hyattsville, Md.: Public Health Service. (June).
 1998   *Healthy People 2010 Objectives: Draft for Public Comment.* Washington, D.C.: U.S. Government Printing Office. (September).
 1996   The History of the U.S. Public Health Service. [online document] www.waisgate.hhs.gov.
Dickey LL and Petitti D
 1992   Patient-held minirecord to promote adult preventive care. *Journal of Family Practice* 34:457–63.
Durch, J
 1999   Section 317 Funding: Patterns of Awards, Expenditures, and Carryover, 1990–1999. Paper prepared for the Institute of Medicine Committee on Immunization Finance Policies and Practices. (April). Washington, D.C.
Ellwood M
 1999   *The Medicaid Eligibility Maze: Coverage Expands, but Enrollment Problems Persist: Findings from a Five State Study.* Mathematic Policy Research, Inc. (September). Washington, D.C.
Fairbrother G
 2000   Immunization Priorities and Impact of 317 Funding Policies in Los Angeles and San Diego Counties. Case study prepared for the Institute of Medicine Committee on Immunization Finance Policies and Practices. (February). Washington, D.C.
 1999   Immunization Priorities and Impact of 317 Funding Policies in New Jersey. Case study prepared for the Institute of Medicine Committee on Immunization Finance Policies and Practices. (December). Washington, D.C.
Fairbrother G and Freed GL
Forthcoming   Measuring immunization coverage. *American Journal of Preventive Medicine*, supplement [Expected 19(3S), October].

Fairbrother G, Friedman S, Hanson KL, and Butts GC
1997   Effect of the Vaccines for Children Program on inner-city neighborhood
            physicians. *Archives of Pediatric and Adolescent Medicine* 151:1229–35.
Fairbrother G, Hanson KL, and Butts G
1996   Medicaid managed care in New York: Problems and promise for child-
            hood immunizations. *Journal of Public Health Management Practice*
            (Winter):59–66.
Fairbrother G, Kuttner H, Miller W, Hogan R, McPhillips H, Johnson KA, and
Alexander ER
Forthcoming Findings from case studies of state and local immunization programs.
            American Journal of Preventive Medicine, Supplement [Expected 19(3S),
            October].
Feikema SM, Klevens RM, Washington ML, and Barker L
2000   Extraimmunization among U.S. children. *Journal of the American Medi-
            cal Association* 283(10):1311–17.
Feikin DR, Schuchat A, Kolczak M, Barrett NL, Harrison LH, Lefkowitz L, McGeer A,
Farley MM, Vugia DJ, Lexau C, Stefonek KR, Patterson JE, and Jorgensen JH
2000   Mortality from invasive pneumococcal pneumonia in the era of
            antibiotic resistance, 1995–1997. *American Journal of Public Health*
            90(2):223–29.
Fielding JE, Cumberland WG, and Pettitt L
1994   Immunization status of children of employees in a large corporation.
            Journal of the American Medical Association 271:525–30.
Fine A
1999   Federal Agency Rules and Responsibilities in Immunization Policies
            and Practices. Paper prepared for the Institute of Medicine Committee
            on Immunization Finance Policies and Practices. (April). Washington,
            D.C.
Findley SE, Irigoyen M, and Schulman A
1999   Children on the move and vaccination coverage in a low-income, ur-
            ban Latino population. *American Journal of Public Health* 89(11):1728–31.
Fleming G
1995   Vaccine administration fee survey. *Child Health Care* 11:6.
Food and Drug Administration
1999   Vaccine adverse event reporting system (VAERS). (November). [online
            document] www.fda.gov/cber/vaers/vaers.htm. Washington, D.C.
Freed GL, Clark SJ, and Cowan AE
1999   State-level Perspectives on Immunization Policies, Practices, and Pro-
            gram Financing. Paper prepared for the Institute of Medicine Commit-
            tee on Immunization Policies and Practices. (November). Washington,
            D.C.
Fronstin P
1996   *Sources of Health Insurance and Characteristics of the Uninsured: Analysis of
            the March Current Population Survey*. Washington, D.C.: Employee Ben-
            efit Research Institute.

General Accounting Office

1996   *CDC's National Immunization Survey: Methodological Problems Limit Survey's Utility.* Washington, D.C. (September).

1995a   *Vaccines for Children: Reexamination of Program Goals and Implementation Needed to Ensure Vaccination.* Washington, D.C. (June).

1995b   *Immunization: HHS Could Do More to Increase Vaccination Among Older Adults.* Washington, D.C. (June).

Health Care Financing Administration

2000a   State Children's Health Insurance Program Now Reaching Two Million. Press release. (January 11). [online document] www.hcfa.gov/init/011100wh.htm.

2000b   State Child Health Insurance Program Plan Activity Map. [online document] www.hcfa.gov/init/chip-map.htm. (January 18).

2000c   National Summary of Medicaid Managed Care Programs and Enrollment. [online document] www.hcfa.gov/medicaid/trends98.htm.

2000d   Medicaid recipients and vendor payments by age. [online document] www.hcfa.gov/medicaid/2082-6.htm.

1999a   Administrative Data. [online document] www.hcfa.gov.

1999b   The State Children's Health Insurance Program Annual Enrollment Report, October 1, 1998–September 30, 1999. [online document] www.hcfa.gov/init/20000111.htm.

Health Research and Educational Trust

1999   *Employer Health Benefits: 1999 Annual Survey.*

Health Resources Services Administration

2000a   National Vaccine Injury Compensation Program. [online document] www.hrsa.dhhs.gov/bhpr/vicp/dvicprog.htm.

2000b   National Vaccine Injury Compensation Program. Monthly Statistics Report. [online document] www.hrsa.dhhs.gov/bhpr/vicp/monthly.htm.

2000c   Commonly Asked Questions About the National Vaccine Injury Compensation Program. [online document] www.hrsa.dhhs.gov/bhpr/vicp/qanda.htm.

Horne PR, Saarlas KN, and Hinman AR

Forthcoming   *Costs of Immunization Registries: Experiences from the All Kids Count II Projects.* Baltimore, MD: Annie E. Casey Foundation.

Huse DM, Meisser HC, Lacey MJ, and Oster G

1994   Childhood vaccination against chickenpox: An analysis of benefits and costs. *Journal of Pediatrics* 124(6):869–74.

Hutchins SS, Rosenthal J, Eason P, Swint E, Guerrero H, and Hadler S

1999   Effectiveness and cost-effectiveness of linking the special supplemental program for women, infants, and children (WIC) and immunization activities. *Journal of Public Health Policy* 20(4):408–26.

Institute of Medicine

2000   *Managed Care Systems and Emerging Infections. Challenges and Opportunities for Strengthening Surveillance, Research, and Prevention.* Workshop Summary. Washington, D.C.: National Academy Press.

1999a   *Preliminary Considerations Regarding Federal Investments in Vaccine Pur-*
            chased and Immunization Services: Interim Reports on Immunization Finance
            Policies and Practices. (May).

1999b   *Vaccines for the 21st Century: A Tool for Decisionmaking.* Washington, D.C.:
            National Academy Press.

1998a   *Antimicrobial Resistance: Issues and Options.* Washington, D.C.: National
            Academy Press.

1998b   *From Generation to Generation: The Health and Well-Being of Children in*
            Immigrant Families. Washington, D.C.: National Academy Press.

1997   *Improving Health in the Community.* Washington, D.C.: National Acad-
            emy Press.

1994a   *Research Strategies for Assessing Adverse Events Associated with Vaccines:*
            A Workshop Summary. Washington, D.C.: National Academy Press.

1994b   *Overcoming Barriers to Immunization.* Washington, D.C.: National Acad-
            emy Press.

1993   *Adverse Events Associated with Childhood Vaccines: Evidence Bearing on*
            Causality. Washington, D.C.: National Academy Press.

1992   *Emerging Infections: Microbial Threats to Health in the United States.* Wash-
            ington, D.C.: National Academy Press.

1991   *Adverse Effects of Pertussis and Rubella Vaccines.* Washington, D.C.:
            National Academy Press.

1988   *The Future of Public Health.* Washington, D.C.: National Academy Press.

Janes GR, Blackman GK, Bolen JC, Kamimoto LA, Rhodes L, Caplan LS, Nadel MR,
Tomar SL, Lando JF, Greby SM, Singleton JA, Strikas RA, and Wooten KG

1999   Surveillance for use of preventive health-care services by older adults,
            1995–1997. *Morbidity and Mortality Weekly Report* 48(SS08):51.

Johnson KA, Sardell A, and Richards B

Forthcoming Federal immunization policy and funding: A history of responding to
            crises. *American Journal of Preventive Medicine*, supplement. [Expected
            19(3S), October].

Kelley DK, Barnow BS, Gold WA, and Aron LY

1993   *An Analysis of the Federal and State Roles in the Immunization of Preschool*
            Children. Lewin-VHI, Inc. (January 18).

Kenyon TA, Matuck MA, and Stroh G

1998   Persistent low immunization coverage among inner-city preschool chil-
            dren despite access to free vaccine. *Pediatrics* 101(4):612–16.

Kilbourne EM

1998   *Immunization Registries: Current Status and Issues.* (December).

Kominski R and Adams A

1991   *Social and Economic Characteristics of Students.* Current Population Re-
            port Series. Washington, D.C.: U.S. Department of Commerce, Bureau
            of the Census. (October 1).

KPMG Peat Marwick

1998   Employer Health Benefits: 1998 Annual Survey.

Kuttner H

1999   Immunization Priorities and Impact of 317 Funding Policies in Michigan. Case study prepared for the Institute of Medicine Committee on Immunization Finance Policies and Practices. (January).

Lieu T, Smith M, and Newacheck P

1994   Health insurance and preventive care sources of children at public immunization clinics. *Pediatrics* 93:373–78.

Lieu TA, Ray GT, Black SB, Butler JC, Klein JO, Breiman RF, Miller MA, and Shinefield HR

2000   Projected cost-effectiveness of pneumococcal conjugate vaccination of healthy infants and young children. *Journal of the American Medical Association* 283(11):1460–68.

Linkins RW and Feikema SM

1998   Immunization registries: The cornerstone of childhood immunization in the 21st century. *Pediatric Annals* 27(6):349–54.

Mainous AG III and Hueston WJ

1995   Medicaid free distribution programs and availability of childhood immunizations in rural practices. *Family Medicine* 27:166–69.

Marquis S and Long SH

1997   Federalism and health system reform. *Journal of the American Medical Association* 278(6):514–17.

Midani S, Ayoub EM, and Rathore MH

1995   Cost-effectiveness of *Haemophilus influenzae* type b conjugate vaccine program in Florida. *Journal of the Florida Medical Association* 82(6):401–02.

Mountain K

1999   Presentation to the Institute of Medicine Workshop on Financing Immunization Services for High-Risk Groups (September 7) Washington, D.C.

Mullen F

1999   Sam Ho, MD: Idealist, Innovator, Entrepreneur. *Journal of the American Medical Association* 281(10):947–51.

National Association of City and County Health Officers

1999   The Impact of Cuts on Local Health Departments' Immunization Programs and Infrastructure. (July). Unpublished paper. Washington, D.C.

National Center for Health Statistics

1997   National Health Interview Survey. Unpublished. As cited in Poland G and Miller S.

National Foundation for Infectious Disease

1999   Facts about adult immunization. [online document] www.nfid.org/factsheets/adultfact.html.

National Vaccine Advisory Committee

1991   The measles epidemic: The problems, barriers, and recommendations. *Journal of the American Medical Association* 266(11):1547–52.

1999a   Strategies to sustain success in childhood immunizations. *Journal of the American Medical Association* 282(4):363–70.

1999b   *Development of Community- and State-Based Immunization Registries.* (January 12).

Nichol KL, Mendelman PM, Mallon KP, Jackson LA, Gorse GJ, Belshe RB, Glezen WP, and Wittes J
  1999   Effectiveness of live, attenuated intranasal influenza virus vaccine in healthy, working adults: A randomized controlled trial. *Journal of the American Medical Association* 282(2):137–44.
Orenstein WA and Bernier RH
  1990   Surveillance—information for action. *Pediatric Clinics of North America* 37:709–34.
Orenstein WA, Hinman AR, and Rodewald LE
  1999   Public Health Considerations—United States. In *Vaccines*, 3rd ed., SA Plotkin and WA Orenstein (eds.) Philadelphia: W.B. Saunders.
Ortega AN, Andrews SF, Katz SH, Dowshen SA, Curtice WS, Cannon ME, Stewart DC, and Kaiser K
  1997   Comparing a computer-based childhood vaccination registry with parental vaccination cards: A population-based study of Delaware children. *Clinical Pediatrics* (April):217–21.
Poland GA and Miller SM
  2000   Funding Mechanisms and Infrastructure for Delivery of Adult Vaccines in the United States: The Undeclared Public Health Emergency. Paper prepared for the Institute of Medicine Committee on Immunization Policies and Practices. Washington, D.C.
Poland GA and Couch R
  1999   Intranasal influenza vaccine: Adding to the armamentarium for influenza control. *Journal of the American Medical Association* 282(2):182–84.
Polzer K
  2000   ERISA Health Plan Liability: Issues and Options for Reform. Paper presented to the National Health Policy Forum (January). Washington, D.C.
Preston R
  1999   The demon in the freezer. *The New Yorker* (July 12):44–60.
Richardson SK
  1999   Letter to State Health Officials. Health Care Financing Administration. (May 11). Baltimore, MD.
Richardson SK and Orenstein WA
  1999   Letter to State Health Officials. Health Care Financing Administration. (June 25). Baltimore, MD.
Robert Wood Johnson Foundation
  1996   *Childhood Immunization Registry Systems: A General Definition of Terms, Scope, and Components.* (January). Philadelphia, PA.
Rosenbaum S, Johnson K, Sonosky C, Markus A, and DeGraw C
  1999   The children's hour: The State Children's Health Insurance Program. *Health Affairs* 7(1):75–89.
Rosenbaum S, Smith B, Shin P, Zakheim M, Shaw K, Sonosky C, and Repasch L
  1998   *Negotiating the New Health System: A Nationwide Study of Medicaid Managed Care Contracts.* Washington, D.C.: Center for Health Services Research and Policy, The George Washington University Medical Center, School of Public Health and Health Services.

Rosenbaum S, Spernak S, and Wehr E

1992   *Immunization in the United States: A Compendium of Federal Immunization Laws and Programs*. (November). Washington, D.C.: Center for Health Services Research and Policy, The George Washington University Medical Center, School of Public Health and Health Services.

Ruch-Ross HS and O'Connor KG

1994   Immunization referral practices of pediatricians in the United States. *Pediatrics* 94:508–13.

Santoli JM

1999   Health Department Clinics as Immunization Providers for Pediatric Patients: A 1998 National Survey. Paper presented before the Institute of Medicine Workshop on Financing Immunization Services for High-Risk Groups (September 7). Washington, D.C.

Santoli JM, Setia S, Rodewald LE, O'Mara D, Gallo B, and Brink E

Forthcoming   Immunization pockets of need: Science, policy, and program. *American Journal of Preventive Medicine*, supplement [Expected 19(3S), October].

Santoli JM, Szilagyi PS, and Rodewald LE

1998   Barriers to immunization and missed opportunities. *Pediatric Annals* 27(6):366–74.

Schauffler HH, Brown C, and Milstein A

1999   Raising the bar: The use of performance guarantees by the Pacific Business Group on Health. *Health Affairs* 18(2):134–42.

Selden TM, Banthin JS, and Cohen JW

1999   Waiting in the wings: Eligibility and enrollment in the State Children's Health Insurance Program. *Health Affairs* 18(2):126–33.

1998   Medicaid's problem children: Eligible but not enrolled, *Health Affairs* 17(3):192–200.

Shaheen MA, Frerichs RR, Alexopoulos N, and Rainey JJ

2000   Immunization coverage among predominantly Hispanic children, aged 2–3 years, in central Los Angeles. *Annals of Epidemiology* 10(3):160–8.

Singleton JA, Greby SM, and Wooten, KG

Forthcoming   *Influenza, Pneumococcal and Tetanus Toxoid Vaccination of Adults—United States, 1993–1997*.

Sisk J, Moskowitz A, Whang W, Lin JD, Fedson DS, McBean AM, Plouffe JF, Cetron MS, and Butler JC

1997   Cost-effectiveness of vaccination against pneumococcal bacteremia among elderly people. *Journal of the American Medical Association* 278(16):1333–39.

Slifkin RT, Freeman VA, and Biddle A

1999   *The Cost of Immunization Registries: Four Case Studies*. A Report to the Robert Wood Johnson Foundation. (April).

St. Peter RE, Newacheck PW, and Halfon N

1992   Access to care for poor children: Separate and unequal? *Journal of the American Medical Association* 267:2760–64.

Stolberg SG

2000   FDA approves costly meningitis shots. *New York Times* (February 18):A18.

Szilagyi PG
1999   Where Can Immunization Program Investments Achieve High Pay-offs for High Risk Groups? Paper presented before the Institute of Medicine Workshop on Financing Immunization Services for High Risk Groups. (September 7). Washington, D.C.

Szilagyi PG, Rodewald LE, Savageau J, Yoos L, and Doane C
1992   Improving influenza vaccination rates in children with asthma: A test of a computerized reminder system and an analysis of factors predicting vaccination compliance. *Pediatrics* 90(6):871–75.

Tatande M, Dietz V, Lewin M, and Zell E
1996   Health care characteristics and their association with the vaccination status of children. *Archives of Pediatric and Adolescent Medicine* 150(Suppl 4):abstract 161.

Taylor JA, Darden PM, Slora E, Hasemeier CM, Asmussen L, and Wasserman R
1997   Influence of provider behavior, parental characteristics, and a public policy initiative on the immunization status of children followed by private pediatricians: A study from pediatric research in office settings. *Pediatrics* 99:209–15.

Thompson FE
1998   Letter to Department of Health and Human Services Secretary Donna E. Shalala. (December 31). Association of State and Territorial Health Officers. Washington, D.C.

U.S. House of Representatives
2000   *Autism: Present Challenges, Future Needs—Why Increased Rates?* Committee on Government Reform Hearing. The Honorable Dan Burton (R-IN), Chairman. Washington, D.C.: U.S. Government Printing Office. (April 6).

1999a   To amend title XXI of the Social Security Act to permit children covered under a State child health plan (SCHIP) to continue to be eligible for benefits under the Vaccines for Children program. Bill H.R. 2976. (September 29).

1999b   *Vaccines—Finding the Balance Between Public Safety and Personal Choice.* Committee on Government Reform Hearing. The Honorable Dan Burton (R-IN), Chairman. Washington, D.C.: U.S. Government Printing Office. (August 3).

1996   *Departments of Labor, Health and Human Services, and Education, and Related Agencies Appropriation Bill, 1997.* Committee on Appropriations. Report 104-659. Washington, D.C.: U.S. Government Printing Office. (July 8).

1992   *Departments of Labor, Health and Human Services, and Education, and Related Agencies Appropriation Bill, 1993.* Committee on Appropriations. Report 102-708. Washington, D.C.: U.S. Government Printing Office. (July 23).

1991   *Departments of Labor, Health and Human Services, and Education, and Related Agencies Appropriation Bill, 1992.* Committee on Appropriations. Report 102-121. Washington, D.C.: U.S. Government Printing Office. (June 20).

1989   *Departments of Labor, Health and Human Services, and Education, and Related Agencies Appropriation Bill, 1990.* Committee on Appropriations. Report 101-172. Washington, D.C.: U.S. Government Printing Office. (July 25).

U.S. Senate
1999   To amend title XXI of the Social Security Act to permit children covered under a State child health plan (SCHIP) to continue to be eligible for benefits under the Vaccines for Children program. Bill S. 1656. (September 28).

1998   *Departments of Labor, Health and Human Services, and Education, and Related Agencies Appropriation Bill, 1998.* Committee on Appropriations. Report 105-300. Washington, D.C.: U.S. Government Printing Office. (September 3).

1995   *Departments of Labor, Health and Human Services, and Education, and Related Agencies Appropriation Bill, 1996.* Committee on Appropriations. Report 104-145. Washington, D.C.: U.S. Government Printing Office. (September 15).

1994   *Departments of Labor, Health and Human Services, and Education, and Related Agencies Appropriation Bill, 1995.* Committee on Appropriations. Report 103-318. Washington, D.C.: U.S. Government Printing Office. (July 20).

1993   *Departments of Labor, Health and Human Services, and Education, and Related Agencies Appropriation Bill, 1994.* Committee on Appropriations. Report 103-143. Washington, D.C.: U.S. Government Printing Office. (September 15).

1992   *Departments of Labor, Health and Human Services, and Education, and Related Agencies Appropriation Bill, 1993.* Committee on Appropriations. Report 102-397. Washington, D.C.: U.S. Government Printing Office. (September 10).

Vivier, PM
1996   National Policies for Childhood Immunization in the United States: A Historical Perspective. Unpublished dissertation. Ann Arbor, Michigan: UMI Dissertation Services.

Watson, Jr. WC, Saarlas KN, Hearn R, and Russell R
1997   The All Kids Count National Program: A Robert Wood Johnson Foundation initiative to develop immunization registries. Pp. 3–6 in JF Cordero, FA Guerra, and KN Saarlas, eds., *Preventive Medicine* Supplement to 13(2)(March/April).

Watt J, Kahane S, Smith N, Newell K, Kellam S, Wight S, Reingold A, and Adler R
1998   The Difference Between Measured and Estimated Vaccination Coverage Among Private Physicians in California. California Department of Health Services, University of California-Berkeley. Paper presented before the Pediatric Academic Societies meeting. (May 1). New Orleans.

Webster's Dictionary
1996   *Webster's II New Riverside Dictionary, Revised Edition.* Office Edition. Boston, Mass.: Houghton Mifflin Company.

Wharton M and Strebel PM
1994   Vaccine preventable diseases. Pp. 281–90 in LS Wilcox and JS Marks, eds., *From Data to Action: CDC's Public Health Surveillance for Women, Infants, and Children.* Atlanta, Ga.: U.S. Department of Health and Human Services, Public Health Service, Centers for Disease Control and Prevention.

White CC, Koplan JP, and Orenstein WA
1985   Benefits, risks, and costs of immunization for measles, mumps, and rubella. *American Journal of Public Health* 75(7):739–44.

Wilton R and Pennisi AJ
1994   Evaluating the accuracy of transcribed computer-stored immunization data. *Pediatrics* 94(6):902–06.

Wood D, Saarlas KN, Inkelas M, and Matyas BT
1999   Immunization registries in the United States: Implications for the practice of public health in a changing health care system. *Annual Review of Public Health* 20:231–55.

Zablocki E
1996   Collaborating on a statewide immunization registry. *Health System Leader* (December):17–19.

Zimmerman RK, Medsger AR, Ricci EM, Raymund M, Mieczkowski TA, and Grufferman S
1997   Impact of free vaccine and insurance status on physician referral of children to public vaccine clinics. *Journal of the American Medical Association* 278:996–1000.

Other References

American Association of Health Plans
2000   Report of the AAHP immunization task force members' responses to the IOM inquiry on immunization finance policies and practices. (January). Washington, D.C.

Freed GL, Clark SJ, and Cowan AE
Forthcoming   State-level perspectives on immunization policies, practices, and program financing in the 1990s. *American Journal of Preventive Medicine,* supplement. [Expected 19(3S), October].

Hogan R
1999   Immunization Policies and Funding in Alabama. Case study prepared for the IOM Committee on Immunization Finance Policies and Practices (December).

1999   Immunization Policies and Funding in Texas. Case study prepared for the IOM Committee on Immunization Finance Policies and Practices (October).

Johnson, K
2000   Immunization Policies and Funding in Maine. Case study prepared for the IOM Committee on Immunization Finance Policies and Practices (November).

McPhillips H, and Alexander R
    2000   Immunization Policies and Funding in Washington. Case study prepared for the IOM Committee on Immunization Finance Policies and Practices (May).

Miller VJ
    1999   Federalism, Entitlements, and Categorical Grants: The Fiscal Context of National Support for Immunization Programs. Paper prepared for the IOM Committee on Immunization Finance Policies and Practices. (July).

    Forthcoming   Federalism, entitlements, and discretionary grants: The fiscal context of national support for immunization programs. *American Journal of Preventive Medicine*, supplement. [Expected 19(3S), October].

Miller W
    1999   Immunization Polices and Funding in North Carolina. Case study prepared for the IOM Committee on Immunization Finance Policies and Practices (November).

Rand R, Sylvia L, and Rosenbaum, S
    1999   Chapter 2 supplement to *Law and the American Health System*, New York, NY: Foundation Press.

Appendixes

Appendix A

Public Health Services Act, Section 317

PROJECT GRANTS FOR PREVENTIVE HEALTH SERVICES

SEC. 317. [247b] (a) The Secretary may make grants to States, and in consultation with State health authorities, to political subdivisions of States and to other public entities to assist them in meeting the costs of establishing and maintaining preventive health service programs.

(b) No grant may be made under subsection (a) unless an application therefor has been submitted to, and approved by, the Secretary. Such an application shall be in such form and be submitted in such manner as the Secretary shall by regulation prescribe and shall provide—

(1) a complete description of the type and extent of the program for which the applicant is seeking a grant under subsection (a);

(2) with respect to each such program (A) the amount of Federal, State, and other funds obligated by the applicant in its latest annual accounting period for the provision of such program, (B) a description of the services provided by the applicant in such program in such period, (C) the amount of Federal funds needed by the applicant to continue providing such services in such program, and (D) if the applicant proposes changes in the provision of the services in such program, the priorities of such proposed changes, reasons for such changes, and the amount of Federal funds needed by the applicant to make such changes;

(3) assurances satisfactory to the Secretary that the program which will be provided with funds under a grant under subsection (a) will

be provided in a manner consistent with the State health plan in effect under section 1524(c) and in those cases where the applicant is a State, that such program will be provided, where appropriate, in a manner consistent with any plans in effect under an application approved under section 315;

(4) assurances satisfactory to the Secretary that the applicant will provide for such fiscal control and fund accounting procedures as the Secretary by regulation prescribes to assure the proper disbursement of and accounting for funds received under grants under subsection (a);

(5) assurances satisfactory to the Secretary that the applicant will provide for periodic evaluation of its program or programs;

(6) assurances satisfactory to the Secretary that the applicant will make such reports (in such form and containing such information as the Secretary may by regulation prescribe) as the Secretary may reasonably require and keep such records and afford such access thereto as the Secretary may find necessary to assure the correctness of, and to verify, such reports;

(7) assurances satisfactory to the Secretary that the applicant will comply with any other conditions imposed by this section with respect to grants; and

(8) such other information as the Secretary may by regulation prescribe.

(c) (1) The Secretary shall not approve an application submitted under subsection (b) for a grant for a program for which a grant was previously made under subsection (a) unless the Secretary determines—

(A) the program for which the application was submitted is operating effectively to achieve its stated purpose,

(B) the applicant complied with the assurances provided the Secretary when applying for such previous grant, and

(C) the applicant will comply with the assurances provided with the application.

(2) The Secretary shall review annually the activities undertaken by each recipient of a grant under subsection (a) to determine if the program assisted by such grant is operating effectively to achieve its stated purposes and if the recipient is in compliance with the assurances provided the Secretary when applying for such grant.

(d) The amount of a grant under subsection (a) shall be determined by the Secretary. Payments under such grants may be made in advance on the basis of estimates or by the way of reimbursement, with necessary adjustments on account of underpayments or overpayments, and in such installments and on such terms and conditions as the Secretary finds necessary to carry out the purposes of such grants.

(e) The Secretary, at the request of a recipient of a grant under subsection (a), may reduce the amount of such grant by—

(1) the fair market value of any supplies (including vaccines and other preventive agents) or equipment furnished the grant recipient, and

(2) the amount of the pay, allowances, and travel expenses of any officer or employee of the Government when detailed to the grant recipient and the amount of any other costs incurred in connection with detail of such officer or employee. When the furnishing of such supplies or equipment or the detail of such an officer or employee is for the convenience of and at the request of such grant recipient and for the purpose of carrying out a program with respect to which the grant under subsection (a) is made. The amount by which any such grant is so reduced shall be available for payment by the Secretary of the costs incurred in furnishing the supplies or equipment, or in detailing the personnel, on which the reduction of such grant is based, and such amount shall be deemed as part of the grant and shall be deemed to have been paid to the grant recipient.

(f) (1) Each recipient of a grant under subsection (a) shall keep such records as the Secretary shall by regulation prescribe, including records which fully disclose the amount and disposition by such recipient of the proceeds of such grant, the total cost of the undertaking in connection with which such grant was made, and the amount of that portion of the cost of the undertaking supplied by other sources, and such other records as will facilitate an effective audit.

(2) The Secretary and the Comptroller General of the United States, or any of their duly authorized representatives, shall have access for the purpose of audit and examination to any books, documents, papers, and records of the recipient of grants under subsection (a) that are pertinent to such grants.

(g) (1) Nothing in this section shall limit or otherwise restrict the use of funds which are granted to a State or to an agency or a political subdivision of a State under provisions of Federal law (other than this section) and which are available for the conduct of preventive health service programs from being used on connection with programs assisted through grants under subsection (a).

(2) Nothing in this section shall be construed to require any State or any agency or political subdivision of a State to have a preventive health service program which would require any person, who objects to any treatment provided under such a program, to be treated or to have any child or ward treated under such program.

(h) The Secretary shall include, as part of the report required by section 1705, a report on the extent of the problems presented by the diseases and conditions referred to in subsection (j) on the amount of funds obligated under grants under subsection (a) in the preceding fiscal year for each of the programs listed in subsection (j); and on the effectiveness of the activities assisted under grants under subsection (a) in controlling such diseases and conditions.

(i) The Secretary may provide technical assistance to States, State health authorities, and other public entities in connection with the operation of their preventive health service programs.

(j) (1) Except for grants for immunization programs the authorization of appropriations for which are established in paragraph (2), for grants under subsections (a) and (k)(1) for preventive health service programs to immunize without charge children, adolescents, and adults against vaccine-preventable diseases, there are authorized to be appropriated such sums as may be necessary for each of the fiscal years 1998 through 2002. Not more than 10 percent to the total amount appropriated under the preceding sentence for any fiscal year shall be available for grants under subsection (k)(1) for such fiscal year.

(2) For grants under subsection (a) for preventive health service programs for the provision without charge of immunizations with vaccines approved for use, and recommended for routine use, after October 1, 1997, there are authorized to be appropriated such sums as may be necessary.

(k) (1) The Secretary may make grants to States, political subdivisions of States, and other public and nonprofit private entities for—

(A) research into the prevention and control of diseases that may be prevented through vaccination;

(B) demonstration projects for the prevention and control of such diseases;

(C) public information and education programs for the prevention and control of such diseases; and

(D) education, training, and clinical skills improvement activities in the prevention and control of such diseases for health professionals (including allied health personnel).

(2) The Secretary may make grants to States, political subdivisions of States, and other public and nonprofit private entities for—

(A) research into the prevention and control of diseases and conditions;

(B) demonstration projects for the prevention and control of such diseases and conditions;

(C) public information and education programs for the prevention and control of such diseases and conditions; and

(D) education, training, and clinical skills improvement activities in the prevention and control of such diseases and conditions for health professionals (including allied health personnel).

(3) No grant may be made under this subsection unless an application therefor is submitted to the Secretary in such form, at such time, and containing such information as the Secretary may by regulation prescribe.

(4) Subsections (d), (e), and (f) shall apply to grants under this subsection in the same manner as such subsections apply to grants under subsection (a).

Appendix B

Immunization Time-Line

1955   Poliomyelitis Vaccination Assistance Act
           (President Eisenhower)

- Start of federal funding for immunization (primarily vaccine purchase)
- Public Health Service begins to collect data on national immunization rates (polio)

1962–1964   Vaccination Assistance Act *(President Kennedy)*

- Adoption of Section 317 of the Public Health Service Act and creation of the National Immunization Program at CDC (1963)
- Federal funds targeted for vaccine purchase for polio, diphtheria, pertussis, and tetanus (measles added to federal purchase plan in 1965)
- National data collection efforts expanded to include vaccine coverage rates for diphtheria, pertussis, tetanus, and measles (rates increased from 68% in 1962 to mid to high 70% range by the end of the decade)
- Major outbreak of rubella affecting pregnant women (1964—no vaccine available)

1966–1968   Partnership for Health Initiative *(President Johnson)*

- Part of broader effort to reduce growing number of federal categorical programs in health
- Section 317 program replaced with state block grants
- Disease reports decline in four key categories (measles, polio, pertussis, and diphtheria)
- Federal resources shifted away from state grants and measles vaccine to support purchase of rubella vaccine when license was approved (1969)
- Compulsory school laws adopted by half of the states

1970   New Section 317 authority restored *(President Nixon)*

- Reported measles cases increased sharply (1969–1971)
- Reports of insufficient state funds, personnel, and activity in immunization programs other than rubella
- Earlier block grant effort seen as weakening of federal effort, leading to disease outbreaks

1976–1978   National Childhood Immunization Initiative
(President Carter)

- Second measles outbreak in 1977
- New initiative stimulated by Mrs. Betty Bumpers, wife of Arkansas Governor Dale Bumpers
- Federal commitment made to increase and maintain immunization levels among school-aged children to 90% and above (coverage rates reported as 95%)
- Growth occurred in federal grants for state immunization budgets ($5 million in 1976 to $35 million in 1979)

1986–1988   Continued Federal Support for State and Local Grantees
(President Reagan)

- Level of federal support remained stable but did not grow
- New vaccines added to immunization schedule
- Public health delivery system remained unchanged
- National Childhood Vaccine Injury Act (1986) adopted

1991   **Federal Request for State Immunization Action Plans**
          (President Bush)

- Measles epidemic in 1989–1991
- Announced federal goal of raising national immunization levels among preschool children to 90% by year 2000
- Immunization Action Plans formulated by all states and 28 metropolitan areas
- Federal grant funds authorized for direct delivery of immunization services as well as vaccine purchase (new awards for state grants tripled from $37.0 million in 1991 to $98.2 million in 1993)

1993–1995 **Childhood Immunization Initiative** *(President Clinton)*

- Major infusion of federal funds for service delivery and immunization programs, including surveillance, assessment, and registry activities (peak of $261 million in state and local awards in 1995)
- 90% coverage rate for most vaccines for preschool children achieved by 1996
- Vaccines for Children Program adopted as amendment to Medicaid (1994), providing >$500 million in federal funds for vaccine purchase and delivery

1996–1998 **New Federal–State Partnerships in Health Care Services**
          (President Clinton)

- State Children's Health Insurance Program (1997) adopted as a major new block grant program for the states to ensure access to health care services, including immunization services for uninsured children (<18 years)
- Childhood immunization coverage rates reached record highs
- Influenza coverage for adults reached new high rates
- State immunization grants within Section 317 budget decreased significantly
- States reported cutbacks in vaccine administration services, outreach programs, and data collection efforts

SOURCE: Adapted from Vivier, 1996.

Appendix C

List of Contributors

**CENTERS FOR DISEASE CONTROL AND PREVENTION
NATIONAL IMMUNIZATION PROGRAM**

Walter Orenstein, Director
Jose Cordero, Deputy Director
Martin Landry, Associate Director for Planning, Evaluation, and Legislation
Angie Bauer, Program Analyst, Office of the Director, Office of Planning, Evaluation, and Legislation
Nicole Smith, Program Analyst, Office of the Director, Office of Planning, Evaluation, and Legislation
Bill Gallo, Associate Director for Policy, Planning and Legislation, Immunization Services Division/Office of the Director

William Nichols, Associate Director for Management and Operations
Kim Lane, Deputy Associate Director for Management and Operations
Joel Kuritsky, Director, Immunization Services Division
Tami Kicera, Deputy Director, Immunization Services Division
Lance Rodewald, Associate Director for Science and Acting Director, Health Services Research and Evaluation Branch, Immunization Services Division

James Mize, Deputy Public
Health Advisor, Health
Services Research and
Evaluation Branch,
Immunization Services
Division

Jeanne Santoli, Medical Officer,
Health Services Research and
Evaluation Branch,
Immunization Services
Division

Abigail Shefer, Medical Officer/
Epidemiologist, Health
Services Research and
Evaluation Branch,
Immunization Services
Division

Robert Deuson, Visiting Scientist,
Health Services Research and
Evaluation Branch,
Immunization Services
Division

Dean Mason, Chief, Program
Support Branch,
Immunization Services
Division

Kristin Brusuelas, Public Health
Advisor, Los Angeles County
Health Department, on detail
to Program Support Branch,
Immunization Services
Division

Nancy Fenlon, Public Health
Analyst, Program Support
Branch, Immunization
Services Division

Lisa Galloway, Computer
Specialist, Program Support
Branch, Immunization
Services Division

Alison Johnson, Public Health
Analyst, Program Support
Branch, Immunization
Services Division

Dianne Ochoa, Public Health
Analyst, Program Support
Branch, Immunization
Services Division

Paula Rosenberg, Public Health
Analyst, Program Support
Branch, Immunization
Services Division

Robert Snyder, Public Health
Advisor, Program Support
Branch, Immunization
Services Division

Dennis O'Mara, Chief, Program
Operations Branch,
Immunization Services
Division

Glen Koops, Deputy Chief,
Program Operations Branch,
Immunization Services
Division

Ken Sharp, Public Health
Advisor, Program Operations
Branch, Immunization
Services Division

Russell Havlak, Public Health
Analyst, NCHSTP, on detail
to Immunization Services
Division/Office of the
Director

Robert Chen, Chief, Vaccine
Safety and Development
Activity, Epidemiology and
Surveillance Division

Charles Lebaron, Child Vaccine
Preventable Diseases Branch,
Epidemiology and
Surveillance Division

Roger Burr, Preventive Medicine Resident, Child Vaccine Preventable Diseases Branch, Epidemiology and Surveillance Division

Mark Papania, Chief, Measles Elimination Activity, Child Vaccine Preventable Diseases Branch, Epidemiology and Surveillance Division

Sandy Roush, Epidemiologist, Child Vaccine Preventable Diseases Branch, Epidemiology and Surveillance Division

Jim Singleton, Acting Chief, Adult Vaccine Preventable Diseases Branch, Epidemiology and Surveillance Division

Melinda Wharton, Chief, Child Vaccine Preventable Diseases Branch, Epidemiology and Surveillance Division

Edward Maes, Associate Director for Science, Data Management Division

Victor Coronado, Visiting Scientist, Assessment Branch, Division of Data Management

Jim Harrison, Public Health Advisor, Systems Development Branch, Division of Data Management

Monina Klevens, Chief, Assessment Branch, Division of Data Management

Phil Smith, Mathematical Statistician, Assessment Branch, Division of Data Management

Gary Urquhart, Program Analyst, Systems Development Branch, Division of Data Management

Michael Washington, Prevention Effectiveness Fellow, Statistical Analysis Branch, Division of Data Management

Allyson Shoe, Contract Specialist, Office of Program Support, Procurement and Grants Office

Margie Usry, Contract Specialist, Office of Program Support, Procurement and Grants Office

Ellen Cooper, Funding Resource Specialist, Office of the Director

Kelly Correll, Funding Resource Specialist, Office of the Director

Patrick Flaherty, Public Health Prevention Specialist, Office of the Director

Elizabeth Spears, Program Analyst, Office of the Director

Patricia Smith, Visual Information Specialist, Office of Health Communications

SITE VISIT PARTICIPANTS

Los Angeles County, California

Kristin Brusuelas, Immunization Program, LA County Department of Health Services, Los Angeles, CA

Helen DuPlessis, LA Care Health Plan, Los Angeles, CA

Stephen Feig, Children's Comprehensive Medical Group, Los Angeles, CA

Lloyd Hunter, Children's Comprehensive Medical Group, Los Angeles, CA

Mitch Mellman, Immunization Program, LA County Department of Health Services, Los Angeles, CA

Paula Packwood, LA Care Health Plan, Los Angeles, CA

Lizz Romo, Women, Infants, and Children Clinic, Los Angeles, CA

Cathy Schellhase, Immunization Program, LA County Department of Health Services, Los Angeles, CA

Kathy Stroup, UCLA Research and Education Institute, Los Angeles, CA

San Diego County, California

Nancy Fink, County of San Diego Health and Human Services Agency, Department of Immunizations, San Diego, CA

John Fontanesi, Kaiser Permanente and UCSD Partnership of Immunization Providers, San Diego, CA

Kathleen Gustafson, County of San Diego Health and Human Services Agency, Department of Immunizations, San Diego, CA

Larry Hansley, North County Health Services, San Marcos, CA

Mickey Keil, North County Health Services, San Marcos, CA

Kenneth Morris, North County Health Services, San Marcos, CA

Nathan Rendler, Valle Verde Pediatrics, San Marcos, CA

Sandy Ross, County of San Diego Health and Human Services Agency, Department of Immunizations, San Diego, CA

Detroit, Michigan

Ann Casadei, Child Health Network, Henry Ford Health System, Detroit, MI

Ronald Davis, Center for Health Promotion and Disease Prevention, Henry Ford Health System, Detroit, MI

Paul T. Giblin, Department of Pediatrics, Wayne State University School of Medicine, Detroit, MI

Rebecca Guzman, Child Health Network Immunization Project, Detroit, MI

Richard Kallenbach, Department
of Community Medicine,
Wayne State University
School of Medicine, Detroit,
MI

Sheryl Weir, Child Health
Network Immunization
Project, Detroit, MI

Newark, New Jersey

Kate Aquino, Vaccine Preventable
Disease Program, New Jersey
Department of Health and
Human Services, Newark NJ

Sandra Bernard, New Jersey
Department of Health and
Human Services, Newark, NJ

Christine Grant, New Jersey
Department of Health and
Social Services, Trenton, NJ

Stephanie Harris-Kuiper,
Immunization Program,
Newark Department of
Health and Human Services,
Newark, NJ

Marsha McGowan, Newark
Department of Health and
Human Services, Newark, NJ

Kenyatta O'Bryant, Newark
Department of Health and
Human Services, Newark, NJ

Monique Smalls, Newark
Department of Health and
Human Services, Newark, NJ

Altagracia Trinidad, Newark
Community Health Center-
Ludlow, Newark, NJ

Loretta Uy, Private Physician,
Newark, NJ

Houston, Texas

Kathy Barton, Houston
Department of Health and
Human Services, Houston

James Boland, Kelsey-Seybold
Clinic, Houston, TX

Mary des Vignes-Kendrick,
Houston Department of
Health and Human Services,
Houston, TX

Jean Galloway, Houston
Department of Health and
Human Services, Houston, TX

Orin Gill, Houston Department of
Health and Human Services,
Houston, TX

Mark Guidry, Texas Department
of Health, Houston, TX

Celine Hanson, Baylor College of
Medicine, Houston, TX

Brock Lamont, Houston
Department of Health and
Human Services, Houston, TX

Mary Jane Lowrey, Houston
Department of Health and
Human Services, Houston, TX

Sharon Marsh, Houston
Department of Health and
Human Services, Houston,
TX

Maureen Moore, Houston
Department of Health and
Human Services, Houston, TX

Antonia Stewart, La Nueva Casa
De Amigos Health Center,
Houston, TX

OTHER CONTRIBUTORS

Kathleen Barnett, Texas Department of Health, Austin, TX

Jack Blane, Immunization Education Action Committee, Highland Park, IL

Craig Carlson, American Association of Health Plans, Washington, DC

Linda Cole, Texas Department of Health, Austin, TX

Richard Curtis, Institute for Health Policy Solutions, Washington, DC

Mary Dingrando, National Association of State Budget Officers, Washington, DC

Catherine Ehlen, American Association of Health Plans, Washington, DC

William Evans, Department of Economics, University of Maryland, College Park, MD

David Fedson, Pasteur Merieux MSD, Lyon, France

Denise Ferris, West Virginia Women, Infants, and Children Program, Charleston, WV

Cathy Franklin, National Association of Women, Infants, and Children Directors, Immunization Task Force, Olympia, WA

Victoria Freeman, C.G. Sheps Center for Health Services Research, Chapel Hill, NC

Steven Friedman, New York City Health Dept, New York, New York

Lisa German, Office of Senator Jack Reed, Washington, DC

Paula Gola, Texas Department of Health, Austin, TX

Paula Gomez, Brownesville Community Health Center, Brownesville, TX

Rita Goodman, Bureau of Primary Health Care, Health Resources and Services Administration, Bethesda, MD

Randolph Graydon, Division of Advocacy, Health Care Financing Administration, Baltimore, MD

Douglas Greenaway, National Association of Women, Infants, and Children Directors, Washington, DC

Fernando Guerra, San Antonio Metropolitan Health District, San Antonio, TX

James Hadler, Connecticut Department of Health, Hartford, CT

Claire Hannan, Association of State and Territorial Health Officials, Washington, DC

Daniel Hawkins, Jr., National Association of Community Health Centers, Washington, DC

Karen Hendricks, American Academy of Pediatrics, Washington, DC

Joan Henneberry, Health Policy Studies Divison, National Governors' Association, Washington, DC

Catherine Hess, Association of Maternal and Child Health Programs, Washington, DC

Gary Higginbotham, Alabama Department of Public Health, Montgomery, AL

Alan Hinman, Task Force for Child Survival and Development, Decatur, GA

Philip Horne, Independent Scholar, Tucker, GA

Kerry Howard, Texas Department of Health, Austin, TX

Babatunde Jinadu, Kern County Department of Public Health, Bakersfield, CA

David Johnson, Michigan Department of Community Health, Lansing, MI

Donald Johnson, National Association of Women, Infants, and Children Directors, Washington, DC

Stephen Keith, North American Vaccine, Inc., Columbia, MD

Akiko Kimura, LA County Department of Public Health, Los Angeles, CA

Neva Klotz, Texas Department of Health, Austin, TX

Virginia Lewis, Blue Cross Blue Shield of Tennessee, Chattanooga, TN

Alan Lifson, Minnesota Department of Health, Minneapolis, MN

Ruth Watson Lubic, District of Columbia Developing Families Center, Washington, DC

Patricia MacTaggart, Quality and Performance/CMSO, Health Care Financing Administration, Baltimore, MD

Joan Mahanes, Medicaid Immunization Liaison, Health Care Financing Administration, Baltimore, MD

Adolfo Mata, Bureau of Primary Health Care, Health Resources and Services Administration, Bethesda, MD

Ella McDowell, National Association of Women, Infants, and Children Directors, Washington, DC

Kathy McNamara, National Association of Community Health Centers, Washington, DC

Patti Mitchell, Supplemental Food Program Division, U.S. Department of Agriculture, Alexandria, VA

Karen Mountain, Migrant Clinicians Network, Austin, TX

Elka Munizaga, Montefiore Medical Center, New York, NY

Kelly O'Brien, Office of Senator Dick Durbin, Washington, DC

J.P. Passino, Women, Infants, and Children Program, U.S. Department of Agriculture, Alexandria, VA

James Pearson, Division of
Consolidated Laboratory
Services, Richmond, VA

Jay Petillo, Office of the Assistant
Secretary for Management
and Budget, Department of
Health and Human Services,
Washington, DC

Cynthia Phillips, National
Association of County and
City Health Officials,
Washington, DC

Amy Pisani, Every Child By Two,
Washington, DC

Brad Prescott, Texas Department
of Health, Austin, TX

John Quinley, New York State
Peer Review Organization,
New York, NY

Edd Rhoades, Oklahoma State
Department of Health,
Oklahoma City, OK

Pat Ford Roegner, Heidepriem &
Mager, Inc, Washington, DC

William Roper, School of Public
Health, University of North
Carolina, Chapel Hill, NC

Charles Rotan, Texas Department
of Health, Austin, TX

Eleni Sfakianaki, Dade County
Health Department, Miami,
FL

Amy Sheahan, National Coalition
for Adult Immunization,
Bethesda, MD

Winkler Sims, Alabama
Department of Public Health,
Montgomery, AL

Natalie Smith, Immunization
Branch, California
Department of Health,
Berkeley, CA

Peter Szilagyi, Department of
Pediatrics, University of
Rochester, Rochester, NY

Edward Thompson, Jr.,
Mississippi State Department
of Health, Jackson, MS

Joseph Thompson, Pediatrics
Care Department, University
of Arkansas for Medical
Sciences, Little Rock, AR

Mary Tierney, Department of
Pediatrics, Public Benefits
Corporation of the District of
Columbia, Washington, DC

Denia Varrasso, William F. Ryan
Community Health Center,
New York, NY

Kathy Vincent, Alabama
Department of Public Health,
Montgomery, AL

Timothy Westmoreland, Federal
Legislation Clinic,
Georgetown University Law
Center, Washington, DC

Scott Williams, Utah Department
of Health, Salt Lake City, UT

Donald Williamson, Alabama
Department of Public Health,
Montgomery, AL

Charles Woernle, Alabama
Department of Public Health,
Montgomery, AL

David Woods, International
Shriners Headquarters,
Tampa, FL

Beth Zahn, Texas Department of
Health, Austin, TX

Appendix D

Overview of State Survey

In May 1999, the Institute of Medicine Committee on Immunization Finance Policies and Practices commissioned a 50-state survey from Gary L. Freed, Sarah J. Clark, and Anne Cowan at the Division of General Pediatrics, University of Michigan.

The University of Michigan team conducted the survey via phone and mail during the period May–October 1999 with the immunization program managers and project directors in each of the 50 states and the District of Columbia. The names of the program managers and project directors were provided by CDC.

Each state project director was asked to designate a respondent who could provide information regarding immunization policies and practices within the state. The respondents were asked to identify other individuals within the state who could provide insights, experience, and data describing how federal, state, and local funds are used to support immunization efforts. These individuals included the state Medicaid director, the chief fiscal officer for state health efforts, and the state director for maternal and child health, among others. CDC also provided state-level data, including copies of the state immunization grant awards and core functions site visit data.

In separate, individual interviews, respondents were asked to address a number of topics, including the major outreach campaigns in the 1990s; the state's response to CDC's pockets-of-need approach; the structure of the state health department and the relationship of the immunization program within the department; the scope of child health services delivered in health departments through the 1990s; immunization-related "hot issues" with the state legislature; the experience with seeking funding for immunization within the state; the current status of the state's immunization registry; the state's role in assessing day care and school immunization coverage levels; enforcement of immunization requirements; exemptions, penalties, and sanctions in the school requirements; and state mandates for insurance coverage of immunizations.

Responses were received from all 50 states. A summary of the survey findings is scheduled for publication (forthcoming, *American Journal of Preventive Medicine*, supplement, 19[3S], October 2000).

Appendix E

Overview of Case Studies and Site Visits

This overview describes the purpose and the methodology of the committee's case studies and site visits. Information gathered through these efforts is incorporated in the body of the report, often featured in the boxes accompanying the text. A more detailed presentation of the findings of the individual case studies and site visits is contained in a forthcoming special issue of the *American Journal of Preventive Medicine*, (v. 19 [3S], October 2000) devoted to the research conducted in the development of this report.

The committee undertook eight state or locality-specific case studies in order to deepen the picture of local policy choices and performance of immunization programs and spending over the past decade. The state survey conducted for the committee by Dr. Gary Freed and associates provides a comprehensive view of the significant programmatic features and issues regarding immunization across the country (see Appendix D for a brief description of this survey). The individual case studies were designed to:

- trace program changes, development, and performance over time,
- collect detailed information on state- (and in the case of Los Angeles and San Diego, county-) level spending for immunization-related activities, and
- document the impact of federal policy directions and funding levels on state programs over the past decade.

The sampling of states and localities is far too small to be statistically representative, and the findings of the case studies cannot be used by themselves to make national generalizations, at least as regards state-level program models and policy choices. Nevertheless, the case studies and site visits allowed the committee to pursue questions about the implementation of national program and funding policies across an array of states. They also gave committee members, staff, and consultants the opportunity to communicate directly with state and local immunization and health program managers in a sustained fashion on several occasions, which provided much insight into the impact and importance of federal policies.

The sites chosen were Maine; New Jersey; North Carolina; Alabama; Michigan; Texas; Washington; and, in California, Los Angeles and San Diego Counties. These states and counties were selected because they vary demographically, and because their immunization policies and program structures reflect distinctive choices that convey a sense of the variety among all the states in immunization strategies, challenges, and achievements. Table E-1 displays notable demographic statistics for these states (California data are used for Los Angeles and San Diego Counties), Table E-2 shows immunization-related public policies and programmatic features; and Table E-3 displays Section 317, VFC, and state-source immunization spending for 1995 and 1998.

The framework for developing profiles of individual states and the data elements to be collected for all cases were designed by staff and reviewed by the committee. A subcommittee to oversee the conduct of the case studies was formed, and members of this subcommittee, as well as members of the committee at large, participated in site visits and were involved in both the written and oral presentation of findings to the rest of the committee.

Four site visits were conducted to large metropolitan areas known to have pockets of need and/or overall low immunization coverage rates:

- Detroit, Michigan;
- Newark, New Jersey;
- Houston, Texas; and
- Los Angeles and San Diego, California (a combined visit).

Interviews with and visits to operating programs included the following in each of the sites:

- county and municipal immunization program and health directors,
- managed care organizations serving Medicaid and SCHIP clients,
- persons using or developing immunization registries,

- WIC clinics or coordinators,
- private-practice physicians, and
- managers and practitioners in federally qualified health care centers.

The information gathered during the site visits was incorporated into each state's case study.

The case study reports were developed through interviews with state health department officials, including the immunization program directors, Medicaid agency staff, budget analysts, and CDC public health advisors to the state, among others. These interviews were, in most cases, coordinated with the initial telephone interview conducted by the research team for the state survey to minimize the imposition on the state respondent's time and avoid duplication. In addition to the interviews with key program managers, the case study sites were asked to provide detailed information on state spending from all revenue sources for immunization activities for the period 1992 through 1998:

- federal grants,
- state revenues (in the case of Los Angeles and San Diego, county revenues as well), and
- foundation grants.

Reconstruction of this historical information, broken out by category of spending (e.g., personnel, contracts, aid to counties) was extraordinarily difficult and labor-intensive for the state health departments, involving the efforts of their own budget analysts and sometimes state budget office staff. The cooperation the committee received from all of the studied states in retrieving and reporting this information was extraordinary as well. The detailed reports of spending on immunization activities comprise an essential element of the information base used by the committee in developing its findings and recommendations.

Finally, the respective state grant applications to CDC for Section 317 funds for 1992, 1995, 1999, and 2000 were reviewed, providing another source of information over time for the case studies.

TABLE E-1 Demographic Characteristics of Case Study States

State	Child Pop (thousands)[a]	Birth Cohort (% National Cohort) [b]	Region	Fiscal Capacity Index (national rank)[c]
Maine	297	13,669 (.35)	New England	111 (19)
New Jersey	1,987	113,279 (2.9)	Mid-Atlantic	186 (1)
North Carolina	1,873	107,015 (2.8)	South	92 (31)
Alabama	1,071	60,914 (1.6)	South	68 (40)
Michigan	2,506	133,714 (3.4)	Midwest	88 (33)
Texas	5,577	333,974 (8.6)	South	62 (42)
Washington	1,455	78,190 (2.0)	North West	114 (17)
California	8,952	524,840 (13.5)	West	73 (38)
Los Angeles	2,518[g]	175,000		
San Diego		45,000		
National	69,528	3,880,894		100

[a]Population data from 1997. Cited in *Kids Count Data Book*. The Annie E. Casey Foundation, 1999.
[b]Cited in *National Vital Statistics Reports, 1997*. 47(18):April 29, 1999.
[c]State per capita income divided by number of poor children in state, 1995 data. Toby Douglas and Kimura Flores, Urban Institute, March 1998.

TABLE E-2 State Program Characteristics

State	% in Medicaid Managed Care[a]	FMAP[b]	SCHIP Program[c]	State Vaccine Purchase
Maine	11	66%	Mixed	UP[e]
New Jersey	59	50%	Mixed	non-UP
North Carolina	69	63%	Sep. plan	UP
Alabama	71	69%	Mixed	non-UP
Michigan	68	54%	Mixed	Partial state purchase (for uninsured)
Texas	25	62%	Mixed	Partial state purchase (for uninsured)
Washington	91	52%	Sep. plan	UP
California	46	51%	Mixed	non-UP
Los Angeles				
San Diego				

[a]1998 Managed Care Enrollment, www.hcfa.gov/medicaid/mcstat98.htm.
[b]FMAP = Federal Medical Assistance Percentage, or federal matching rate for Medicaid service expenditures, at www.hcfa.gov.medicaid.
[c]SCHIP Plan Activity Map, 4/24/2000, at www.hcfa.gov/init/chip-map.htm.

% Children w/Medicaid[d]	% Children Uninsured[e]	% Non-White Births	% Children <100% FPL[f]
20	13	7	14
16	14	42	14
27	15	35	19
22	15	35	24
25	8	30	19
24	24	59	25
25	9	28	15
29	18	66	35
25	14	40	20

[d]Percentage data from 1996. Cited in *Kids Count Data Book*. The Annie E. Casey Foundation, 1999.
[e]Cited in *Kids Count Data Book*. The Annie E. Casey Foundation, 1999.
[f]FPL = federal poverty level.
[g]Population data for Los Angeles County from U.S. Bureau of the Census, July 1, 1995.

Medicaid Vaccine Admin. Fee	First $ Coverage Required for Private Insurers	1998 Statewide Immunization Rates	1998 Metro Area Immunization Rates for Children ≤ FPL[d]
$5.00	No	89%	
$11.50 in MCO[f] rates, passed thru	Yes	85%	Newark: 71.4%
$13.71/1 dose; double for > 2	No	84%	
$8.00/dose	No	84%	Jefferson County: 90.5%
$7/injection; $3/oral	HMOs only	79%	Detroit: 72%
$5.00	Yes for plans since 1/98; no small employers	75%	Houston: 55%; Dallas: 69%
$5.00	No	81%	
$7.50/dose	Yes	78%	
			67%
			73.5%

[d]FPL = federal poverty level.
[e]UP = universal purchase.
[f]MCO = managed care organization.

TABLE E-3 Section 317, VFC, and State Immunization Spending (dollars in millions [dollar per birth cohort member])

	Vaccine Purchase					
	317 DA 1995	317 DA 1998	VFC DA 1995	VFC DA 1998	State Revs 1995	State Revs 1998
Maine	0.682	1.883	1.26	1.592	included in infrastructure	
($/birth cohort)	[47.23	137.76	87.25		116.47]	
New Jersey	1.673	1.916	2.654	3.259	0.02	0.02
	[14.24	16.91	22.59	28.77	0.17	0.18]
North Carolina	1.985	3.154	4.129	10.92	7.875	10.737
	[19.57	29.47	40.71	102.04	77.65	100.33]
Alabama	3.54	2.265	4.941	7.06	1	0.4
	[58.09	37.18	81.08	115.9	16.41	6.57]
Michigan	4.987	10.463	9.071	12.742	3.911	0.101
	[36.13	78.25	65.72	95.29	28.33	0.76]
Texas	6.476	9.098	28.023	34.524	19.863	13.731
	[20.17	27.24	87.27	103.37	61.86	41.11]
Washington	2.512	3.266	3.106	6.008	3.534	7.082
	[32.47	41.77	40.15	76.84	45.68	90.57]
California	6.987	9.241	51.319	72.555		
	[13.31	17.61	97.78	138.24]		
Los Angeles						0.099
						[0.57]
San Diego						0.05
						[1.11]
National	96.304	135.562	247.692	399.974		
	[24.36	34.93	62.65	103.06]		

NOTE: Los Angeles and San Diego include county as well as state spending. Texas includes separate 317 grants to Houston and San Antonio.

SOURCES: CDC, National Immunization program data for 317 and VFC. IOM case study data for state and local immunization spending. 1994 and 1997 birth cohorts: National Center for Health Statistics, Vital Health Statistics.

Infrastructure

317 FA 1995	317 FA 1998	VFC FA 1995	VFC FA 1998	State Revs 1995	State Revs 1998
1.228	1.665	0.233	0.495	0.1	0.5
[85.04	121.81	16.13	34.28	$6.92	36.58]
2.502	4.071	1.692	1.505	0.482	0.94
[21.29	35.94	14.4	13.29	4.1	8.3]
5.765	4.14	0.334	0.375	1.639	1.482
[56.84	38.69	3.29	3.5	16.16	13.85]
2.97	3.194	0.387	0.439	0.6	0.6
[48.74	52.43	6.35	7.21	9.85	9.85]
6.376	6.2	2.453	1.435	0.647	4.046
[46.19	46.37	17.77	10.73	4.69	30.26]
8.58	13.925	0.965	2.07	16.251	8.779
[26.72	41.69	3.01	6.2	50.61	26.29]
4.52	3.231	0.285	0.87	0.352	0.423
[58.43	41.32	3.68	11.13	4.55	5.11]
23.427	18.312	1.205	1.974		
[44.64	34.89	2.3	3.76]		
				0.426	2.308
					[13.19]
				1.992	3.374
					[74.98]
195.405	186.149	23.288	29.475		
[49.42	47.97	5.89	7.59]		

BOX E-1
Case Study Summary

The following authors prepared the eight case studies discussed in this report:

- **Alabama**—Roy Hogan, M.P.A., Consultant, Austin, Texas
- **Maine**—Kay Johnson, Ed.M., M.P.H., Johnson Group Consultants, Inc., Hinesburg, Vt.
- **Michigan**—Hanns Kuttner, M.A., School of Public Policy Studies, University of Chicago
- **New Jersey**—Gerry Fairbrother, Ph.D., Associate Professor of Epidemiology and Social Medicine, Montefiore Medical Center, New York City, and Paul Meissner, M.S.P.H., and Alana Balaban, B.Sc., Division of Epidemiology and Social Medicine, Montefiore Medical Center, New York City
- **North Carolina**—Wilhelmine Miller, M.S., Ph.D., Program Officer, Institute of Medicine
- **Texas**—Roy Hogan, M.P.A., Consultant, Austin, Texas
- **Washington**—Heather McPhillips, M.D., M.P.H., Department of Pediatrics, University of Washington, and E. Russell Alexander, M.D., M.P.H., Professor Emeritus, School of Public Health, University of Washington
- **Comparison of Los Angeles and San Diego Counties, California**—Gerry Fairbrother, Ph.D., Associate Professor of Epidemiology and Social Medicine, Montefiore Medical Center, New York City, and Elka Munizaga, Division of Epidemiology and Social Medicine, Montefiore Medical Center, New York City

The case studies are available on line at **www.books.nap.edu/catalog/9836.html.**

A summary article of the case study findings appears in the *American Journal of Preventive Medicine* (Fairbrother et al., forthcoming).

Appendix F

Annual Section 317 Awards to States, 1995–1999

1995

Grantee	SECTION 317 DA FUNDS			SECTION 317 FA FUNDS		
	New DA Award	Total DA Award	Expenditure	New FA Award	Total FA Award	Expenditure
Alabama	$1,650,262	$3,938,587	$3,540,138	$3,977,361	$5,136,403	$2,969,856
Alaska	$817,405	$1,753,597	$1,774,232	$1,233,094	$2,062,985	$1,824,421
Arizona	$1,280,647	$1,280,655	$1,188,916	$4,278,816	$5,005,364	$4,475,828
Arkansas	$1,209,665	$1,308,511	$1,308,465	$2,452,187	$3,994,230	$2,708,365
California	$6,543,678	$10,727,534	$3,740,132	$33,491,094	$35,004,219	$23,426,701
Colorado	$1,350,130	$2,312,254	$1,273,939	$3,529,847	$4,907,869	$3,095,531
Connecticut	$903,005	$2,971,562	$781,108	$3,513,742	$4,271,038	$1,744,008
Delaware	$408,315	$1,049,831	$66,957	$1,048,865	$1,585,559	$977,166
DC	$116,274	$1,570,075	$90,777	$599,514	$1,417,726	$207,849
Florida	$3,313,636	$7,019,910	$6,654,342	$11,761,066	$20,803,979	$14,804,736
Georgia	$1,853,602	$5,265,562	$3,634,201	$8,085,025	$9,831,103	$8,257,503
Hawaii	$595,642	$825,507	$678,362	$2,179,035	$2,179,035	$1,035,919
Idaho	$591,097	$779,840	$767,211	$1,158,388	$1,158,388	$830,292
Illinois	$3,737,675	$6,151,847	$3,250,033	$7,712,545	$8,152,545	$3,920,240
Chicago				$3,883,175	$4,661,828	$3,936,049
Indiana	$1,638,462	$2,050,585	$2,102,636	$4,982,526	$5,570,782	$4,141,547
Iowa	$934,414	$1,766,356	$462,521	$2,712,386	$4,008,262	$1,923,994
Kansas	$887,301	$2,078,224	$1,966,564	$2,705,244	$2,705,244	$1,961,411
Kentucky	$1,262,731	$2,715,173	$2,048,869	$3,575,772	$5,003,172	$3,694,344
Louisiana	$1,452,722	$3,790,882	$1,086,308	$3,781,858	$3,858,843	$1,814,984
Maine	$400,000	$685,192	$682,014	$1,368,855	$1,921,172	$1,227,985
Maryland	$1,456,887	$2,833,824	$2,422,288	$5,314,159	$6,701,139	$2,831,171
Massachusetts	$1,539,035	$2,866,130	$2,487,730	$6,971,957	$10,038,841	$6,843,982
Michigan	$4,961,243	$4,964,221	$4,986,546	$7,279,851	$7,459,851	$6,375,851
Minnesota	$1,232,798	$3,482,960	$1,403,831	$4,340,255	$7,622,292	$3,613,184

Mississippi	$1,498,765	$1,574,043	$1,573,963	$3,205,154	$6,010,840	$4,472,359
Missouri	$1,548,831	$1,761,839	$1,719,429	$4,263,028	$6,977,763	$5,023,502
Montana	$578,110	$1,066,491	$747,444	$978,169	$1,528,117	$881,215
Nebraska	$604,621	$1,587,656	$1,058,670	$1,526,156	$1,866,058	$1,334,800
Nevada	$732,172	$989,796	$891,777	$1,579,370	$2,122,734	$1,525,649
New Hampshire	$727,302	$733,257	$538,979	$1,287,518	$1,687,471	$1,113,639
New Jersey	$1,680,375	$3,527,959	$1,673,040	$6,725,480	$7,667,749	$2,502,488
New Mexico	$961,946	$3,044,993	$1,532,070	$1,505,150	$1,745,606	$1,071,906
New York State	$2,783,564	$2,783,586	$3,052,886	$10,228,040	$16,825,960	$7,883,408
New York City	$2,112,247	$5,342,888	$2,399,461	$8,141,971	$11,399,242	$2,169,562
North Carolina	$2,064,844	$3,183,353	$1,985,189	$7,334,474	$10,299,421	$5,765,227
North Dakota	$581,064	$2,424,892	$475,863	$918,944	$1,093,753	$689,366
Ohio	$2,536,266	$4,764,235	$3,945,545	$9,071,919	$10,315,969	$5,991,584
Oklahoma	$1,314,742	$1,314,770	$1,211,308	$3,326,412	$4,127,917	$3,221,699
Oregon	$531,087	$1,709,134	$907,354	$2,961,538	$3,057,538	$2,270,495
Pennsylvania	$500,000	$11,517,736	$1,262,676	$6,346,625	$8,005,436	$2,871,683
Philadelphia	$1,468,982	$1,468,982	$675,074	$3,771,755	$3,771,755	$2,446,111
Rhode Island	$750,859	$751,074	$751,066	$1,589,147	$2,772,578	$1,066,311
South Carolina	$1,438,900	$1,625,574	$1,653,322	$4,161,507	$7,327,998	$3,759,412
South Dakota	$730,942	$1,085,931	$767,679	$773,065	$853,065	$437,407
Tennessee	$1,643,058	$2,087,926	$1,125,107	$4,597,568	$4,597,568	$3,336,483
Texas	$5,259,029	$5,262,197	$5,262,182	$15,907,918	$15,907,918	$5,186,660
Houston	$0	$425,862	$425,742	$2,167,742	$3,364,292	$2,217,677
San Antonio	$703,746	$788,317	$788,205	$1,240,851	$1,535,789	$1,175,291
Utah	$1,247,796	$3,317,436	$1,034,772	$2,146,888	$2,723,972	$1,740,424
Vermont	$486,838	$1,233,556	$637,110	$853,994	$1,112,563	$641,175
Virginia	$1,008,973	$2,928,237	$1,006,619	$5,221,036	$5,221,036	$2,872,068
Washington	$1,421,766	$2,653,556	$2,512,096	$5,367,128	$8,714,152	$4,519,757
West Virginia	$992,801	$992,845	$916,278	$1,902,002	$3,275,900	$1,599,662
Wisconsin	$1,523,330	$6,509,254	$3,684,240	$4,325,975	$5,824,465	$2,941,017
Wyoming	$494,000	$606,835	$595,706	$775,001	$775,001	$497,998

continued

1996

Grantee	SECTION 317 DA FUNDS			SECTION 317 FA FUNDS		
	New DA Award	Total DA Award	Expenditure	New FA Award	Total FA Award	Expenditure
Alabama	$1,727,733	$2,116,788	$783,540	$3,351,217	$6,962,523	$5,685,092
Alaska	$3,301,953	$3,301,953	$1,371,653	$914,204	$989,204	$989,204
Arizona	$1,056,843	$1,091,491	$1,067,703	$3,117,387	$3,509,504	$3,456,126
Arkansas	$3,111,761	$3,111,761	$2,131,287	$1,841,265	$3,082,330	$2,087,123
California	$5,640,842	$6,414,895	$3,985,356	$21,397,231	$43,241,964	$31,193,644
Colorado	$1,568,845	$1,568,845	$655,325	$2,600,857	$4,491,438	$3,524,524
Connecticut	$347,459	$581,719	$326,884	$878,450	$5,523,033	$2,608,285
Delaware	$630,117	$630,117	$447,072	$887,034	$1,059,097	$635,452
DC	$110,379	$428,459	$111,920	$19	$1,266,802	$405,324
Florida	$5,812,848	$6,825,376	$6,091,147	$8,915,195	$15,937,858	$14,275,209
Georgia	$4,103,144	$4,103,144	$2,521,644	$6,913,692	$8,754,692	$8,009,054
Hawaii	$2,083,856	$2,083,856	$1,373,372	$792,312	$3,821,690	$2,178,222
Idaho	$672,785	$676,007	$672,768	$684,344	$1,454,692	$791,985
Illinois	$4,388,250	$6,799,197	$4,550,757	$4,689,653	$17,045,615	$7,170,181
Chicago	$0	$0	$0	$2,984,530	$3,817,094	$3,736,494
Indiana	$3,486,497	$3,486,497	$1,266,751	$1,415,974	$5,677,415	$2,578,207
Iowa	$1,481,358	$1,481,358	$1,455,854	$2,032,808	$4,117,076	$3,592,781
Kansas	$1,535,874	$1,535,874	$1,116,519	$1,948,754	$4,369,664	$2,797,700
Kentucky	$1,404,612	$1,404,612	$1,316,060	$2,466,829	$3,995,392	$3,093,909
Louisiana	$2,395,798	$2,395,798	$2,201,230	$0	$4,635,756	$1,813,128
Maine	$2,331,393	$2,331,393	$1,304,206	$726,119	$2,017,225	$1,215,740
Maryland	$2,930,753	$3,437,853	$2,545,816	$3,600,950	$9,108,886	$6,477,969
Massachusetts	$3,933,952	$4,126,977	$4,395,050	$5,652,950	$8,847,809	$6,970,822
Michigan	$7,747,107	$7,747,107	$7,738,498	$5,579,148	$10,476,969	$10,472,951
Minnesota	$3,689,297	$3,986,629	$3,055,214	$2,949,614	$7,226,076	$7,194,196

Mississippi	$3,107,460	$3,107,460	$2,666,638	$2,816,920	$4,125,367	$2,589,811
Missouri	$2,071,563	$2,071,563	$2,012,767	$3,951,232	$6,111,174	$2,962,818
Montana	$299,326	$299,326	$64,488	$712,242	$1,185,256	$932,062
Nebraska	$1,240,469	$1,240,469	$650,540	$969,050	$2,501,337	$1,531,562
Nevada	$792,002	$892,712	$791,952	$1,198,950	$2,121,921	$1,466,403
New Hampshire	$433,348	$529,764	$524,642	$664,976	$1,397,723	$1,315,692
New Jersey	$2,366,859	$2,366,859	$1,238,197	$4,786,441	$11,577,515	$5,819,672
New Mexico	$663,882	$1,313,691	$947,595	$1,276,376	$2,430,781	$2,031,099
New York State	$2,761,377	$2,761,377	$2,761,138	$7,107,055	$15,304,112	$10,985,547
New York City	$3,152,949	$3,152,949	$3,152,818	$5,611,414	$12,826,159	$4,363,843
North Carolina	$3,006,333	$3,088,393	$3,088,327	$4,767,829	$10,045,349	$5,834,196
North Dakota	$1,011,818	$1,192,140	$734,674	$678,233	$1,146,234	$756,162
Ohio	$4,952,801	$4,952,801	$4,870,242	$6,361,600	$13,890,410	$8,758,492
Oklahoma	$2,710,831	$2,710,831	$2,446,091	$3,210,767	$4,355,406	$4,300,406
Oregon	$368,061	$693,675	$329,705	$2,096,197	$3,115,977	$2,662,752
Pennsylvania	$3,125,791	$3,125,791	$468,128	$5,736,273	$13,508,044	$4,514,892
Philadelphia	$933,242	$1,145,802	$974,060	$1,827,612	$2,921,321	$2,634,418
Rhode Island	$778,138	$779,442	$778,067	$1,308,272	$3,014,538	$2,066,077
South Carolina	$3,718,699	$3,729,108	$1,627,823	$3,001,684	$7,509,841	$5,243,123
South Dakota	$750,270	$1,078,377	$865,415	$627,449	$1,687,259	$1,277,009
Tennessee	$1,064,385	$2,027,203	$1,909,253	$3,071,188	$5,322,713	$2,879,530
Texas	$9,020,526	$9,020,526	$9,018,686	$8,300,103	$14,893,411	$9,504,047
Houston		$0	$0	$1,451,938	$3,159,531	$2,612,900
San Antonio	$513,294	$513,294	$494,148	$1,058,618	$1,215,729	$973,762
Utah	$1,597,571	$2,138,664	$1,331,376	$1,462,023	$2,632,433	$1,440,178
Vermont	$486,632	$1,060,403	$920,983	$633,234	$1,104,622	$672,235
Virginia	$1,694,666	$1,694,666	$1,125,637	$5,865,736	$10,857,366	$6,203,271
Washington	$5,004,877	$5,004,877	$4,697,396	$3,963,789	$8,119,503	$6,267,790
West Virginia	$579,775	$581,999	$573,529	$1,629,293	$3,322,792	$1,879,366
Wisconsin	$2,524,672	$2,524,672	$2,410,390	$3,136,770	$7,850,965	$6,280,782
Wyoming	$1,143,855	$1,143,855	$598,753	$697,255	$993,977	$433,863

continued

	SECTION 317 DA FUNDS			SECTION 317 FA FUNDS		
Grantee	New DA Award	Total DA Award	Expenditure	New FA Award	Total FA Award	Expenditure
Alabama	$2,000,000	$3,106,301	$962,691	$3,362,824	$4,640,933	$4,270,568
Alaska	$312,229	$2,242,970	$542,369	$932,828	$1,110,117	$1,110,117
Arizona	$983,768	$983,768	$966,929	$1,746,013	$2,684,660	$2,684,660
Arkansas	$1,800,000	$2,758,049	$2,118,801	$1,862,543	$3,284,191	$2,452,921
California	$6,370,920	$8,434,264	$8,246,683	$20,964,189	$27,349,485	$24,670,438
Colorado	$780,844	$1,810,083	$1,695,935	$2,709,531	$3,677,937	$3,677,937
Connecticut	$300,000	$653,256	$650,424	$1,793,682	$4,624,891	$3,066,445
Delaware	$650,000	$942,705	$515,536	$623,622	$1,232,317	$788,112
DC	$125,000	$125,000	$120,520	$683,539	$1,632,403	$547,376
Florida	$4,500,000	$5,195,827	$4,932,103	$7,670,232	$9,321,637	$8,106,170
Georgia	$3,340,600	$5,130,199	$3,996,313	$6,998,034	$7,866,915	$7,697,809
Hawaii	$1,650,000	$1,650,000	$1,612,119	$1,024,304	$2,667,771	$2,425,635
Idaho	$700,000	$700,000	$676,670	$587,905	$1,353,043	$1,068,776
Illinois	$3,391,691	$5,481,546	$5,411,841	$2,386,426	$10,694,571	$6,934,159
Chicago	$0	$59,419	$0	$3,872,272	$3,952,040	$3,589,632
Indiana	$1,795,846	$3,984,596	$3,796,309	$3,899,072	$5,399,072	$5,398,844
Iowa	$1,370,000	$1,525,862	$1,366,874	$1,967,906	$2,492,201	$2,179,933
Kansas	$1,100,000	$1,448,475	$1,448,296	$1,948,857	$2,579,753	$2,492,092
Kentucky	$2,000,000	$2,308,951	$2,302,780	$2,486,090	$3,387,573	$3,043,685
Louisiana	$1,537,537	$2,021,617	$2,029,331	$0	$2,618,565	$1,699,450
Maine	$577,846	$1,639,481	$1,621,922	$2,031,482	$2,832,972	$2,832,927
Maryland	$3,300,000	$3,988,969	$3,573,070	$3,457,392	$6,170,719	$5,094,067
Massachusetts	$6,224,036	$6,224,036	$5,792,597	$4,525,137	$6,402,125	$6,188,746
Michigan	$8,958,457	$9,028,632	$9,028,568	$5,953,064	$5,953,064	$5,953,064
Minnesota	$3,245,975	$4,092,208	$3,691,166	$2,855,347	$2,888,698	$2,888,698

Mississippi	$2,800,000	$2,983,149	$2,019,117	$2,321,219	$4,092,732	$3,612,320
Missouri	$2,800,000	$2,818,408	$2,318,807	$3,830,765	$6,979,122	$6,979,122
Montana	$348,316	$652,482	$554,968	$705,566	$1,134,790	$925,317
Nebraska	$1,000,000	$1,714,376	$1,193,280	$1,003,937	$1,973,712	$1,648,805
Nevada	$1,000,000	$1,119,387	$1,119,288	$1,441,636	$2,097,154	$2,061,749
New Hampshire	$700,000	$737,296	$737,182	$397,924	$812,605	$790,213
New Jersey	$2,000,000	$3,291,328	$1,263,742	$4,302,980	$9,508,053	$6,327,007
New Mexico	$1,000,000	$1,347,058	$1,347,055	$1,280,044	$1,328,295	$1,238,703
New York State	$3,679,228	$3,937,948	$2,163,615	$7,950,847	$12,919,894	$12,315,730
New York City	$2,000,000	$2,318,589	$2,257,365	$4,390,324	$17,151,926	$15,383,539
North Carolina	$4,068,583	$4,305,973	$4,204,909	$4,172,649	$8,534,602	$8,534,602
North Dakota	$889,675	$1,601,732	$883,714	$507,776	$972,392	$821,617
Ohio	$3,946,884	$4,342,938	$3,993,785	$4,492,942	$8,833,274	$7,187,854
Oklahoma	$2,655,816	$3,040,584	$3,076,824	$3,300,371	$3,345,371	$3,345,371
Oregon	$507,944	$507,944	$507,740	$1,866,392	$2,319,616	$2,019,616
Pennsylvania	$2,000,000	$5,763,275	$1,986,497	$1,511,350	$8,808,451	$4,684,457
Philadelphia	$750,000	$750,000	$750,064	$1,209,061	$1,551,270	$1,468,646
Rhode Island	$1,065,450	$1,101,816	$984,579	$1,193,096	$2,141,558	$1,929,580
South Carolina	$1,181,562	$3,239,298	$480,989	$2,798,095	$4,910,413	$3,271,924
South Dakota	$1,274,184	$1,274,184	$1,237,932	$467,469	$890,134	$720,341
Tennessee	$1,509,098	$1,634,797	$1,263,220	$424,164	$3,564,378	$2,904,149
Texas	$8,293,769	$8,310,784	$4,115,690	$2,488,214	$11,580,593	$11,030,593
Houston	$44,065	$70,079	$0	$1,646,564	$2,227,508	$2,146,362
San Antonio	$900,000	$914,296	$913,860	$950,368	$1,395,722	$1,208,721
Utah	$2,500,000	$2,978,030	$1,295,811	$1,405,478	$2,477,448	$2,174,247
Vermont	$815,386	$815,386	$597,509	$607,886	$1,040,273	$1,040,273
Virginia	$1,460,000	$1,460,000	$1,391,749	$4,514,758	$7,514,758	$5,860,180
Washington	$5,088,938	$5,408,325	$5,408,285	$3,305,555	$4,983,227	$4,237,476
West Virginia	$1,339,614	$1,361,486	$1,348,015	$1,965,166	$3,412,643	$2,244,669
Wisconsin	$4,000,000	$4,344,642	$4,355,493	$3,224,022	$4,969,163	$4,088,175
Wyoming	$699,637	$1,243,988	$1,051,906	$691,310	$1,051,178	$926,609

continued

1998

Grantee	SECTION 317 DA FUNDS			SECTION 317 FA FUNDS		
	New DA Award	Total DA Award	Expenditure	New FA Award	Total FA Award	Expenditure
Alabama	$50,000	$2,522,486	$2,265,257	$3,011,520	$3,543,929	$3,193,929
Alaska	$0	$1,756,775	$1,753,157	$861,608	$861,608	$861,608
Arizona	$1,103,316	$1,103,469	$1,228,421	$2,367,375	$2,367,375	$2,367,375
Arkansas	$2,150,408	$2,739,846	$2,739,761	$1,172,697	$2,003,966	$1,768,966
California	$9,183,203	$9,328,281	$9,240,626	$9,719,898	$20,711,874	$18,311,874
Colorado	$789,562	$918,073	$865,486	$3,502,495	$3,502,495	$3,502,495
Connecticut	$257,021	$406,907	$406,469	$748,906	$2,439,235	$2,439,235
Delaware	$50,000	$477,168	$196,472	$267,999	$963,491	$963,491
DC	$1,036,584	$1,146,036	$417,291	$21,255	$976,876	$626,876
Florida	$1,112,720	$1,178,988	$1,178,930	$6,228,394	$7,455,104	$6,730,104
Georgia	$1,244,479	$2,351,967	$2,350,451	$5,947,314	$6,116,421	$6,116,421
Hawaii	$1,700,727	$1,727,034	$881,108	$708,336	$1,045,522	$1,045,522
Idaho	$541,250	$544,624	$544,509	$406,572	$710,867	$685,683
Illinois	$12,172,047	$12,746,843	$12,952,791	$232,267	$3,866,106	$3,716,106
Chicago	$0	$35,000	$0	$3,398,433	$3,953,572	$3,953,572
Indiana	$2,999,823	$3,897,360	$3,698,076	$1,435,141	$3,437,486	$3,437,486
Iowa	$1,558,203	$1,717,191	$1,657,533	$1,556,738	$1,869,006	$1,739,006
Kansas	$830,883	$831,061	$831,727	$1,177,798	$2,206,527	$2,156,527
Kentucky	$3,142,468	$3,148,131	$3,120,240	$2,440,718	$2,784,606	$2,784,606
Louisiana	$2,492,412	$2,540,231	$2,485,031	$80,110	$1,944,998	$1,944,998
Maine	$1,881,977	$1,926,401	$1,883,251	$1,664,873	$1,664,918	$1,664,918
Maryland	$928,567	$1,908,215	$1,848,541	$2,766,682	$3,843,334	$3,843,334
Massachusetts	$4,327,602	$4,465,937	$4,417,378	$4,311,680	$4,525,058	$4,515,058
Michigan	$10,595,105	$10,597,904	$10,463,341	$6,196,307	$6,200,235	$6,200,325
Minnesota	$1,586,367	$2,081,418	$1,985,005	$3,083,698	$3,083,698	$3,083,698

Mississippi	$1,187,242	$2,422,125	$1,616,938	$1,911,607	$2,427,575	$2,427,575
Missouri	$1,657,512	$2,314,727	$2,295,983	$4,085,213	$4,085,213	$4,085,213
Montana	$466,270	$563,783	$517,766	$456,122	$669,119	$659,119
Nebraska	$785,790	$1,268,926	$1,243,565	$1,134,768	$1,301,960	$1,301,960
Nevada	$1,409,386	$1,409,386	$1,409,266	$1,507,467	$1,542,872	$1,542,872
New Hampshire	$1,550,902	$1,550,902	$1,548,822	$592,155	$696,576	$696,576
New Jersey	$0	$2,050,684	$1,916,207	$305,187	$4,721,393	$4,071,393
New Mexico	$1,507,540	$1,507,540	$1,507,491	$650,161	$1,153,000	$1,053,000
New York State	$777,992	$2,569,740	$1,801,092	$8,079,792	$9,309,866	$9,309,866
New York City	$2,043,750	$2,441,252	$2,434,227	$2,263,534	$7,443,441	$7,349,931
North Carolina	$3,261,616	$3,269,997	$3,154,047	$4,289,886	$4,289,887	$4,139,887
North Dakota	$138,016	$1,012,124	$1,003,350	$465,737	$616,512	$600,552
Ohio	$6,062,233	$6,411,704	$5,824,549	$2,126,433	$6,357,650	$5,957,650
Oklahoma	$5,624,961	$5,656,017	$5,574,055	$2,659,342	$2,669,342	$2,669,342
Oregon	$467,856	$773,375	$758,131	$1,608,410	$1,908,411	$1,908,411
Pennsylvania	$0	$3,641,372	$3,091,389	$0	$8,222,538	$8,001,026
Philadelphia	$600,276	$785,274	$766,264	$1,791,847	$1,874,471	$1,874,471
Rhode Island	$931,121	$1,051,733	$1,051,607	$995,507	$1,207,485	$1,207,485
South Carolina	$0	$2,805,659	$2,159,258	$853,407	$2,646,297	$2,502,145
South Dakota	$414,612	$802,374	$648,005	$472,015	$659,383	$659,383
Tennessee	$1,573,338	$2,108,214	$2,098,407	$1,132,531	$2,801,348	$2,401,348
Texas	$4,705,879	$8,690,254	$8,690,998	$2,668,044	$11,619,197	$11,319,197
Houston	$0	$57,014	$0	$1,469,834	$1,549,067	$1,534,067
San Antonio	$410,284	$410,720	$407,266	$884,695	$1,071,697	$1,071,697
Utah	$100,000	$2,370,274	$2,055,948	$898,774	$1,476,476	$1,401,476
Vermont	$483,208	$877,490	$873,823	$706,867	$706,867	$706,867
Virginia	$247,469	$1,152,150	$983,526	$1,169,834	$4,478,507	$3,728,507
Washington	$3,238,082	$3,238,082	$3,266,174	$2,409,986	$3,230,718	$3,230,718
West Virginia	$530,372	$541,631	$533,942	$330,032	$1,448,458	$1,085,458
Wisconsin	$2,784,888	$2,784,888	$2,651,043	$2,934,890	$3,771,786	$3,751,786
Wyoming	$206,157	$374,973	$301,141	$328,765	$666,921	$666,921

continued

1999

Grantee	SECTION 317 DA FUNDS		SECTION 317 FA FUNDS	
	New DA Award	Total DA Award	New FA Award	Total FA Award
Alabama	$1,174,078	$1,479,161	$3,080,389	$3,351,982
Alaska	$1,493,960	$1,493,960	$750,056	$750,056
Arizona	$4,106,677	$4,128,998	$2,369,814	$2,369,814
Arkansas	$1,955,091	$1,958,657	$1,310,710	$1,486,960
California	$14,557,598	$14,648,839	$4,518,567	$11,943,591
Colorado	$1,466,053	$1,473,964	$2,208,205	$2,208,205
Connecticut	$2,034,733	$2,037,676	$1,427,603	$1,427,603
Delaware	$48,037	$336,522	$699,264	$699,264
DC	$336,949	$1,043,277	$503,864	$916,180
Florida	$1,839,676	$2,106,409	$5,643,876	$6,187,626
Georgia	$965,782	$996,695	$3,862,512	$3,862,512
Hawaii	$935,477	$1,781,709	$1,080,214	$1,080,214
Idaho	$406,153	$429,353	$367,057	$415,807
Illinois	$7,682,160	$7,682,160	$1,283,872	$3,090,234
Chicago	$253,876	$253,876	$2,246,787	$2,246,787
Indiana	$2,760,360	$2,907,942	$2,042,123	$2,042,123
Iowa	$1,143,202	$1,155,745	$1,240,695	$1,338,195
Kansas	$1,345,321	$1,345,342	$1,841,445	$1,878,945
Kentucky	$3,038,099	$3,085,076	$2,269,309	$2,269,309
Louisiana	$2,377,521	$2,377,841	$2,270,886	$2,319,560
Maine	$1,931,545	$1,976,702	$1,307,211	$1,307,211
Maryland	$1,093,785	$1,130,916	$3,431,873	$3,431,873
Massachusetts	$7,319,796	$7,388,927	$3,486,388	$3,493,888
Michigan	$7,409,349	$7,409,349	$5,624,450	$5,624,450
Minnesota	$2,082,956	$2,090,386	$2,487,520	$2,487,520
Mississippi	$764,562	$1,378,011	$1,614,406	$1,614,406

Missouri	$3,642,897	$3,701,436	$2,574,361	$2,574,361
Montana	$354,117	$395,034	$456,215	$463,715
Nebraska	$961,180	$1,025,314	$897,619	$1,055,334
Nevada	$1,811,514	$1,851,209	$1,300,195	$1,300,195
New Hampshire	$1,053,536	$1,056,533	$635,886	$635,886
New Jersey	$1,430,134	$1,519,834	$0	$2,340,009
New Mexico	$759,145	$759,193	$854,108	$929,108
New York State	$798,841	$1,469,852	$6,505,771	$6,505,771
New York City	$1,527,521	$1,527,521	$3,816,484	$3,886,617
North Carolina	$3,940,888	$4,157,214	$3,502,557	$3,615,057
North Dakota	$742,862	$752,713	$598,463	$610,433
Ohio	$4,995,223	$5,582,377	$1,058,241	$1,358,241
Oklahoma	$2,039,306	$2,053,971	$2,200,988	$2,200,988
Oregon	$731,449	$731,449	$1,407,936	$1,407,936
Pennsylvania	$1,849,893	$2,435,829	$2,062,843	$5,056,665
Philadelphia	$718,980	$723,163	$1,545,991	$1,545,991
Rhode Island	$1,071,635	$1,075,294	$862,299	$862,299
South Carolina	$754,948	$1,302,937	$2,282,908	$2,391,022
South Dakota	$596,132	$755,628	$542,919	$582,761
Tennessee	$2,464,388	$2,474,195	$2,069,796	$2,369,796
Texas	$8,903,058	$9,113,777	$6,269,763	$6,494,763
Houston	$186,215	$230,280	$782,154	$795,316
San Antonio	$839,505	$839,571	$904,379	$904,379
Utah	$635,293	$833,645	$1,034,460	$1,090,710
Vermont	$906,490	$909,496	$636,174	$636,174
Virginia	$301,387	$470,011	$2,775,703	$3,338,203
Washington	$4,113,825	$4,114,136	$2,124,649	$2,262,390
West Virginia	$641,941	$651,841	$763,228	$1,085,026
Wisconsin	$2,169,770	$2,259,622	$3,033,452	$3,102,277
Wyoming	$850,179	$953,624	$309,335	$309,335

NOTE: DA = direct assistance; FA = financial assistance.

Appendix G

State Immunization Requirements for School Children

State	Minimum Doses Required		New or Planned Requirements[c]
	Kindergarten[a]	Middle School[b]	
AL	4 DTP 2 M, 1 MR 3 Polio	Td booster (10 yr)	
AK	4 DTP 2 M, 1 R 3 Polio		
AZ	4 DTP 2 MMR 3 Polio 3 Hep B		Phase in 3 Hep B and 2 MMR for K–12 by 2005
AR	4 DTP 2 Me[d], 1 R 3 Polio		In process of requiring mumps and Hep B for K, 7th, and transfer students, and Varicella for K
CA	4 DTP 2 M, 1 MR 3 Polio 3 Hep B	2 Me 3 Hep B	Varicella and Hep A have been proposed in the legislature
CO	4 DTP 1 MMR 3 Polio 3 Hep B	2 MMR 3 Hep B	Effective July 1, 2000, for K, ≥4 DTP, ≥3 Polio, 2 MMR, 1 Varicella

continued

282

| State | Minimum Doses Required | | New or Planned Requirements[c] |
	Kindergarten[a]	Middle School[b]	
CT	4 DTP 1 MMR 3 Polio 3 Hep B	2 Me	Proposed law for Varicella (6th–7th graders and all born after 1/1/97 without proof of immunity)
DE	4 DTP 2 MMR 3 Polio		Varicella will become a requirement in 2000
DC	4 DTP 2 MMR 3 Polio 3 Hep B 1 Varicella	2 MMR 1 Varicella	
FL	4 DTP 2 M, 1 MR 3 Polio 3 Hep B	2 M, 1 MR 3 Hep B	
GA	3 DTP 1 MMR 3 Polio 3 Hep B	2 MMR	
HI	4 DTP 2 M, 1 MR 3 Polio 3 Hep B		
ID	4 DT 1 MMR 3 Polio 3 Hep B		
IL	4 DTP 2 M, 1 MR 3 Polio	Td booster (10 yr) 3 Hep B (5th)	
IN	4 DTP 2 M, 1 MR 3 Polio 3 Hep B	2 Me	
IA	3 DTP 2 MeR 3 Polio 3 Hep B		
KS	4 DTP 2 MMR 3 Polio		
KY	4 DTP 2 M, 1 MR 3 Polio 3 Hep B	Td booster (10 yr) 2 Me	

continued

| State | Minimum Doses Required | | New or Planned Requirements[c] |
	Kindergarten[a]	Middle School[b]	
LA	4 DTP 2 M, 1 MR 3 Polio 3 Hep B		Effective fall 2003, Varicella
ME	4 DTP 2 MMR 3 Polio		
MD	4 DTP 2 M, 1 MR 3 Polio		
MA	5 DTP 2 M, 1 MR 4 Polio 3 Hep B 1 Varicella	Td booster 2 Me 3 Hep B 1 Varicella	
MI	4 DTP 2 M, 1 MR 3 Polio	Td booster (10 yr)	Effective 2000, 3 Hep B for new school entries; effective January 1, 2002, Varicella for K–12
MN	4 DTP 1 MMR 3 Polio	Td booster 2 MMR	Effective 2000, 3 Hep B for K; effective 2001, 3 Hep B for 7th
MS	4 DTP 2 M, 1 MR 3 Polio		
MO	4 DTP 2 M, 1 MR 3 Polio 3 Hep B		
MT	4 DTP 2 MMR 3 Polio	2 MMR	
NE	3 DTP 2 MMR 3 Polio 3 Hep B	2 MMR	Effective July 1, 2000, 3 Hep B for 7th
NV	4 DTP 2 MMR 3 Polio		
NH	4 DTP 1 MMR 3 Polio 3 Hep B	Td booster (10 yr) 2 Me	
NJ	4 DTP 2 M, 1 MR 3 Polio		Immunization program plans to propose Hep B

continued

| State | Minimum Doses Required | | New or Planned Requirements[c] |
	Kindergarten[a]	Middle School[b]	
NM	4 DTP 2 M, 1 MR 3 Polio	3 Hep B	Effective September 1, 2002, 3 Hep B for K and new entries
NY	3 D (NYC: 4 DTP) 2 M, 1 MR 3 Polio 3 Hep B		Pending legislation for Varicella and adolescent Hep B
NC	4 DTP 2 M, 1 MR 3 Polio 3 Hep B		
ND	4 DTP 2 MMR 3 Polio		
OH	4 DTP 2 MMR 3 Polio 3 Hep B	2 MMR	
OK	4 DTP 2 MMR 3 Polio 3 Hep B 2 Hep A 1 Varicella	3 Hep B 2 Hep A	
OR	4 DT 2 M, 1 MR 3 Polio 3 Hep B		Effective 2000 for adolescents, 2 Measles, 3 Hep B, Varicella; effective 2000 for K, Varicella
PA	4 DT 2 M, 1 MR 3 Polio 3 Hep B	(Philadelphia: 3 Hep B)	Effective 2000 K–12, 2 Measles
RI	4 DTP 2 M, 1 MR 3 Polio 3 Hep B 1 Varicella	Td booster (7th)	Effective August 1, 2000, 3 Hep B for 7th, 1 Varicella, with phase-in of Hep B and Varicella completed for all grades by August 1, 2005; in August 2001, 2 M required K–12
SC	3 DTP 2 M, 1 MR 3 Polio 3 Hep B	3 Hep B	
SD	4 DTP 2 MMR 3 Polio		

continued

State	Minimum Doses Required		New or Planned Requirements[c]
	Kindergarten[a]	Middle School[b]	
TN	4 DTP 2 MMR 3 Polio 3 Hep B	2 MMR	
TX	4 DT 2 M, 1 MR 3 Polio 3 Hep B	Td booster (10 yr)	Effective fall 2000 for K, 1 Varicella; 3 Hep B, 1 Varicella for 7th
UT	4 DTP 2 M, 1 MR 3 Polio 3 Hep B		
VT	3 DTP 2 Me, 1 R 3 Polio	3 Hep B	
VA	3 DTP 2 M, 1 MR 3 Polio 3 Hep B	2 Me	
WA	4 DTP 1 MMR 3 Polio 3 Hep B	2 Me	
WV	3 DTP 2 Me, 1 R 3 Polio		
WI	4 DTP 2 MMR 4 Polio 3 Hep B	3 Hep B	
WY	4 DTP 2 MMR 4 Polio 3 Hep B	2 MMR 3 Hep B	

[a]Includes any requirements that begin in kindergarten (K), including those applicable to new entrants, K–12, and K–1.
[b]Only those requirements that specifically begin in middle school (e.g., 6th–8th grades).
[c] May not be a comprehensive listing.
[d]Me = Measles.

SOURCE: Freed et al., 1999.

Appendix H

Committee and Staff Biographies

BERNARD GUYER, M.D., M.P.H. (*Chair*), is chairman of the Department of Population and Family Health Sciences in the Johns Hopkins School of Hygiene and Public Health. He also holds joint appointments in Pediatrics in the Johns Hopkins School of Medicine and in International Health in the Vaccines Sciences Program. Dr. Guyer previously served as the director of the Division of Family Health Services for the Massachusetts Department of Public Health (1979–1986) and was also a Centers for Disease Control and Prevention (CDC) medical epidemiologist assigned to Cameroon, Africa (1974–1977). He is a member of the Institute of Medicine and has served on several IOM committees, including the IOM Committee on Injury Prevention and Control (1997–1998), the Committee on a Maternal and Child Health Perspective on Health Care Reform (1991–1993), the Quality Initiative Coordinating Committee, and the Committee to Study Outreach for Prenatal Care (1986–1988). He is a former member of the IOM-National Research Council Board on Children, Youth, and Families (1993–1997). He is the coeditor (with H. Grason) of the text *Assessing and Developing Primary Care for Children: Reforms in Health Systems* (National Center for Education in Maternal and Child Health, 1995).

DAVID R. SMITH, M.D. (*Vice-Chair*), was appointed President of the Texas Tech University Health Sciences Center in 1996, following a 5-year term as Commissioner of the Texas Department of Health. He previously served as senior vice president of Parkland Memorial Hospital in Dallas and chief executive officer and medical director of Parkland's Community Oriented Primary Care Program. He has been a member of the U.S. Department of Health and Human Services' National Vaccine Advisory Committee and the U.S. Environmental Protection Agency's Good Neighbor Environmental Board. Dr. Smith also serves in a national leadership conference organized by the Surgeon General to find solutions that will eliminate racial and ethnic disparities in six health areas by the year 2010. He is a pediatrician, former president of the Association of State and Territorial Health Officers, and a past member of the National Vaccine Advisory Committee. Dr. Smith has been a member of two previous IOM committees: the Committee on the Health and Adjustment of Immigrant Children and Families (1996–1998) and the Committee to Study Outreach for Prenatal Care (1984–1986).

E. RUSSELL ALEXANDER, M.D., is a pediatrician who recently retired as Chief of Epidemiology with the Seattle-King County Health Department (1990–1998). He previously served in CDC's Division of Sexually Transmitted Diseases (1983–1989) and was an epidemic intelligence service officer for CDC in 1955–1957 and 1959–1960. Dr. Alexander is also professor emeritus, having served as professor and chair of the Department of Epidemiology and International Health for the University of Washington School of Public Health (1969–1979 and 1990–1998). He was professor of pediatrics at the University of Arizona 1979–1983. He serves on the IOM Vaccine Safety Forum (1994–present) and was a member of the IOM Vaccine Safety Committee (1992–1994) and the IOM Committee on Human Health Hazards of Antibiotics in Animal Feed (1979–1980).

GORDON BERLIN, M.A., has worked since 1990 with the Manpower Demonstration Research Corporation (a social policy research and demonstration intermediary that develops and manages large-scale, multisite demonstration projects designed to test new social policies in the areas of work, training, income support, and social services for at-risk populations). He also was the founding executive director of the Social Research and Demonstration Corporation, a sister organization operating in Canada. In addition to his responsibility for corporate strategic planning and project management, Mr. Berlin oversees all of the corporation's evaluation and demonstration projects concerned with state welfare-to-work programs and work incentive projects for the working poor. Previously he was the executive deputy administrator for management, budget, and policy for the New York City Human Resources Administration. Mr. Berlin has also served as program officer and deputy director of the Urban Poverty Program of the Ford Foundation. He was previously a member of the NRC Panel on High-Risk Youth (1992–1993).

STEVE BLACK, M.D., is codirector of the Kaiser Pediatric Vaccine Study Center in Oakland, California. The Center was established in 1984 for the prelicensure and postlicensure evaluation of adult and pediatric vaccine safety, immunogenicity, efficacy, and cost-effectiveness. Dr. Black is also a pediatric infectious disease specialist at the Kaiser Permanente Medical Center in Oakland. In addition, he is an associate clinical professor of pediatrics at the University of California, San Francisco. Dr. Black is a member of the Pediatric Infectious Disease Society, the European Society for Pediatric Infectious Disease, and the Society for Pediatric Research. He is a fellow of the Infectious Disease Society of America and a member of the European Society for Pediatric Research. Dr. Black received a B.S. degree in biochemistry and molecular biology and a B.A. degree in chemistry from the University of California, Santa Barbara, as well as a medical degree from the University of California, San Diego. He completed a fellowship in pediatric infectious disease at the University of California, San Francisco. Dr. Black has authored or coauthored more than 30 articles on vaccine issues, including pre- and post-licensure evaluations of combination vaccines.

SHEILA BURKE, M.P.A, R.N., F.A.A.N., is the executive dean and a lecturer in public policy at the John F. Kennedy School of Government at Harvard University. She served as the chief of staff to former Senate Majority Leader Bob Dole (1986–1996), and was also elected to serve as Secretary of the Senate in 1995. Ms. Burke served as deputy chief of staff to the Senate Majority Leader (1985–1986), and was a professional staff member of the Senate Finance Committee (1979–1980) and deputy staff director of the Senate Finance Committee (1981–1985). She is a member of the board of the Center for Health Care Strategies, Inc. in Princeton, NJ; the Kaiser Commission on the Future of Medicaid; and the national advisory committee for the Robert Wood Johnson Foundation's Covering Kids initiative. Ms. Burke is a member of the IOM-NRC Board on Children, Youth, and Families (1998–present). She is also a member of the Boards of Trustees of Marymount University and the University of San Francisco.

BARBARA DeBUONO, M.D., M.P.H., is a public health consultant in New York City. She served as commissioner of health for New York State (1995–1998) and was subsequently appointed as chief executive of the New York Presbyterian Healthcare Network and executive vice president of the New York Presbyterian Healthcare System until December 1999. Prior to joining the New York State Department of Health, Dr. DeBuono was director of health for the State of Rhode Island (1991–1995), also serving as a medical and state epidemiologist and medical director in that state (1986–1991). She has previously served on the medical and public health school faculties of Brown University Medical School and the State University of New York in Albany. In her role as Commissioner of Health, Dr. DeBuono shaped New York State's comprehensive Medicaid Managed Care program, with particular emphasis on quality improvement in managed care and primary care access.

GORDON H. DeFRIESE, Ph.D., is professor of social medicine, epidemiology, and health policy and administration at the University of North Carolina at Chapel Hill. For the past 25 years, he has also held an appointment as Director of the Cecil G. Sheps Center for Health Services Research at the university. He is a member of the Global Advisory Group on Health Systems Research of the World Health Organization in Geneva, past president of the Association for Health Services Research and the Foundation for Health Services Research, and a fellow of the New York Academy of Medicine. Since 1994 he has served as president and CEO of the North Carolina Institute of Medicine. Dr. DeFriese is a past president and distinguished fellow of the Association for Health Services Research. He was also the editor (1983–1996, now editor emeritus) of the journal *Health Services Research*. He is a founder of the Partnership for Prevention, a coalition of private-sector business and industry organizations, voluntary health organizations, and state and federal public health agencies based in Washington, D.C., that have joined together to work toward the elevation of disease prevention among the nation's health policy priorities. Dr. DeFriese is a member of IOM and has served on the IOM Committee on Maintaining Privacy and Security in Healthcare Applications of the National Information Infrastructure (1995–1997) and the Forum on Emerging Infections (1996–1999).

R. GORDON DOUGLAS, Jr., M.D., is former president, Merck Vaccine Division, Merck Co. Inc. (from which he retired in May 1999). In that position, he was responsible primarily for the research, development, and manufacturing and marketing of Merck's vaccine products. Prior to joining Merck in 1989, Dr. Douglas had a distinguished career as a physician and academician, specializing in infectious diseases. From 1982 to 1990, he was professor of medicine and chairman, Department of Medicine, Cornell University Medical College and physician-in-chief, The New York Hospital. He also served as head of the Infectious Disease Unit at the University of Rochester School of Medicine. Dr. Douglas is a graduate of Princeton University and Cornell University Medical College. He received his medical staff training at The New York Hospital and Johns Hopkins Hospital. He is a member of IOM, the Association of American Physicians, the Infectious Diseases Society of America, and numerous other organizations, and has served on the National Vaccine Advisory Committee.

WALTER FAGGETT, M.D., is a pediatric consultant in the Washington, D.C., area and chairs the pediatric section of the National Medical Association. He also serves as NMA's liaison to the Advisory Committee on Immunization Practices. He has extensive experience in working with managed care organizations that serve disadvantaged families. He recently served as medical director for Grady Health Care, Inc. in Atlanta; medical director for Omnicare HMO in Memphis, Tennessee; and assistant medical director and pediatrician for Medlink Hospital's Primary Care Center in Washington, D.C. He is a retired United States Army colonel, having served 21 years.

SAMUEL L. KATZ, M.D., is chairman of the Board of the Burroughs Wellcome Fund and Wilburt C. Davison Professor and chairman emeritus of pediatrics at Duke University Medical Center. For 22 years (ending in 1990), Dr. Katz was chairman of the Department of Pediatrics at Duke University School of Medicine. His career has been devoted to infectious disease research, focusing principally on vaccine research and development. Dr. Katz's research included an extensive collaborative effort with Nobel Laureate John F. Enders, during which they developed the attenuated measles virus vaccine now used throughout the world. Dr. Katz has chaired the Committee on Infectious Diseases of the American Academy of Pediatrics (the Redbook Committee), CDC's Advisory Committee on Immunization Practices, and several World Health Organization and Children's Vaccine Initiative panels on vaccines and human immunodeficiency virus infections. He has been president of the American Pediatric Society and of the Association of Medical School Pediatric Department Chairmen. He is coeditor (with A. Gershon and P. Hotez) of a textbook (now in its 10th edition) on infectious diseases. Dr. Katz is a member of IOM and serves on the IOM Committee on Establishing Vaccine Development Priorities for the United States (1995–1999). He has been a member of many other IOM committees, including the Forum on Emerging Infections (1996–1999), the Committee on Child Health in the Former Yugoslavia (1995), the Committee for the Children's Vaccine Initiative—Continuing Activities (1995), the Committee for a Study of Public/Private Sector Relations in Vaccine Innovation (1985), and the Committee on Issues and Priorities for New Vaccine Development (1982–1986). Currently he co-chairs, with Dr. Louis Sullivan, the Vaccine Initiative of the Infectious Diseases Society of America and the Pediatric Infectious Diseases Society.

SARA ROSENBAUM, J.D., is director of the Center for Health Services Research and Policy and professor in the Department of Health Services Management and Policy in the School of Public Health and Health Services at The George Washington University. She also holds appointments in the Schools of Law and Medicine and Health Sciences. Ms. Rosenbaum has worked extensively in the areas of health law for the poor, health care financing and managed care, and maternal and child health. During 1993 and 1994, she worked with the White House Domestic Policy Council and the U.S. Department of Health and Human Services, directing the legislative drafting of the Health Security Act for the President. She has served on policy advisory boards for the Congressional Office of Technology Assessment, the U.S. Public Health Service, and the Health Care Financing Administration. She also holds positions on technical and expert advisory boards including the Committee on Performance Measures of the National Committee on Quality Assurance (NCQA), and since 1992 has served as the public member of the American Board of Pediatrics. She has co-authored (with R. Rosenblatt and S. Law) *Law and the American Health Care System*. Prior to joining the Center, Ms. Rosenbaum was on the staff of the Children's Defense Fund, where she served as director of both the Health Division and the Department of Programs and Policy.

CATHY SCHOEN, M.A., joined The Commonwealth Fund in September 1995 as director of research and evaluation. Prior to joining the Fund, she was director of special projects at the University of Massachusetts Labor Relations and Research Center. She also serves as program director of the Fund's Health Care Coverage and Quality Program, a policy and research grant program established to help inform national and state health insurance and delivery system policy decisions. During the 1980s, Ms. Schoen directed the Service Employees International Union's Research and Policy Department in Washington, D.C. She went to SEIU after serving as a member of President Carter's national health insurance task force, where she was responsible for national reform issues and research and policy related to Medicaid and ambulatory care payment policies. She also served as a senior health advisor during the 1988 presidential campaign. Prior to her federal government service, she was a research associate at the Brookings Institution. She is the author and coauthor of many publications on health care coverage and quality issues.

JANE E. SISK, Ph.D., is professor of health policy, Mount Sinai School of Medicine, New York. Her current research is focusing on the cost-effectiveness of health care interventions, including pneumococcal vaccination for elderly people, implementation of evidence-based guidelines, and evaluation of Medicaid managed care. Before coming to Mount Sinai in 1999, Dr. Sisk was professor of public health, Columbia University School of Public Health, where she developed and directed the Master's Program in Effectiveness and Outcome Research. She previously directed health policy projects at the Congressional Office of Technology Assessment, where she was a senior associate and project director in the Health Program. Her reports addressed such topics as information for consumers on the quality of medical care, Medicare payment for physician services, and the cost-effectiveness of preventive services. Dr. Sisk is currently a member of the IOM/NRC National Cancer Policy Board (2000). She has previously served on IOM's Committee on Evaluating Telemedicine: Clinical, Economic, and Policy Issues (1995–1996); the Committee on the Children's Vaccine Initiative (1992–1993); the Committee to Advise the National Library of Medicine on Information Center Services (1990–1991); the Committee on Public/Private Sector Relations in Vaccine Innovation (1985); and the Committee on Issues and Priorities for New Vaccine Development (1982–1986). Dr. Sisk received a Ph.D. in economics from McGill University and a B.A. with honors in international relations from Brown University, where she graduated Phi Beta Kappa and magna cum laude. She is an elected fellow in the Association for Health Service Research.

BARBARA WOLFE, Ph.D., is director of the Institute for Research on Poverty and professor of economics, public affairs, and preventive medicine, University of Wisconsin-Madison. She teaches courses in health economics and public economics, and is the coauthor of *Succeeding Generations: On the Effects of Investments in Children*. She has been a Fellow at the Netherlands Institute for Advanced Study, a Research Associate for the National Bureau of Economics Research, a member of IOM's Board on International Health, and a scholar at the Russell Sage Foundation. Dr. Wolfe received a Ph.D. and M.A. in economics at the University of Pennsylvania, and a B.A. in economics at Cornell University.

STAFF

ROSEMARY CHALK is study director for the IOM Committee on Immunization Finance Policies and Practices. She has served as a study director or senior program officer for several projects within both IOM and NRC since 1986, including studies on family violence, child abuse and neglect, research ethics, and education finance. Prior to that time she was a consultant for science and society research projects in Cambridge, Massachusetts. She was program head of the Committee on Scientific Freedom and Responsibility of the American Association for the Advancement of Science, 1976–1986. Ms. Chalk has a B.A. in foreign affairs from the University of Cincinnati.

TRACY McKAY is a senior program assistant in the IOM Division of Health Care Services. She has worked on several projects, including the National Roundtable on Health Care Quality; Children, Health Insurance and Access to Care; Quality of Health Care in America; and a study on non-heart-beating organ donors. She is currently providing assistance for the National Quality Report on Health Care Delivery and a new project on the health consequences of being uninsured in America. Ms. McKay received her B.A. in sociology from Vassar College in May 1996.

SUZANNE MILLER is a senior program assistant in the IOM Division of Health Care Services. She graduated with a B.A. in history and biology from Harvard College in 1999 and will begin studies at the Harvard Medical School in fall 2000.

WILHELMINE MILLER, M.S., Ph.D., is a senior program officer in the Division of Health Care Services. Prior to joining IOM, Dr. Miller was an adjunct professor of philosophy at Georgetown University and Trinity College, teaching political philosophy, ethics, and public policy. She received her doctorate in philosophy from Georgetown, with studies and research in bioethics and issues of social justice. In 1994–1995, Dr. Miller was a consultant to the President's Advisory Committee on Human Radiation Experiments, evaluating the implementation of current protections for federal human research subjects by federal agencies. Dr. Miller was a program analyst in the Department of Health and Human Services for 14 years, responsible for policy development and regulatory review in areas including hospital and HMO payment, prescription drug benefits, and child health. Her M.S. from Harvard University is in health policy and management.

Index

295

N